DENTAL
ANATOMY

DENTAL ANATOMY

A Self-Instructional Program

Ninth Edition

TEACHING RESEARCH

A Division of
The Oregon State System of Higher Education

APPLETON-CENTURY-CROFTS/Norwalk, Connecticut

93 94 95 / 10

Prentice-Hall International, Inc., London
Prentice-Hall of Australia, Pty. Ltd., Sydney
Prentice-Hall of India Private Limited, New Delhi
Prentice-Hall of Japan, Inc., Tokyo
Prentice-Hall of Southeast Asia (Pte.) Ltd., Singapore
Whitehall Books Ltd., Wellington, New Zealand
Editora Prentice-Hall Do Brasil LTDA., Rio de Janeiro

Library of Congress Cataloging in Publication Data
   Main entry under title:

   Dental anatomy.

      Includes index.
      1. Teeth.   [DNLM: 1. Tooth—Anatomy and histology—
   Programmed texts.   WU 18 D414]
   RK280.D36   1982   611'.314   82-13838
   ISBN 0-8385-1567-3

Cover design: Lynn M. Luchetti
Text design: Gloria Moyer
Production: Judith Warm Steinig

PRINTED IN THE UNITED STATES OF AMERICA

CONTENTS

CHAPTER 2   PERMANENT ANTERIOR TEETH

CHAPTER 3   THE PERMANENT PREMOLARS

PREFACE

This ninth edition represents the latest refinement of the Teaching Research dental anatomy program. The efforts of dental educators and instructional designers for over two decades are invested in the dental anatomy program. Continuous development, pilot testing, evaluation, and validation have characterized the program, and hard data from field tests show that it is successful.

Contributors to this program are noted elsewhere in this volume, but three persons merit special recognition for their investment in this work: Casper F. Paulson, Ed. D., for his guidance in the early project development; William A. Richter, D.M.D., M.S., for his continuing attention to program accuracy; and most notably Gale H. Roid, Ph.D., for his extensive professional and personal commitment to the constant improvement of the Dental Anatomy Program as an efficient learning aid.

ACKNOWLEDGMENTS

The combined efforts of many instructional designers and countless dental educators have been felt in the more than two decade history of the dental anatomy self-instructional program. A complete listing would run to several pages and even this would not include the thousands of students in community colleges, colleges, and universities who have tested and validated this program. We would be remiss though, not to acknowledge our appreciation to those whose contributions have been especially important.

The early development was achieved through the cooperation of staff of the Teaching Research Division of the Oregon State System of Higher Education, including Charles Frye, Richard Schultz, Robert Lange, and Thomas Haines, under the direction of Casper F. Paulson, Jr., and faculty of the University of Oregon Dental School including Drs. Bruce Burns, Duane Paulson, Robert Watkins, James Mock, Frank Everett, Hiroshi Ueno, and notably Drs. Robert L. Lang, William A. Richter, and James Grenfell.

Major content revision and reorganizations in the late 1960s evidenced Teaching Research's commitment to the program. Content advisors from around the country who contributed to this updating included Drs. Robert Canfield, Bruce Jones, Edmund Vanden Bosche, Lowell Whitsett, Erlinda Benedicto, Henry Junemann and Barbara Schulze. Major responsibility, however, rightfully belongs to Gale H. Roid, Ph.D., of Teaching Research, and William A. Richter, D.M.D., M.S., then of the University of California, Los Angeles.

In the middle 1970s, additional updating and streamlining were combined with completion of a coordinated student study and self-test guide. Substantial field testing was undertaken and involved students and faculty at Schools of Dentistry at the University of Missouri at Kansas City, the University of Southern California, and the University of Illinois, as well as dental hygiene departments at East Tennessee State University, Yakima Valley College, Owens Technical College, and Chemeketa Community College. Major content review was provided by Drs. Lawrence G. Wilson and J. Henry Clarke of the University of Oregon Health Sciences Center and Dr. Robert P. Scapino, of the University of Chicago Medical Center and University of Illinois. Thomas Haladyna, Linda Chevraux and Casper Paulson of Teaching Research assisted the program editor with programming changes and field test work.

The early 1980s have seen this continuing commitment to program excellence evidenced through additional program reformatting and streamlining. This work is the effort of Gale Roid, Robert M. Olsen, and Jacqueline D. Olsen, of the Teaching Research Division of the Oregon State System of Higher Education.

DIRECTIONS FOR THE STUDENT

The objective of this text is to help you learn the terminology and basic facts of dental anatomy. This self-instructional text has been tested on a large number of students over many years. This experience shows that when students use the text according to directions and diligently answer the embedded questions and tests, they effectively learn dental anatomy.

Because this is a self-instructional volume, you will find that it is different from ordinary textbooks in many ways. First, in addition to reading you will be answering questions that are in the text. Second, you will make a "mask" from a 3×5 or 5×7 note card. Hold this mask in one hand and use it to cover up the answers to the questions in the text. Questions appear in nearly every "frame" of the text. Frames are separated by black lines and answers to questions are usually printed below these lines. Move the mask down the page until you can read a frame and question, but are still shielding the answer to that question. Using a mask in this way helps to prevent you from just reading both the questions and their answers. Research has shown that significant learning will take place if you use the mask and respond *before* revealing the answer. (It is not necessary to actually write your response in the book; just "say it to yourself.")

Third, you will be able to check your understanding continuously by comparing your responses with correct answers. You will only be able to accurately check your understanding if you use a mask.

Fourth, you will not read all of the pages of the book consecutively. The text has been designed to present review and repetition only as each student demonstrates a need for it. Thus, at a number of points you will be directed to different pages depending on your answer to a question. It is important that you follow directions exactly to avoid getting lost or missing needed instruction. Directions appear at the bottom of each page or at the end of a frame.

Fifth, you are given review tests at regular intervals throughout the volume to help you check your understanding of each section of material presented. There are also tests which appear in table or matrix form ("Matrix Tests"). These tests will help you to measure whether you have mastered each section and can go on to the next section or whether you need to review. Mastery of each section is important because later parts of the volumes rely on your knowledge of earlier parts. Also, these tests help you to prepare for exams in school.

Now turn to Page 1 and begin.

DENTAL ANATOMY

1
INTRODUCTION TO DENTAL ANATOMY

SECTION 1.0   CROWN AND ROOT

Every tooth has two basic parts, a **crown** and a **root.** The part of a tooth which is visible in the mouth is the **clinical crown.** The part which is not visible in the mouth is the **clinical root.**

To the clinician, then, the supportive soft tissue that surrounds the tooth forms the boundary between the _____ and the _____ of a tooth.

Crown

Root

---

clinical crown, clinical root

When examining a tooth outside of the mouth, a clinical crown and root cannot be defined because there is no soft tissue to form a boundary. However, an **anatomical crown** and **anatomical root** can be defined by the type of hard tissue covering the tooth. **Enamel** is a very hard, whitish, translucent tooth tissue which covers and defines the anatomical crown. Another hard tooth tissue called **cementum,** covers and defines the anatomical _____.

---

root

The part of a tooth covered with cementum, which connects the tooth to surrounding tissue, is termed the _____ root.

The boundary between the anatomical crown and root is the **cervical line** (SIR vik ul—the word is related to "cervix," the neck). On actual teeth, the cervical line is the division between the enamel and cementum and it may be faint or distinct. You will see it drawn as a line separating the crown and root in illustrations in this text. Identify the cervical line in the drawing at the right—is it A, B, or C? _____.

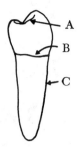

B

Eruption is the movement of the tooth through the surrounding tissues so that gradually more of the tooth becomes visible in the mouth.

If a tooth in the mouth of a child is *partially* erupted, then which of the following is true? _____

a. the clinical crown includes all of the anatomical crown.

b. part of the anatomical crown may not be included in the clinical crown.

b

If you said *a,* you were not correct. If a tooth is partially erupted, only a small portion would be visible and the clinical crown would not include all of the anatomical crown. Some of the anatomical crown would be still covered by supportive soft tissues.

If you said *b,* you were correct. Note the distinction between the boundaries of the anatomical and clinical crowns. The boundary of the anatomical crown never changes. However, the boundary of the clinical crown and clinical root can change with the position of the tooth and position of the supportive soft tissues around the tooth.

An adult with a normally developed **dentition** (full set of teeth) has 32 teeth. Each of these 32 teeth has a crown. However, the crowns may not resemble each other. Teeth are classified into four groups, **incisors** (in SIZE urs), **canines**, **premolars** and **molars**. Teeth in each classification have similarities of form, location and functions.

SECTION 1.1   INCISORS

In the adult dentition, <u>8 of the 32 teeth</u> have crowns with relatively straight edges which are well designed to *cut* through foods. A term similar to "<u>cut</u>" is "incise." The associated noun is *incisor*. An instrument used to make an incision could be called an incisor. Teeth that have this shape are called _____.

incisors

Those *eight* teeth whose crowns are so well adapted to cutting are the *incisors*. Their cutting edges are termed **incisal** (in SIZE ul) **edges.** Identify the incisal edge in this drawing of an incisor (A or B or C?):

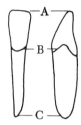

A

SECTION 1.2   CANINES

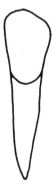

Canines are another classification of teeth. Of the 32 teeth in an adult dentition, <u>4 are canines</u>. We associate the word "canine" with the dog family. We can use this association to aid our memory. In dogs, the canine is usually a prominent tooth. The long, pointed canine of a snarling dog can be frightening.

These teeth are often called "<u>eye teeth</u>" or "<u>cuspids</u>," but the preferred term is *canine*.

In humans, the <u>canine is somewhat pointed.</u> The incisal edge is not straight like the incisors, <u>but spear-shaped.</u> The point is called a **cusp.** A cusp is <u>a pointed projection or mound on a tooth's crown.</u>

The cusp shape and the well-developed root of the canines make them very powerful teeth, able to concentrate forces into a small area. The canines can function as wedges, to <u>pierce and hold foods.</u> The strength and shape of canines aids the tearing and breaking action accomplished by the coordination of the teeth with the movement of fingers, wrist and arm. In eating a crisp apple, for instance, we grasp or hold the apple with our teeth, then, with a motion of the fingers, wrist and arm, we break or tear the food into pieces of a size suitable for chewing. Another example of canines in action would be in the eating of a tough steak where the canines would help to _____ and _____ the meat.

The piercing and holding function of the canine teeth is made easy by the pointed shape of their crowns. The point on the crown of these teeth is called a _____.

Both the cutting edge of an incisor and the piercing edge of the canine cusp are termed _____ edges.

The process of chewing food is called **mastication** (mass tuh KAY shun). The incisal edge of a canine and its pointed _____ are involved in mastication.

The cusp of a canine tooth provides an example of a convex surface. All tooth surfaces are either **flat, concave,** or **convex.**

    Some students have trouble with the terms "convex" and "concave." Convex means bulging or arching outward like the surface of a ball. Concave means being shaped like a hollow or recess. A mental clue is that the word con*cave* suggests something *cave*like.

Which figure has a convex top? _____

Which figure has a concave top? _____

A   **B**

Therefore, when we say that the incisal edge or cusp of the canine is convex, we mean that it bulges or arches _____ (toward/away from) the root.

The overall crown and root length of canines make them the longest teeth in an adult's mouth. The long root gives the canines pronounced stability. Because of their firm anchorage and location in the mouth, the canines contribute importantly to the stability of all the teeth.

The tissue that surrounds the root structure receives its contours from the shape of the root and in turn affects the contours in the person's face, particularly around the "corners" of the mouth. Thus, canine teeth have a major influence on a person's facial appearance.

The two classifications of teeth which have been discussed in the program so far are _____ and _____.

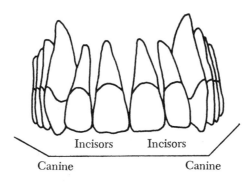

Incisors   Incisors

Canine   Canine

The incisors and the canines, two of the four classifications of teeth, are both wedge-shaped in appearance from a side view of their crowns.

Both incisors and canines have edges suitable for cutting or piercing food. The incisal edges of both are involved in the process of chewing, which is called _____.

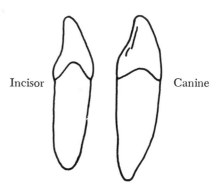

Incisor   Canine

The incisors and the canines have two of the following four characteristics in common:

_____

(Choose the pair of letters of the two correct statements)

a.	Both have incisal edges.	a and b
b.	The incisal edge on each is relatively straight and sharp.	b and c
c.	There are four teeth in each classification.	a and c
d.	Both are relatively wedge-shaped in appearance when viewing the crown from the side.	a and d
		c and d

a and d

If you chose another answer, go back and review beginning at page 1. For your own benefit and increased learning, you should evaluate your answers to questions in this text in a critical and honest way. You should now be able to describe the differences between incisors and canines on the basis of what has been presented so far. If you can do this it will help you identify these teeth and communicate with other professional people. If you can not yet do this, please review from page 1.

The next classification of teeth to be considered consists of as many teeth as the incisors. These teeth are called *premolars*. There are how many premolars? _____.

eight

SECTION 1.3   PREMOLARS

Eight teeth of the adult dentition are premolars. These teeth are sometimes called *bicuspids*, because they generally have two _____.

The term "bicuspid" has been used because these teeth usually have only two cusps. However, since two of the eight premolars vary in that they may have either two or three cusps, the term "bicuspid" is not technically accurate. While this program will use the term *premolar*, the student should be aware of other common terms so that he can recognize and identify the appropriate teeth from any typical word usage.

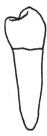

In the drawing on the right, the premolars and molars are identified. We use the name *pre*molars because these teeth are _____ (in front of/behind) the molars.

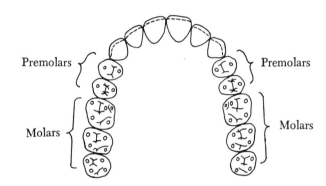

The premolars and molars have larger masticating surfaces than do the incisors and canines to facilitate the crushing and grinding of foods. Premolars have similarities to molars but they differ from molars in the number of cusps, their form, and arrangement. Premolars have smaller masticating surfaces and more pointed cusps which concentrate the forces exerted on foods. In this respect, premolar cusps resemble the form of the cusps on _____ teeth.

SECTION 1.4   MOLARS

There are twelve molars. The molars have more cusps and a larger masticating surface than the other classifications of teeth. They are located in the back of the mouth where the muscles of the jaw can apply strong forces, making the molars effective in crushing and grinding.

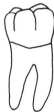

Molars are distinguished from one another by their position in the mouth, the shape of the crown, and the number of cusps. Molars may have from three to five cusps, depending on their location in the mouth and normal variations which occur. The apex or point of each cusp is called a **cusp tip.** The number of cusps may easily be determined by counting the *cusp tips* (marked as small circles in the illustration). How many cusps are there on the tooth marked with the arrow? _____

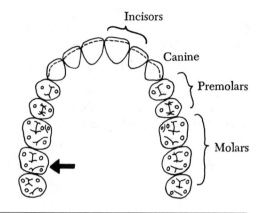

Four is correct

REVIEW TEST 1

1. Supply the name for the teeth corresponding to the following anatomical forms:

Tooth name   **Form**

a. _____ one cusp
b. _____ usually, two cusps
c. _____ straight incisal edge

2. During the development of teeth in adolescence, the clinical crowns of teeth gradually become longer. What is the name for this process?
   a. mastication
   b. eruption
   c. cusp development

3. How many teeth in the adult dentition are molars (expressed as a fraction of the total number of teeth)?
   a. 1/4   c. 3/8
   b. 1/8   d. 1/2

4. Which two classifications of teeth have a wedge-shaped crown from a side view?
   a. Incisor   c. Premolar
   b. Canine   d. Molar

5. Which of the following would never be seen in a visual inspection of the mouth, by definition?
   a. anatomical crown
   b. anatomical root
   c. clinical root

MAKE A NOTE OF YOUR ANSWERS AND TURN TO PAGE 47.

SECTION 2.0 ARRANGEMENT OF TEETH

Each tooth is fixed in its relative position in the supporting bone to form the dentition. The dentition is divided into two **arches,** the **upper** and **lower.** The teeth belonging to the upper arch are supported in the maxilla (MAX uh luh) or maxillary (MAX uh larry) bone. They are therefore called _____ teeth.

maxillary

The maxillary teeth account for one half of the total number of teeth. The total number of teeth in the adult maxillary arch is _____.

sixteen

The upper jaw is the maxilla. Another name for the maxillary set of teeth is the _____ set of teeth.

upper

The lower jaw is the **mandible** (MAN duh bull), and therefore the set of teeth attached to the mandible makes up the mandibular (man DIB u lur) arch.
   Mandre means to chew. The mandible is the movable jaw used for chewing.
   As the mandible is raised, the teeth in the mandibular arch are brought into contact with those of the _____.

maxillary arch

The incisors and canines are positioned in the *front* part of the mouth and are called **anterior teeth**. Premolars and molars are located in the *back* of each dental arch and are called _____ teeth.

posterior

The grinding or chewing surfaces of maxillary and mandibular **posterior** teeth come into contact when the mouth is closed. These surfaces are termed **occlusal** (ah CLUE zul) surfaces. Which two classifications of teeth have occlusal surfaces? _____ and _____.

The teeth with incisal edges are collectively called anterior teeth. The teeth with occlusal surfaces are collectively called _____ teeth.

Which group of teeth have masticating surfaces called incisal edges? _____

The masticating surfaces of the posterior teeth are termed _____ surfaces.

Which of the following are anterior teeth? _____

    a.   incisors and canines
    b.   premolars and molars

To identify a tooth as a maxillary canine, for example, is not sufficient to identify a specific tooth since two such teeth are normally present. Not only is the dentition divided into maxillary and mandibular arches but also into right and left **quadrants.**

The technical term for the dividing line between the right and left sides of the body is *mid-saggital* (mid SAHJ juh tull) *plane.* Dentally, this is called the **midline** or *median line* of the dental arches. The midline equally divides both the maxillary and mandibular arches, falling between the central incisors. Each half of each segment then be-comes a quadrant, or one-fourth of the complete dentition. Normally, there are eight permanent teeth in a quadrant.

The order of arrangement of the eight teeth is identical in each of the four quadrants. The diagram below shows the maxillary arch as seen if you were looking into a patient's mouth. Indicating either the right or left quadrant is always in reference to the patient's right or left, *not* in reference to the viewer's right or left.

The labeled teeth in the diagram below represent an occlusal view of the maxillary _____ (right/left) quadrant.

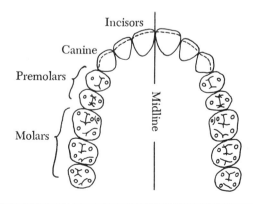

Incisors
Canine
Premolars
Molars
Midline

The human dentition is composed of several kinds of teeth, serving a variety of functions. The term to denote this is **heterodont** dentition (*hetero* means "different"; *-odont* means "tooth," thus heterodont means literally "different teeth"). It is used to refer to "having teeth of different shapes."

In some species, only one type of tooth is found throughout the arches. This is known as **homodont** dentition (*homo* means "the same").

Human dentition is also described as **diphyodont** (die FI oh dont; *di* – "two"; phyo – to produce; *-odont* – "tooth," meaning "to produce two sets of teeth"), because during

his lifetime, man has two different sets of teeth, the **primary** (**deciduous**) teeth, and the **permanent** teeth. In contrast, fishes, amphibians and reptiles continue to replace teeth throughout their lifetime, so with respect to replacement, their dentition is described as **polyphyodont** (*poly* – "many"; meaning "to produce many sets of teeth").

We have discussed two terms that describe human dentition. When we speak of the variety of teeth in a dental arch, we use the term _____. When we speak of the fact that humans have primary teeth and then permanent teeth, we use the term _____.

heterodont, diphyodont

The first set of teeth may properly be called primary, which obviously means first; or deciduous, which means falling away and refers to the fact that, like the leaves of deciduous trees, they will fall away when their function has been fulfilled.

These teeth are also often called the

"baby," "temporary," or "milk teeth," but these terms are technically unacceptable.

A complete set of the primary dentition includes only twenty teeth. Each arch of primary dentition therefore contains how many teeth? _____.

Ten

Ten is correct. This means that there are six less teeth in an arch of primary dentition than in the same arch of permanent dentition. As the skull grows and develops along with the development and growth of the body, the increased size of the maxilla and mandible accommodates the eruption of three permanent molar teeth in each quadrant posterior to the primary molars.

In each *quadrant*, five permanent teeth, the incisors, canine, and premolars, succeed or take the place of the five primary teeth. They are therefore called **succedaneous** (SUCK sa DANE nee us; *suc-cedo* means "to

follow") teeth. Three permanent molars do not succeed deciduous teeth (in each quadrant); therefore, they are **nonsuccedaneous** teeth.

Each quadrant of the primary dentition includes two incisors (2 I), one canine (1 C), and two molars (2 M). There are no primary premolars. Since there are four quadrants, the primary dental formula is 2 I plus 1 C plus 2 M = 5; 5 × 4 = 20. There is also a permanent dentition dental formula. Try it on scratch paper and compare your answer with the one in the next frame.

(In each quadrant, two incisors plus one canine plus two premolars plus three molars, totaling eight, times four quadrants, totaling 32 teeth.)

Teeth are identified by their arrangement relative to the median line. In the primary dentition beginning at the midline, the teeth are arranged in the following order: **central incisor, lateral incisor, canine, first molar,** and **second molar.** In the permanent dentition, following the same order relative to the median line, the arrangement of the teeth is **central incisor, lateral incisor, canine, first premolar, second premolar, first, second,** and **third molars.** Because man has two different sets of teeth during his lifetime, human dentition is described as _____.

diphyodont dentition .... GO TO TOP OF PAGE 14.

heterodont dentition ... GO TO NEXT FRAME.

▶ From preceding frame

heterodont is incorrect

Human dentition *is* described as heterodont, but you were asked to choose the term that describes the fact that humans have two sets of teeth during their lifetime—diphyodont.

The prefixes are the clue to help in remembering terms. Heterodont, for instance, has what prefix? _____.

---

hetero

Hetero is also the prefix of heterogeneous, heterozygus, and several other words, each of which refer to instances where *(similar/different)* kinds are present _____.

---

different

Hetero means different or different kinds. *Heterodont* means different kinds of teeth, such as incisors, canines, etc.

Diphyodont, on the other hand, has what prefix? _____.

Di

This prefix is found in such words as divide and dioxide, referring to quantity, simply indicating the presence of _____ of a kind.

---

two

SECTION 2.1 TOOTH NAMING AND CODING

We have covered several items of tooth arrangement. By putting these together, one is able to identify a particular tooth with accuracy, confident of being understood by a colleague.

For example, permanent mandibular left first molar or primary mandibular left lateral incisor. When identifying a specific tooth, we list the **dentition, arch, quadrant,** and **tooth name** in that order. The order in which these have been given has become standard and should be learned in that manner.

Rearrange the description of the following tooth by placing the words in proper order.

right   maxillary   primary   canine

_____   _____   _____   _____

primary   maxillary   right   canine

Which terms name the dentition? _____ _____

primary, permanent

Which terms name the arch? _____

and _____

maxillary, mandibular

Which terms name the quadrant? _____ _____

right, left

List the eight permanent teeth in order starting at the midline (anterior to posterior order).

_____

_____

_____

_____

_____

_____

_____

_____

central incisor, lateral incisor, canine, first premolar, second premolar, first molar, second molar, third molar

Throughout this text, the drawings will be labeled with the correct names, in the correct order, for the tooth or teeth shown in the drawings.

To communicate with colleagues and to keep records of patients' teeth, a coding system for designating teeth is helpful and widely used. There are several different coding systems. One of the most commonly used systems in the United States is the military or **universal coding system.** This code will be used throughout the remainder of this program.

Arabic numbers one through thirty-two (1-32) are used for permanent teeth; letters A through T are used for the twenty primary teeth. Assuming the two arch segments form an elliptical circle, then a diagram can represent the complete dentition, and the pattern for the number and letter code can be readily seen.

Try to use some key numbers to help you remember these codes. For example, 8 and 9 are the maxillary central incisors and 24 and 25 are the mandibular central incisors. You might think of the groups of eight teeth in each quadrant and use 1, 8, 9, 16, 17, 24, 25, and 32 as landmark numbers to help you recall the ones in between.

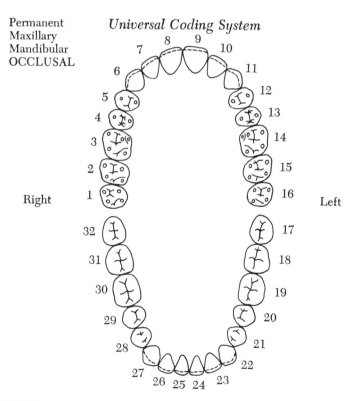

Permanent
Maxillary
Mandibular
OCCLUSAL

Universal Coding System

Right

Left

Notice that the right and left is in reference to the patient, not the viewer. When coding the teeth, you always begin lettering or numbering with the posterior tooth in the _____ _____ quadrant. (Be sure your answer words are in the correct order.)

Universal Coding System

Primary
Maxillary
Mandibular
OCCLUSAL

Right

Left

maxillary right

List the code letter or number for each of the following teeth.

_____ primary maxillary right canine

_____ permanent mandibular left second premolar

_____ permanent maxillary left third molar

_____ primary maxillary left second molar

_____ primary mandibular right central incisor

C, 20, 16, J, P

Which one of the following tooth identifications uses the correct order?

    a.   Permanent mandibular left central incisor.
    b.   Permanent left mandibular central incisor.

a is correct

For each of the following code letters and numbers write the name of the tooth, being careful to place the terms in standard order.

5 ______________________________

30 ______________________________

K ______________________________

26 ______________________________

D ______________________________

9 ______________________________

Q ______________________________

16 ______________________________

5, Permanent maxillary right first premolar;

30, Permanent mandibular right first molar;

K, Primary mandibular left second molar;

26, Permanent mandibular right lateral incisor;

D, Primary maxillary right lateral incisor;

9, Permanent maxillary left central incisor;

Q, Primary mandibular right lateral incisor;

16, Permanent maxillary left third molar

There are several other coding systems used to identify teeth.

There are three main types:

1. *Quadrant symbols:* Symbols for quadrants, (⌐) maxillary right, (¬) maxillary left, (⌐) mandibular left, (¬) mandibular right, are combined with numbers (1-8 for the teeth in each permanent quadrant), or letters (a-h), beginning with the central incisor. Known as "Palmer notation."

2. *Quadrant abbreviations:* Abbreviations for upper and lower, right and left quadrants (UL, UR, LL, LR) are combined with numbers or letters.

3. *International system:* A system that is useful for computer processing and foreign language translation of tooth codes has been approved by the International Federation of Dentistry. In this system, each tooth is given two numbers which may be separated by a dash (as 1-8).

The first number identifies the quadrant. The permanent quadrants are numbered from 1 (maxillary right) to 4 (mandibular right) following the standard elliptical diagram of teeth in a clockwise direction. The primary quadrants are numbered from 5 (maxillary right) to 8 (mandibular right) in the same way. The permanent *teeth* are numbered from 1 (central incisor) to 8 (third molar) in each quadrant. The primary teeth are numbered from 1 to 5.

INTERNATIONAL CODING SYSTEM

quadrant, tooth #

PERMANENT TEETH	PRIMARY TEETH
Maxillary right	Maxillary right
1-8 1-7 1-6 1-5 1-4 1-3 1-2 1-1	5-5 5-4 5-3 5-2 5-1
4-8 4-7 4-6 4-5 4-4 4-3 4-2 4-1	8-5 8-4 8-3 8-2 8-1
Mandibular right	Mandibular Right
Maxillary left	Maxillary left
2-1 2-2 2-3 2-4 2-5 2-6 2-7 2-8	6-1 6-2 6-3 6-4 6-5
3-1 3-2 3-3 3-4 3-5 3-6 3-7 3-8	7-1 7-2 7-3 7-4 7-5
Mandibular left	Mandibular Left

The first digit of the international code identifies the quadrant and whether the tooth is permanent or primary. Below is a list of the *first digit* numbers and quadrants. Fill in the missing elements by writing the dentition and quadrant name in the blank space.

First digit of International Code:

1—Permanent maxillary right

2—Permanent maxillary left

3—_____ _____ _____

4—_____ _____ _____

5—Primary maxillary right

6—_____ _____ _____

7—Primary mandibular left

8—Primary mandibular right

The *second digit* of the international code identifies the individual teeth within each quadrant. Below is a list of the second-digit codes with some missing elements. Fill in the missing tooth names.

Second digit of International Code:

1—Permanent or primary central incisor
2—Permanent or primary lateral incisor
3—Permanent or primary canine
4—Permanent first premolar or primary _____

_____

5—Permanent second premolar or primary second molar
6—_____   _____   _____
7—Permanent second molar
8—Permanent third molar

Although the international system is probably the code of the future, it is not currently in wide use in the United States.

Throughout the remainder of this program, the military (universal) code of 1-32 and A-T will be used, because of its popularity and because the introduction of two codes throughout the text would be confusing. From time to time you will be asked to remember the correct universal code for certain teeth. A table of code conversions is included at the end of the book.

SECTION 2.2   TOOTH SURFACES

After having designated a particular tooth, it becomes necessary to be able to designate any one of the surfaces on the tooth. The tooth surfaces receive their name either because of function, relationship to the midline, or anatomical structure.

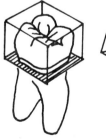
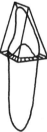

The crown of a tooth may be visualized as a cube or a wedge. One surface is occupied by the root end. Incisors and canines are roughly wedge-shaped with the narrow portion of the wedge corresponding to the incisal edge. Molars and premolars can be visualized as cubes with the top surface of the cube called the _____ surface.

Even though teeth are not exact cubes or wedges, it is helpful to imagine them in this way in order to learn the names of each surface.

The premolars and molars are collectively called _____ teeth, being _____ (*same word*) to the incisors and canines.

The posterior teeth do <u>not</u> have incisal edges. Instead, their masticating surface is in the form of an occlusal "table," with interspaced valleys and projecting mounds called _____.

Two surfaces of each tooth receive their name from the position relative to the midline of the face. The <u>mesial</u> (MEE zee ul) surface is toward or adjacent to the midline. The distal surface is away from the midline.

The dental arch is made up of teeth which contact one another, the mesial surface of one tooth contacting the distal surface of the next tooth in most cases. However, the contact between the central incisors (at the midline) is an exception. Is it mesial-distal, mesial-mesial, or distal-distal?

_____

Teeth contact one another **interproximally** (inter PROCK sim ma lee), except the distal of the third molars. Therefore, each tooth normally has _____ contacting surfaces.

two . . . . GO TO NEXT FRAME

three . . . . GO TO TOP OF PAGE 21

◆ From preceding frame   *two is correct*

You are correct. Of course, you realize that the occlusal surface is a contacting surface also. But for now the contact between teeth belonging to different arches will not be considered. By limiting the use of the words "contacting surface" to those surfaces, where contact remains constant, only the **proximal** (PROCK sim ul) surfaces are contacting surfaces. In this context, the _____ surface of one tooth ordinarily contacts the _____ surface of the adjacent tooth (use the technical words).

GO TO MIDDLE OF PAGE 21.

You are counting the surface contacting the tooth on the mesial side (toward the midline), the surface contacting the tooth on the distal side (away from the midline), and the masticating surface (incisal or occlusal, as the case may be). You are right. These three surfaces normally do make contact with another tooth surface.

For the present time, the contact between teeth belonging to different arches will not be considered. By limiting the use of the words "contacting surfaces" to those surfaces where contact remains constant, only the **proximal** (PROCK sim ul) surfaces are contacting surfaces. Considering one arch only, the _____ surface of one tooth ordinarily contacts the _____ surface of the adjacent tooth (use technical words).

The *distal* surface of one tooth ordinarily contacts the *mesial* surface of the adjacent one, or vice versa. However, there are four teeth whose distal surface does not contact another tooth. These four teeth all belong to the same family; in fact, they are all _____.

Also, there are four teeth whose *mesial* surfaces contact mesial surfaces. These four teeth are all _____.

Except for the mesial surfaces of the central incisors and the distal surfaces of the third molars, the mesial surfaces make contact with adjacent distal surfaces. Surfaces facing toward adjacent teeth are known as **proximal** (PROCK sim ul) surfaces. The term proximal *cannot* be used collectively to describe *all* mesial and distal surfaces because the _____ surface of the third molar does not face an adjacent tooth.

However, both the mesial and distal surfaces of *most* teeth are correctly termed _____ surfaces.

In truth, a proximal surface does not contact the adjacent tooth throughout its entire wall, but instead touches only in a well-defined, distinct _contact area._

If normally developed teeth <u>do not make contact on their proximal surfaces</u>, the resulting space between the proximal surfaces is known as a **diastema** (die ASS tim uh). This condition occurs frequently between the maxillary central incisors.

Which of the following could correctly be termed a diastema? (select _one_ of the following)

a. The space due to a missing central incisor lost in a fight.

b. The space due to the natural loss of a primary tooth.

c. Neither of these.

c

Lingual (LING wull) refers to the tongue (lingua). The lingual surfaces of maxillary and mandibular teeth are those <u>tooth surfaces adjacent to the tongue</u>. **Facial** (FAY shull), of course, refers to the face and names those surfaces opposite the lingual surfaces and <u>adjacent to the face</u>.

While the term "facial" is correct, the facial surfaces are often further distinguished as to whether they are facial surfaces of anterior teeth or posterior teeth. <u>The facial surfaces of anterior teeth (incisors and canines) are sometimes called **labial**</u> (LAY bee ul), or near the lip, while the facial surfaces of the posterior teeth (premolars and molars) are sometimes called **buccal** (pronounced like "buckle"), <u>or near the cheek</u>. The cheek is where a muscle called the _buccinator_ (BUCK sin nate ur) is located. Even though the terms labial and buccal are often used, it is proper (and simpler) to use _facial_ for all teeth. For this reason, the remainder of this program will emphasize _facial_ surfaces. However, the student should remember each term.

Whether the facial surface is called labial or buccal and whether the functional surface is incisal or occlusal corresponds to whether the tooth is _____ or _____.

maxillary or mandibular .... GO TO NEXT FRAME.

anterior or posterior .... GO TO TOP OF PAGE 23.

♦ From preceding frame

maxillary or mandibular is incorrect

The terms maxillary and mandibular are very common terms in dental anatomy. If you are not sure about their meaning, they are defined on frames on page 10. They primarily refer to the upper (maxillary) and lower (mandibular) arches. The other technical words in the item were anterior and posterior. The prefixes "ante" (before) and "post" (after) suggest the usage of the words. Anterior refers to things in front and posterior to things behind.

RETURN TO FRAME ABOVE and answer the last question again

If a tooth is an anterior tooth, labial applies; if it is a posterior tooth, buccal applies. Four tooth surface names are the same for all teeth, whether anterior or posterior. These four are ——————, ——————, ——————, and ——————.

That tooth surface which is positioned toward and adjacent to either the cheek or lip is termed the ——————.

When a person smiles, you will see his teeth from a —————— view.

That tooth surface which is opposite the facial surface and positioned toward the tongue is termed the lingual surface.

The term "lingual" is a Latin-derived word from which also comes the word "linguist." In viewing a tooth from the tongue side, one sees the —————— surface.

A tooth's facial surface is —————— (adjacent to/opposite) its lingual surface.

For precise communication about tooth surfaces, a scheme of division into thirds is used. The figures on the next pages represent the arbitrary division into thirds. The particular third spoken of is designated the facial third, lingual third, occlusal third, cervical third, etc.

Vertical divisions of the crown from a facial view (figure 1) are **distal third, middle third,** and **mesial third** (anterior or posterior teeth). From the proximal view (figure 2), the vertical divisions are **facial third, middle third,** and **lingual third** (anterior or posterior teeth). From the facial view (figure 3), the horizontal divisions are **incisal third, middle third,** and **cervical third** for anterior teeth (**occlusal third, middle third, and cervical third for posterior teeth**).

What name is given to the division labeled "A" in Figure 3? _____.

Permanent
Maxillary
Right
Central Incisor
1. & 3. FACIAL
2. MESIAL

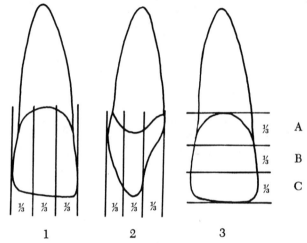

1   2   3

A
B
C

Permanent
Maxillary
Right
Central Incisor
4. & 5. MESIAL
6. FACIAL

In terms of the horizontal divisions of the crown (figure 4), the incisal edge would be located in the _____ third.

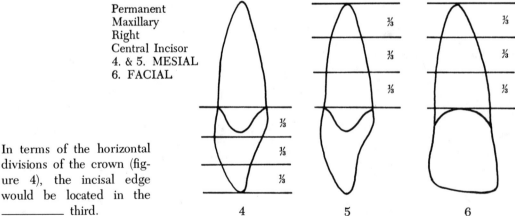

4   5   6

Only horizontal divisions (figures 5,6) are necessary for tooth roots. These are the **cervical third, middle third,** and **apical** (APE ik ul) **third.** The third containing the end of the root would be designated the _____ third.

It should be emphasized that there are no existing anatomical boundary lines for the exact division into thirds. The division is arbitrary.

Review by answering the following:

Vertical divisions of a posterior tooth viewed from the lingual aspect would divide the crown into divisions called the _____, _____, and _____ thirds.

Horizontal divisions of the same tooth viewed from the lingual aspect would divide the crown into divisions called the _____, _____, and _____ thirds.

If the crown of any tooth is divided into thirds horizontally from any view, the cervical line is _____ (always/some-times) in the cervical third.

The root of any tooth is divided into
    a.   vertical thirds
    b.   horizontal thirds
    c.   both vertical and horizontal thirds

REVIEW TEST 2

1. Maxillary and mandibular identify the two _____ of the dentition.
   a. arches
   b. quadrants
   c. diphyodonts

2. Choose the *most correct* statement for normal dentition.
   a. All mesial and distal surfaces are contacting surfaces.
   b. Distal surfaces that contact mesial surfaces are proximal surfaces.
   c. All contacting surfaces are mesial against distal.

3. Which *two* of the following are horizontal divisions of both crowns and roots:
   a. apical third   c. middle third
   b. cervical third   d. lingual third

4. *Two* statements of the following four are *correct*. Identify them.
   a. Lingual surfaces designate the mesial and distal surfaces collectively.
   b. Facial and lingual surfaces are the occlusal surfaces of two different types of teeth.
   c. Every tooth has an occlusal surface.
   d. Some tooth surface names depend on the position of the tooth in the dental arch.

5. Give the full names for the teeth indicated by the universal codes below:

   18 _____

   I _____

   3 _____

   M _____

MAKE A NOTE OF YOUR ANSWERS AND TURN TO PAGE 48

SECTION 3.0   ROOT STRUCTURE OF TEETH

Whereas the crown is the *superstructure* of the tooth, the root is its *substructure*. The basic function of the root is the same for all the teeth; that is, to support the crown so that the tooth may function adequately.

Recall that the *clinical root* is defined as that portion of the tooth which is *not* visible in the mouth. The *anatomical root* is that part of the tooth from the apical end of the root to the _____ line.

cervical

At or near the end or **apex** (A pex) of a root, nerves and blood vessels enter the tooth through one or more openings, the **apical foramen** (pronounced as, foc RAY men, plural: **foramina**, four RAM i na).

When examining a specimen tooth, one could insert a very fine probe through the _____ (apex/apical foramen) located near the _____ (apex/apical foramen) of the tooth.

apical foramen, apex

Some teeth have only one root. Other teeth characteristically have two or three roots. Where there are two roots, the roots are said to be **bifurcated** (BUY fur kate ted; bi- means "two," -*furca* means "to fork"). **Bifur**cation (buy for KAY shun) is the division of one into two branches. Some teeth have **tri**furcated (TRY fur kate ted) roots, a condition where there are _____ roots in number.

three

As shown in the table below, incisors, canines, and some premolars commonly have only one root. The remaining teeth are commonly bifurcated or trifurcated (third molars are variable from one to several roots). Maxillary premolars may be either single-rooted or bifurcated (the maxillary *first* premolar is the one most often bifurcated), and mandibular canines occasionally have bifurcated roots. Maxillary molars are trifurcated and mandibular molars are bifurcated. Which premolar is most often bifurcated? _____

Number of Roots Commonly Found on Permanent Teeth

	INCISORS	CANINES	PREMOLARS	MOLARS*
MAXILLARY	single	single	single or bifurcated	trifurcated
MANDIBULAR	single	single or bifurcated	single	bifurcated

*Third molars are variable

Which of these teeth illus-
trates single roots? _____
Trifurcation?   _____
Bifurcation?   _____

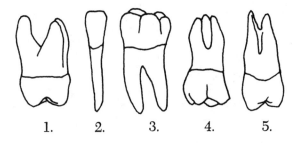

1.   2.   3.   4.   5.

single, 2; trifurcation, 1, 4; bifurcation, 3, 5

For simplification, the anatomical definition for the root of a tooth will be used in the following section of this chapter.

Root anatomy is of particular concern in surgical procedures, fixed and removable bridge design, treatment and maintenance of the supporting tissues, treatment of the root canal, and other dental procedures.

Alveolar (al VEE o lar) **bone** supports the teeth. The bone cavity or socket that holds a root is called an **alveolus** (al VEE oh luss; plural, alveoli, al VEE oh lie). The apex and apical foramen are found at or near the base (deepest point) of the _____.

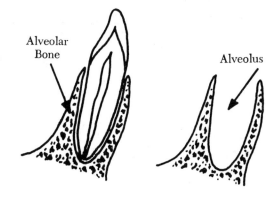

Alveolar
Bone

Alveolus

alveolus

Some of the significant features of root anatomy which you will learn are the number and location of the roots of each tooth, the relative length of the roots, and the usual convex and concave areas on the root surfaces.

Teeth have many variations in their crown and root forms. The greatest variability is found near the end of the root, that is, in the _____ third of the root.

Incisors, most canines and most premolars have a single root. The mandibular canine is infrequently bifurcated. On which of these teeth is a *multiple root* most common (see illustration)?

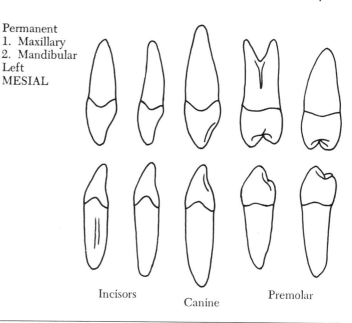

Permanent
1. Maxillary
2. Mandibular
Left
MESIAL

Incisors

Canine

Premolar

——————— ———————
(arch)   (tooth name)

The root of a multi-rooted tooth includes a **root trunk** and two or more **terminal roots.** That portion of a multi-rooted tooth located between the cervical line and the division is called the

——————.

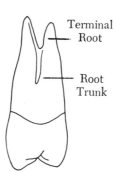

Permanent
Maxillary
Right
1st Premolar
MESIAL

Terminal
Root

Root
Trunk

Maxillary molars generally have three roots. When a tooth has three roots, the root por-

tion of that tooth has one root trunk and three _____.

Permanent
Maxillary
Right
1st Molar
1. DISTAL
2. FACIAL

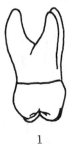 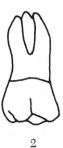

1   2

Although the curved contours of the roots do not present distinct surface boundaries, the terms facial, lingual, mesial, and distal are used to indicate root surfaces and directions.

Of the three terminal roots on maxillary molars, one is located toward the lingual and two toward the _____.

Permanent
Maxillary
Right
1st Molar
1. DISTAL
2. FACIAL

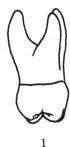 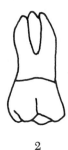

1   2

Terminal roots are named for the position they occupy in relation to the surfaces of the crown. Root A is the distofacial root, B the _____ root, and C the _____ root.

Permanent
Maxillary
1st Molar
Right
1. DISTAL
2. FACIAL

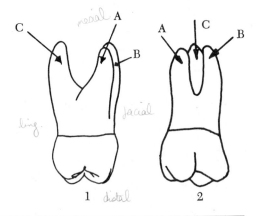

1 distal   2

*Mandibular molars generally have two terminal roots, the _____ and _____.

Permanent
Mandibular
1st Molar
Right
1. FACIAL
2. MESIAL

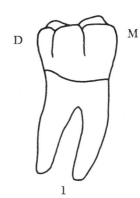 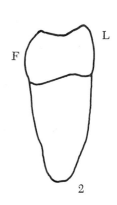

mesial, distal

The maxillary first premolar is usually bifurcated. The terminal roots are named the _____ and _____ roots.

Permanent
Maxillary
1st Premolar
1. FACIAL
2. DISTAL

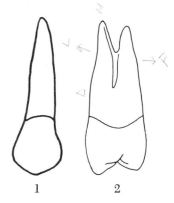

facial, lingual

Of the anterior and premolar teeth, the only tooth that is commonly bifurcated is the _____. The anterior tooth that is less frequently bifurcated is the _____.

Remembering the number and relative position of the roots of the permanent teeth, which one of the following surfaces would *not* generally occur?

    a. The lingual surface of the mesiofacial root of the maxillary second molar ....GO TO NEXT FRAME
    b. The mesial surface of the mesial root of the mandibular first molar........GO TO BOTTOM OF THIS PAGE
    c. The mesial surface of the facial root of the maxillary canine....................GO TO TOP OF PAGE 33.

▶ From preceding frame   *a is incorrect*

A mesiofacial root is usually present on all maxillary molars. Also, there is a distofacial root and a lingual root. Each of these terminal roots has a lingual surface.

Permanent
Maxillary
Right
1st Molar
1. LINGUAL
2. MESIAL

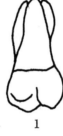 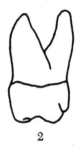

1   2

RETURN TO TOP OF THIS PAGE AND ANSWER AGAIN.

▶ From top of this page   *b is incorrect*

The mandibular first molar has two terminal roots, the mesial and distal. Each of these has a broad mesial surface.

Permanent
Mandibular
Right
1st Molar
FACIAL

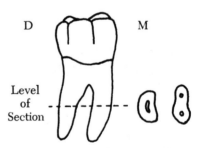

RETURN TO TOP OF THIS PAGE AND ANSWER AGAIN.

◆ From page 32

c *is correct (The maxillary canines are single rooted, and would not have a "facial root")*

Which premolar is frequently multi-rooted, and what are the names of the two roots?

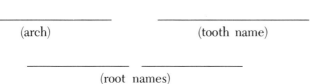

_____   _____
        (arch)   (tooth name)

        _____ _____
              (root names)

---

maxillary first premolar, facial, lingual

Descriptions of teeth involve curvatures in the longitudinal and horizontal directions. For instance, the long dimension of the root (cervical line to apex) is referred to as the **cervicoapical** or **longitudinal** dimension. In the drawing, the longitudinal dimension of the root is indicated by line _____ (A/B/C).

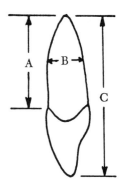

A *is correct*

The width of a tooth is described in either of two directions—**mesiodistal** or **faciolingual.** If you look at the lingual surface of a tooth, the width of the root will be seen in a _____ direction.

Permanent
Maxillary
Right
Central Incisor
1. LINGUAL
2. MESIAL

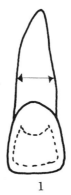
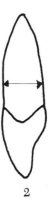

1   2

The three-dimensional form of a tooth is difficult to show in a two-dimensional line drawing, so it is sometimes convenient to illustrate a particular feature of a root by showing either a horizontal or longitudinal **section** of a tooth. Which drawing represents a horizontal section? (sometimes called a cross-section) _____ _____ (Fig. 1/Fig. 2/Fig. 3/Fig. 4)

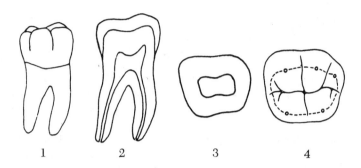

Fig. 3

The concept of horizontal and longitudinal sections is simple, but often the vocabulary is confusing.

A longitudinal section can be taken in two ways: a mesiodistal longitudinal section and a faciolingual longitudinal section. A horizontal section can be taken at different levels but in only one way.

    Permanent
    Maxillary
    Canine
    1. FACIOLINGUAL SECTION
    2. MESIODISTAL SECTION
    3. FACIAL
    4. HORIZONTAL SECTIONS

Which section will show an outline of the mesial surface of the root of the central incisor in the cervicoapical direction?

Faciolingual longitudinal section .... GO TO TOP OF PAGE 35.

Mesiodistal longitudinal section ......GO TO BOTTOM OF PAGE 35.

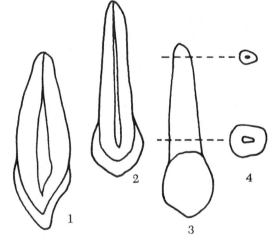

The faciolingual-longitudinal section will show the cervicoapical curvature of the *facial* and *lingual* surfaces. Which longitudinal section will show the cervicoapical curvature of the mesial and distal surfaces? _____.

Permanent
Maxillary
Central Incisor
FACIOLINGUAL LONGITUDINAL
   SECTION

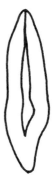

mesiodistal

Which type of section reveals the outline of each of the four root surfaces of the maxillary canine in both the mesiodistal and faciolingual directions? _____.

Permanent
Maxillary
Canine
1. FACIOLINGUAL SECTION
2. MESIODISTAL SECTION
3. FACIAL
4. HORIZONTAL SECTIONS

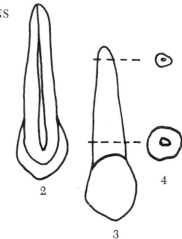

horizontal

TURN TO PAGE 36 AND TAKE REVIEW TEST 3

REVIEW TEST 3

1. The term "alveolus" refers to . . .
   a. a part of the root.
   b. the base of the bone supporting a tooth.
   c. a socket in the bone supporting a tooth.

2. Which list gives the universal code numbers of three teeth that are likely to be bifurcated?
   a. 3, 21, 15
   b. 31, 5, 19
   c. 5, 32, 8

3. Although permanent teeth may have one, two, or three roots, each tooth has only one
   . . .
   a. root trunk.
   b. terminal root.

4. In this volume, the term "root" refers to the anatomical root of a tooth, i.e. that part of a tooth . . .
   a. embedded within the alveolar bone.
   b. between the cervical line and the apex.

5. Which of the following teeth are commonly trifurcated?
   a. lateral incisor
   b. maxillary canine
   c. mandibular molar
   d. maxillary molar
   e. maxillary premolar

6. Which of the following are names of longitudinal sections of roots?
   a. mesiodistal
   b. mesiofacial
   c. faciolingual
   d. distofacial
   e. all of the above

MAKE A NOTE OF YOUR ANSWERS, AND TURN TO PAGE 49

SECTION 4.0   INTRODUCTION TO TOOTH TISSUES

A tooth is composed of both hard and soft tissues. The hard tissues will be discussed first. The hard tissues are **enamel, cementum, and dentin** (DEN tun, not "dentyne"). *Enamel* is the tooth's hardest tissue and forms the shell of the anatomical crown. The enamel ends where it meets the cementum. The *cementum* covers the anatomical root. Where the crown and root join, the cementum and enamel form the **cementoenamel junction,** also called the *cervical line*.

Together, the enamel and cementum form the outer shell of the tooth.

The enamel covers the anatomical _____ of the tooth.

a. FACIAL
b. MESIODISTAL
   LONGITUDINAL
   SECTION

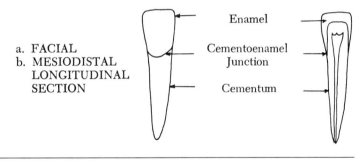

Enamel

Cementoenamel Junction

Cementum

---

crown

The *cementum* covers the anatomical _____ of the tooth.

---

root

The *cementoenamel* junction is found where the _____ and _____ meet.

---

cementum (root), enamel (crown)

Another name for the cementoenamel junction is the _____ line.

37

The *dentin* is the third hard tissue of the tooth. Dentin forms most of the root and a major portion of the crown.

The dentin is covered by the enamel on the crown and the cementum on the root. Within the dentin is a cavity which begins at the apical foramen and terminates in the crown. Within the crown, the cavity is termed **pulp chamber;** within the root, **root canal.** The pulp chamber follows the general contours of the tooth, causing the chambers to terminate in conical-shaped peaks. These are called **pulp horns.** The pulp horns, pulp chamber, and root canal make up the cavity in the _____.

SECTION 4.1   PULP ANATOMY

The cavity in the dentin is filled with soft tissue, called **pulp.** Both the pulp chamber and root canal are filled with pulpal tissue. The pulp chamber is lined with cells called **odontoblasts** (dentin-forming cells). Throughout the pulp is a rich network of blood vessels, and **lymphatic vessels.**

The pulp has several functions. Its primary function is to form dentin throughout the life of the tooth. The pulp also supplies nutrients to the tooth through its network of blood vessels, and responds defensively to any injury to the tooth.

Permanent
Maxillary
1st Premolar
FACIOLINGUAL
    LONGITUDINAL
    SECTION

Permanent
Maxillary
Canine
FACIOLINGUAL
    LONGITUDINAL
    SECTION

— Dentin —

— Pulp —

— Enamel —

The **pulp cavity** is the central cavity within each tooth. The hard tissue that completely surrounds the pulp cavity is the _____ (enamel/dentin/cementum).

Permanent
Mandibular
1st Molar
MESIODISTAL
    SECTION

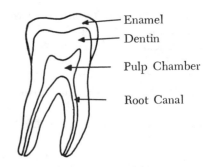

— Enamel
— Dentin
— Pulp Chamber
— Root Canal

The pulp cavity is divided into two major
parts, the *pulp chamber* and the *root canal*.
The pulp chamber occurs in the _____
portion of the tooth.

Permanent
Mandibular
1st Molar
MESIODISTAL
   SECTION

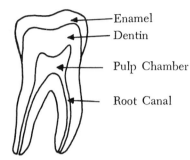

— Enamel

— Dentin

— Pulp Chamber

— Root Canal

The part of the pulp cavity that occurs in the
root is called the _____.

Permanent
Mandibular
1. 1st Molar
2. Canine
MESIODISTAL
   SECTIONS

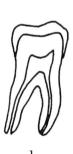 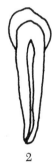

1   2

The two major portions of the pulp cavity are the pulp _____
and the _____.

Permanent
Mandibular
Canine
MESIODISTAL
   SECTION

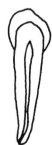

The pulp chamber and root canal are the two parts of the _____.

Permanent
Mandibular
1st Molar
MESIODISTAL
   SECTION

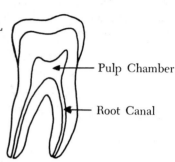

Pulp Chamber

Root Canal

The occlusoapical extremes of the pulp cavity are the **roof** of the pulp chamber and one or more constricted openings over the apex called the apical foramen (pl. foramina). The dentin that forms the most occlusal (incisal) wall of the pulp cavity is called the _____ of the pulp chamber.

The first layer of pulpal tissue within the walls of the pulp cavity is made up of dentin-producing cells called _____.

The openings (one or more) near the apex of each root are called the apical _____ (pl. _____).

The division between the pulp chamber and the root canals in teeth with more than one root canal is usually well defined. In teeth with a single root canal, the division between the pulp chamber and root canal is _____ (distinct/indistinct).

Permanent
Mandibular
1. Lateral Incisor
2. 1st Molar
MESIODISTAL
   SECTIONS

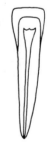 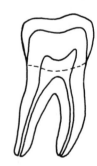

1   2

The division between the pulp chamber and root canal(s) lies at or apical to the division between the anatomical crown and root. In teeth with a more distinct division between the two parts of the pulp cavity, the dentin bounding the pulp chamber and lying somewhat parallel to the roof is called the **floor** of the pulp chamber. A chamber floor is present only when the pulp chamber gives rise to more than one _____.

Permanent
Mandibular
1. Lateral Incisor
2. 1st Molar
MESIODISTAL
    SECTIONS

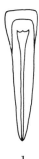
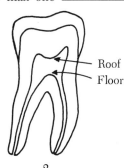

Roof
Floor

1   2

The occlusoapical level of the floor of the pulp chamber lies at or apical to the level of the _____.

Permanent
Mandibular
1. Lateral Incisor
2. 1st Molar
MESIODISTAL
    SECTIONS

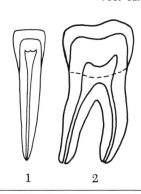

1   2

Each of the openings leading from the pulp chamber to a root canal is called a root canal **orifice.** Therefore, a canal orifice is an opening in the _____ of the pulp chamber.

Permanent
Mandibular
1st Molar
MESIODISTAL
    SECTION

Orifice   Orifice

In teeth with a bifurcation of the pulp cavity at the floor of the chamber, each opening leading from the chamber to a root canal is called a root canal _____.

Permanent
Mandibular
1st Molar
MESIODISTAL
SECTION

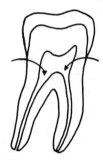

The **walls** of the pulp cavity derive their names from the corresponding walls of the tooth surface. The name of pulp chamber wall A is the _____ wall.

Permanent
Mandibular
1st Molar
MESIODISTAL
SECTION

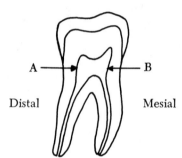

A — Distal   B — Mesial

Name the structures labeled A, B, and C.

A. _____
B. _____
C. _____

Permanent
Mandibular
1st Molar
MESIODISTAL
SECTION

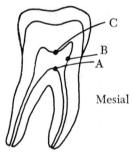

Distal   Mesial

The roof of the pulp chamber is frequently indented by small extensions called **pulp horns,** which generally occur directly beneath each cusp. <u>Each horn is named for its corresponding cusp.</u> Thus, pulp horn A is named the _____ pulp horn.

Permanent
Mandibular
1st Molar
MESIODISTAL SECTION

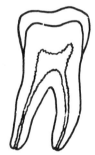

Mesiofacial Cusp

A

Distal

Mesial

mesiofacial

The four-cusped mandibular second molar would have _____ (number) pulp horns, but the two-cusped maxillary first premolar would have only _____ (number) pulp horns.

four, two

Just as there are variations in the external shape of roots, the interior walls of the pulp chamber and root canals are irregular with many small concavities. The drawings in this program show the walls as very smooth, for simplicity, but the reader should think of them as irregular.

In single rooted teeth, the root canal is continuous with the pulp chamber at approximately the _____ line.

Permanent
Mandibular
Canine
MESIODISTAL
SECTION

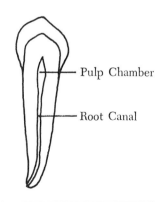

Pulp Chamber

Root Canal

In multi-rooted teeth, the orifice of each root canal is located
on the floor of the _____ .

Permanent
Mandibular
1st Molar
MESIODISTAL
  SECTION

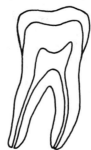

Each root canal terminates
at one or more _____
located near the _____
of the root.

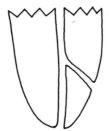 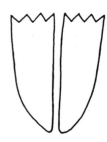

Accessory canals (small branches from the
main root canal) occur almost exclusively in
the _____ third of the root.

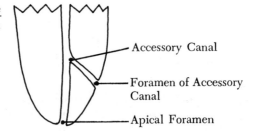

Accessory Canal

Foramen of Accessory
Canal

Apical Foramen

The apical foramen is the opening at (or very near) the apex of
the root shown. A is an _____ ; B is an _____ .

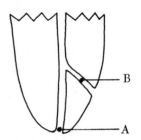

B

A

Foramina and canals may also occur in the middle third rather than the apical third of the root. These canals are called **aberrant canals.** In the illustration, which accessory canal might be called an **aberrant** canal? ——————— (A/B/C)

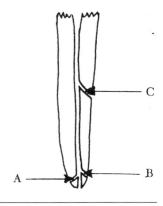

C

The blood vessels and nerves, nourishing and innervating the pulp, enter the pulp cavity primarily through the ———————.

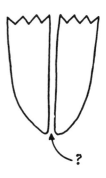

apical foramen (pl. foramina)

Accessory and aberrant canals may also have nerves and blood vessels.

SUMMARY

A tooth is divided into a crown and a root, the crown being covered with enamel and the root with cementum. The cementum and enamel join to form the cementoenamel junction, also called the cervical line. Within this shell of enamel and cementum is the bulk of the tooth, the dentin. A cavity within the dentin is filled with pulpal tissues (odontoblasts, blood vessels, nerves, lymphatic vessels). The pulp cavity is divided into a pulp chamber and one or more root canals. Parts of the pulp cavity include the walls, floor and roof of the pulp chamber, pulp horns, root canal orifices, accessory canals and apical foramina. The walls of the pulp cavity are irregular with many small concavities.

REVIEW TEST 4

Directions: Terms used in this section are listed in Group I (a-m). A set of definitions is given in Group II. In the blank to the right of each definition, write the letter (from Group I) of the term being defined.

Write your answers on scratch paper and turn to Page 50.

Group I

a. aberrant canal	**h.** lymphatic vessels
b. accessory canal	**i.** orifice
c. cementum	**j.** pulp cavity
d. dentin	**k.** pulp chamber
e. floor	**l.** roof
f. apical foramen	**m.** root canal
g. pulp horn	

Group II

1. An outer opening at the apex of the root through which the blood and nerve supply of the pulp enter the tooth. _____

2. An accentuation of the roof of the pulp cavity corresponding to a cusp or lobe. _____

3. An opening in the floor of the pulp chamber leading to a root canal. _____

4. The central cavity within a tooth. _____

5. Lateral branches of the main root canal occurring in the apical third of the root. _____

6. One of the soft pulpal tissues. _____

7. Hard tooth tissue covering the anatomical root. _____

GO TO PAGE 50

TEST ANSWER SECTION

REVIEW TEST 1
(From Page 9)

Correct Answers:

1. *a. canine*
   b. premolar
   c. incisor
2. *b*   3. *c*   4. *a and b*   5. *c*

IF YOU GOT THEM ALL CORRECT, congratulations. STOP right now and take a break to reward yourself for study progress. Do something that is interesting to you and available right now, such as eating or drinking something or taking a walk. This will increase your learning and willingness to study if you DO IT IMMEDIATELY AND CONSISTENTLY AFTER COMPLETING EACH TEST IN THIS PROGRAM. When you return, continue on Page 10.

IF YOU MISSED ONE QUESTION, read the instructions for this question below. Review and then retake the review test (Page 9).

1. IF YOU MISSED QUESTION 1, review the forms and names of the teeth on Pages 3–8.

2. IF YOU MISSED QUESTION 2, review the terms eruption (Page 2) and mastication (Page 4).

3. IF YOU MISSED QUESTION 3, there are 12 molars (Page 7) and use that number as the numerator in the fraction 12/32.

4. IF YOU MISSED QUESTION 4, the wedge-shape of crowns should be reviewed on Page 5.

5. IF YOU MISSED QUESTION 5, note that the anatomical root could in some cases be exposed above surrounding tissue. Review on page 1.

IF YOU MISSED TWO OR MORE QUESTIONS, do not go on until you have reviewed the whole section beginning on page 1. Then, retake the review test (Page 9) until you get all questions correct. Do not be discouraged at being directed to review. It is easier to restudy now than to let it go.

REVIEW TEST 2
(From Page 26)

Correct Answers:

1. *a* 2. *b* 3. *b and c* 4. *a and d* 5. *18, Permanent mandibular left 2nd molar; I, primary maxillary left 1st molar; 3, permanent maxillary right 1st molar; M, primary mandibular left canine.*

IF YOU GOT THEM ALL CORRECT, STOP NOW, and do something rewarding. When you return, continue on Page 27.

IF YOU MISSED ONE QUESTION, read the instructions for that question below. Review and then retake the review test (Page 26).

1. IF YOU MISSED QUESTION 1, review arches (Page 10), quadrants (Page 11) or diphyodont (Page 12).

2. IF YOU MISSED QUESTION 2, review contacting or proximal (Page 20).

3. IF YOU MISSED QUESTION 3, review thirds (Pages 24–25).

4. IF YOU MISSED QUESTION 4, review one or more of the following:
   a. Facial surfaces are labial and buccal surfaces .... Page 22.
   b. Facial and lingual surfaces are not occlusal surfaces .... Pages 10 and 22.
   c. Not every tooth has an occlusal surface, some have incisal .... Page 19.
   d. Tooth surface names, incisal, occlusal, depend on position of the tooth in the arch
   .... Pages 10–11.

5. IF YOU MISSED QUESTION 5, review naming and coding on Pages 14–19.

IF YOU MISSED TWO OR MORE QUESTIONS, return to Page 10, review this section again, and then retake this test (Page 26).

REVIEW TEST 3
(From Page 36)

Correct Answers:

1. *c*   2. *b*   3. *a*   4. *b*   5. *d*   6. *a and c*

IF YOU GOT THEM ALL CORRECT, take a break now . . . you've earned it! Do something to reward yourself, then resume study on the next section (Page 37).

IF YOU MISSED ONE QUESTION, review it using the directions below, and then retake the test on Page 36. A perfect score will advance you to the next section.

1. IF YOU MISSED QUESTION 1, review alveolus on Page 28.

2. IF YOU MISSED QUESTION 2, you may want to review tooth numbering on Page 16. Teeth with bifurcated roots should be reviewed from Page 31.

3. IF YOU MISSED QUESTION 3, review root trunk (Page 30).

4. IF YOU MISSED QUESTION 4, review Page 27, on the definition of the anatomical root.

5. IF YOU MISSED QUESTION 5, review trifurcated roots on Pages 27–31.

6. IF YOU MISSED QUESTION 6, review longitudinal sections on Pages 33–34.

IF YOU MISSED TWO OR MORE QUESTIONS, it would be to your benefit to review this section beginning at Page 27. You will learn more the second time through the section. Retake the review test (Page 36). A perfect score will advance you to the next section.

REVIEW TEST 4
(From Page 46)

Group I

a. aberrant canal
b. accessory canal
c. cementum
d. dentin
e. floor
f. apical foramen
g. pulp horn
h. lymphatic vessels
i. orifice
j. pulp cavity
k. pulp chamber
l. roof
m. root canal

Group II

1. An outer opening of the apex of the root through which the blood and nerve supply of the pulp enter the tooth.

   f.
   Page 45

2. An accentuation of the roof of the pulp cavity corresponding to a cusp or lobe.

   g.
   Page 43

3. An opening in the floor of the pulp chamber leading to a root canal.

   i.
   Page 41

4. The central cavity within a tooth.

   j.
   Page 38

5. Lateral branches of the main root canal generally occurring in the apical third of the root.

   b.
   Pages 44–45

6. One of the soft pulpal tissues.

h.

Page 38

7. Hard tooth tissue covering the anatomical root.

c.

Page 37

IF YOU MISSED TWO OR MORE QUESTIONS, review each question, then, return to Page 37 and go through this section again quickly to be sure you have mastered the material presented. Then, retake this review test (Page 46) until you get all questions correct. When you have finished continue on Page 56.

REVIEW TEST 5
(From Page 66)

Correct Answers:

1. *c* 2. *a* 3. *b*

IF YOU GOT THEM ALL CORRECT, congratulations. TAKE A BREAK NOW and do something that will reward your study progress. Eat or drink something, go somewhere or talk to someone, or whatever. DO IT IMMEDIATELY and it will help you to study and learn. When you return, go to Page 67.

IF YOU MISSED ONE QUESTION, read the instructions for that question below. Review and then retake the review test.

1. IF YOU MISSED QUESTION 1, review cementum on Page 58 or papillary tissue on Pages 64–65, or periodontal ligament on Pages 61–63.

2. IF YOU MISSED QUESTION 2, note that cemento*enamel* junction not the cemento*dental* junction is called the cervical line (see Page 59, then Page 60). If you need to review the term gingival sulcus, see Page 63. If you need to review papillary gingiva, see Pages 64–65.

3. IF YOU MISSED QUESTION 3, if necessary, review secondary dentin on Page 60, or ameloblasts on Page 56, or dentin on Page 58.

IF YOU MISSED TWO OR MORE QUESTIONS, it is to your benefit to review this section again, starting with Page 56. Do not be discouraged at being directed into a preceding part of the program, since it is much easier to correct a misconception early than to let it go.

REVIEW TEST 6
(From Page 81)

Correct Answers:

1. *c*   2. *b*   3. *d*   4. *c*

IF YOU GOT THEM ALL CORRECT, stop and do something to reward your study progress. Do that immediately, then return to Page 82 when you resume studying.

IF YOU MISSED ONE QUESTION, review it by following the directions below, and then retake the test on Page 81. A perfect score will advance you to Page 82.

1. IF YOU MISSED QUESTION 1, review as necessary the following: (a) four or more lobes (Page 69); (b) calcification of crown complete at eruption (Page 74); (c) growth centers (Page 69).

2. IF YOU MISSED QUESTION 2, review as necessary the following: (a) grooves separate the lobes (Page 69); (b) cusp of Carabelli found on the maxillary, not mandibular, first molar (Page 71); (c) lobe arrangement of most premolars similar to incisors (Page 71).

3. IF YOU MISSED QUESTION 3, review the first permanent teeth to erupt (Page 75).

4. IF YOU MISSED QUESTION 4, review as necessary the following: (a) first evidence of development (Page 67); (b) primary eruption sequence (Page 74); (c) active eruption is restrained when antagonists are met, but may continue to compensate for attrition (Page 78).

IF YOU MISSED TWO OR MORE QUESTIONS, you should review beginning on Page 67 so as to master this material before moving on. Retake the review test on Page 81 after you have studied this section again.

REVIEW TEST 7
(From Page 95)

Correct Answers:

1. *b*   2. *b*   3. *c*   4. *b*   5. *a*   6. *b-I, c-II, a-III*   7. *c-I, b-II, a-III*

IF YOU GOT THEM ALL CORRECT, stop, take a break and do something to reward your study progress. Do that immediately and then return to Section 8.0 on Page 97 when you resume studying.

IF YOU MISSED ONE QUESTION, review it by following the directions below. Then retake the review test (Page 95). A perfect score will advance you to the next section.

1. IF YOU MISSED QUESTION 1, review the location of the interdental area on Pages 89–90.

2. IF YOU MISSED QUESTION 2, review Pages 91–92 on embrasures.

3. IF YOU MISSED QUESTION 3, review interdental papilla on Pages 89–90.

4. IF YOU MISSED QUESTION 4, review occlusion on Pages 82–83.

5. IF YOU MISSED QUESTION 5, review centric cusps on Pages 85–87.

6. IF YOU MISSED QUESTION 6, review overlap and classes of occlusion on Pages 83–85.

7. IF YOU MISSED QUESTION 7, review classes of occlusion on Pages 84–85.

IF YOU MISSED TWO OR MORE QUESTIONS, you should review beginning on Page 82 (Section 7.0). It will be important for later work that you master this section before going on. Retake Review Test 7 on Page 95 after reviewing.

REVIEW TEST 8
(From Page 113)

Correct Answers:

1. *c*   2. *a*   3. *a. incisal third, b. middle third, c. incisal third, d. middle third, e. middle third, f. middle third*   4. *a*   5. *b*

IF YOU GOT ALL QUESTIONS CORRECT, congratulations, you have completed this chapter! Take a break now and give yourself a reward (something that *you* enjoy having or doing) for finishing this chapter.

IF YOU MISSED ANY QUESTIONS, review by following the directions below. Then, retake Review Test 8 on Page 113. A perfect score will mean you have completed this chapter.

1. IF YOU MISSED QUESTION 1, review the lingual tipping of mandibular molars on Page 109.

2. IF YOU MISSED QUESTION 2, review Page 104 on the proximal contact areas.

3. IF YOU MISSED QUESTION 3, review the location of proximal contacts in the incisocervical (occlusocervical) dimension on Pages 101–102.

4. IF YOU MISSED QUESTION 4, review the depth of facial embrasures on Pages 98–99.

5. IF YOU MISSED QUESTION 5, review the faciolingual location of contacts of posterior teeth by examining Pages 98–99.

IF YOU MISSED TWO OR MORE QUESTIONS, you should review beginning with Section 8.0 on Page 97. It will be important for later chapters for you to have mastered this material on proximal contacts, embrasures and heights of contour. Retake Review Test 8 on Page 113 after reviewing.

SECTION 5.0 TOOTH TISSUES

Tooth tissues have been previously discussed in regard to anatomical definitions. The junction of the cementum and enamel (cemento-enamel junction) forms the cervical line, separating the tooth into anatomical crown and root portions. The cementum and enamel together form the outer shell of the tooth. The dentin makes up the body or bulk of the tooth. The pulp contains nerve tissues and blood vessels to provide sensation and nutrition to the tooth. Of these four tissues, the first three—enamel, cementum, and dentin—are hard tissues; the fourth—pulp—is soft. These four tissues will be taken up in sequence with a more detailed explanation of their characteristics. The hard tissue that covers the anatomical crown of a tooth is known as _____.

enamel

Beneath the enamel is another tissue, not quite as hard, called the _____.

dentin

The hard outer shell of enamel serves to protect the tooth from wear and prolongs its working life. In fact, the hardest tissue in the body is _____.

enamel

Enamel is translucent but has a bluish-white tint which contributes to the coloration of the tooth. Because of the translucency of the enamel, much of the tooth coloration is due to the _____.

dentin

Enamel is composed of microscopic rods called **enamel rods.** The rods are generally perpendicular to the dentin and are bound together by a cement substance. These rods can be cleaved with cutting instruments. The hardness of enamel makes it susceptible to fracture, especially where it is not supported by dentin. This may occur with dental caries (decay). Despite its hardness, enamel is subject to wear and, over a lifetime, a tooth may lose much of its incisal or occlusal enamel due to wear. The enamel is the only tissue completely formed before the tooth erupts, and once the enamel is laid down by the **ameloblasts** (enamel-producing cells), it *does not* have the ability of self repair. When enamel has been fractured, how is it mended?

By the enamel rods rebonding to each other
.................GO TO TOP OF PAGE 57

By artificial restoration methods ....
..............GO TO MIDDLE OF PAGE 57

◆ From page 56

You missed a small but very important concept. <u>Enamel *does not* have the ability of self repair</u>. After the enamel has initially been laid down, the process will not repeat itself for any type of enamel destruction, whether it is fractured or lost by normal abrasion. While the enamel rods are initially bonded together by a cement-like substance, this natural process cannot be repeated. Therefore, in tooth repair, artificial substances must be used; the correct choice of answers should have been "by artificial restoration methods."

GO TO NEXT FRAME

◆ From page 56

The study of artificial restoration methods would presumably lead to a study of operative or restorative dentistry, which will not be taken up now.

Enamel has at least three unique features: (1) it is complete by the time the tooth erupts; (2) the ameloblasts become inactive, and the tissue ceases to form after the tooth has erupted; and (3) it is the hardest tissue in the human body. Despite its hardness, enamel is subject to considerable _____ during the life of the tooth.

wear

Notice that the enamel layer is thickest on the _____ edge (surface) and tapers toward the _____ line.

Permanent
Maxillary
1. Canine
2. 1st Premolar
FACIOLINGUAL
SECTIONS

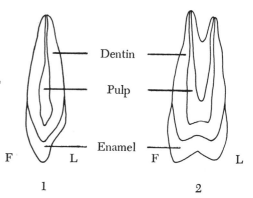

1

2

incisal (occlusal), cervical

Two types of cells that have a role in the formation of tooth tissue have been introduced. The names of these cells have the same suffix (ending). The first layer of pulp tissue that has a role in the formation of dentin is made up of cells called _____. Enamel-producing cells are called _____.

Enamel, the exterior tooth surface, covers the anatomical crown of the tooth.

Cementum is another hard tooth tissue. It is also an exterior tooth tissue covering the anatomical root portion of the tooth. **Cementoblasts, which lay down cementum, are very similar to the osteoblasts which form bone.**

The similarity between cementum and bone is evident histologically, chemically, and in its physiologic behavior. Cementum is continually laid down during the life of the tooth in the areas of the apex and where multiple roots join. The basic difference between cementum and bone tissues is that *bone* undergoes **resorbtion** and formation in cycles. *Cementum continues formation but normally does not resorb.* Because of this process, pressure can be applied to a tooth with an orthodonic appliance ("braces"), and the resorbtion of the _____ allows the tooth to be brought into proper alignment.

We can explain the process which permits orthodonic alignment to occur by studying, in more detail, the cementum and tooth attachment to the alveolar bone. A function of cementum is to attach the tooth root to a ligament called the **periodontal ligament,** which, in turn, attaches to the alveolar bone. A tooth is held in the alveolus by this attachment apparatus composed of three parts: the cementum, the periodontal ligament, and the alveolar bone. Orthodontic bands (or other sustained forces) produce pressure on areas of the periodontal ligament and alveolar bone, resulting in resorption of the bone in those areas. At the same time, tension is produced elsewhere on the periodontal ligament and alveolar bone, resulting in _____ (formation/resorbtion) of new bone tissue in the areas of tension.

Both cementum and enamel are hard tooth tissues, enamel being the hardest tissue in the body. Cementum, a tooth tissue, is also termed a supporting structure, for it serves to attach the tooth to the alveolar bone. Together, enamel and cementum form the outer shell of the tooth.

Within this shell is the dentin, another hard tissue. Although measurements of the hardness of tooth tissues vary with the exact location on the tooth where the measurements are taken, on the average, dentin is found to be not as hard as enamel but harder than cementum. Thus, the order of hardness of the hard tooth tissues is enamel, dentin, and cementum.

Dentin forms the bulk of the tooth, both crown and root, and surrounds the pulp cavity. By making up the bulk of the tooth, dentin gives the tooth its general form and elastic strength. The hard enamel tissue which is laid directly upon the dentin depends upon this elastic strength for support. One can summarize the hard tissue makeup of the tooth as mostly _____ covered with _____ or _____.

The hard tissues of the tooth are the *dentin* which is overlaid on the root with *cementum* and on the crown with *enamel*. Where the under surface of the enamel joins the dentin, a junction is formed. The word that describes this junction, like many other dental terms, has been coined by using the letter "o" resulting in a name for the junction of the dentin and enamel. It is the _____ o _____ junction, also called the D-E junction.

The dentin is thickest in the anatomic crown of a tooth, gradually tapering to thinner and thinner bulk as one approaches the root apex. You might remember that under the dentoenamel junction (in the anatomical crown), the dentin is thicker than in the root. The root, of course, is not covered with enamel. It is covered with _____.

Therefore, the dentoenamel junction does not extend into the anatomical root. Instead, the dentin joins the cementum in this region. The same method for building a descriptive word for this junction holds true— the terms dentin and cementum are connected by an "o." At first everyone has difficulty remembering the correct sequence of words in building such terms. For instance, dentoenamel junction is correct, but enamodental junction is incorrect. The proper order of connecting words is determined by convention and common usage within the dental profession.

What are two words that could be used to describe the junction of the dentin and the cementum? _____ and _____.

The term that is commonly used is *cementodental*.

1. The C-E junction (the junction of the enamel and cementum) is also called the _____ junction which also forms the _____ line.
2. The D-E junction (the junction of the enamel and dentin) is also called the _____ junction.
3. The C-D junction (the junction of the cementum and dentin) is also called the _____ junction.

Because of the translucence of the enamel, the color of the dentin is one of the contributing factors of tooth color, varying from yellow to dark brown in color. Unlike enamel or cementum, dentin is sensitive to touch, thermal change, acids of foods, and the like. Dentin, like cementum, continues to form during the life of the tooth.

Does enamel also continue to form throughout the tooth's lifetime? (Yes? or No?) ——————.

no

Which tooth tissue is usually found to be harder—cementum or dentin? ——————.

dentin

Enamel is the only tooth tissue which is completed upon eruption of the tooth. But, let's study the dentin. It isn't solid inorganic material, but has tube-like structures, called **tubules**, running through it from the pulp to the dentoenamel junction. These tubules contain extensions of the dentin-forming cells, the ——————.

odontoblasts

The structure of the tubules and the presence of living odontoblasts makes dentin a living tissue, permeable to fluids and sensitive to stimuli.

Dentin formation is active during the crown and root formation. We call this dentin the **primary dentin.** Dentin continues to form more slowly after the root is fully formed. This type of dentin differs in morphology from the primary dentin and is called **secondary dentin**.

When irritants act on the tooth, such as hot and cold temperatures, abrasion, dental caries, etc., the pulp and its odontoblasts are stimulated to form secondary dentin over the primary dentin in the pulp chamber and/or root canal to insulate the delicate pulp tissue from the irritation. The effect is to cause recession of the pulp into smaller and smaller confines. Such recession may, in some instances, obliterate the pulp cavity. Dentin also ages and aged dentin tubules may die, becoming *dead tracts,* or the tubules may calcify and become obliterated (*sclerotic dentin*). Sclerotic dentin is more highly mineralized, giving the dentin in the area a translucent appearance somewhat like an agate.

Considering only the dentin which is laid down along the D-E junction, which term properly identifies that dentin? —————— (primary/secondary).

Secondary dentin would be an incorrect answer to the previous question because the tooth forms its dentin from the dentoenamel junction inward towards the pulp cavity. The dentin in the area adjacent to the D-E junction is primary dentin. Secondary dentin is laid down after the tooth is formed, well inwards from the D-E junction. Don't forget that dentin formation is a continual process as long as the pulp provides nutrients to the odontoblasts.

The fourth tooth tissue is *dental pulp*, which is a delicate, soft tissue organ. It is composed of odontoblasts to form dentin, blood vessels for nutrients, nerves for communication to the rest of the body, and connective tissues. The pulp is surrounded by the dentin and is the formative organ of the dentin. Among its functions are the formation of secondary dentin which is a defensive function to protect against irritants. Too much irritation can kill the pulp, ending its odontoblastic activity. Remember that the formation of secondary dentin causes the pulp cavity to become smaller as the tooth ages. What forms secondary dentin? _____.

odontoblasts (in the dental pulp)

Considering the changes in the pulp cavity that occur with age, which patients would generally have larger pulp cavities, younger or older patients? _____.

younger

SECTION 5.1   SUPPORTING STRUCTURES FOR THE TOOTH

The tooth supporting structures, also four in number, are **cementum, periodontal ligament, gingiva** (JIN juh vuh), and **alveolar bone**.

Cementum, as previously noted, is a _____ (hard/soft) tooth tissue as well as being a supporting structure.

ameloblasts
odontoblasts
osteoblasts

Cementum is the hard tissue that bonds the tooth to the periodontal ligament, which is the soft tissue that surrounds the roots of the tooth and attaches to the alveolar bone. The periodontal ligament acts as a shock absorber, cushioning and stabilizing the tooth while transferring forces applied to the tooth into the bone. When severe forces are applied against the tooth, the periodontal ligament may become damaged and pain and inflammation may result. Other functions of the periodontal ligament include sensory and nutritive functions which are fulfilled by nerves and blood vessels within the ligament. Also, located in the area of the periodontal ligament are cementum-forming cells, called _____.

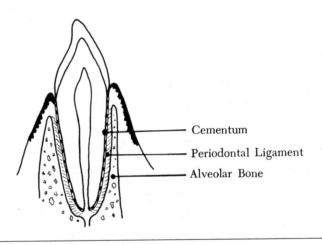

Cementum

Periodontal Ligament

Alveolar Bone

cementoblasts

These items review the subject matter from the previous page. Refer back as necessary until the items are clear.

The tooth is attached to its socket by the _____.

periodontal ligament

The tooth tissue to which the fibers of the periodontal ligament are attached is called the _____.

cementum

The outer ends of these fibers are attached to the _____ bone.

The periodontal ligament functions to protect against forces acting on the tooth by _____.

The outermost of the supporting tissues is the _gingiva_. Healthy gingiva, often incorrectly called "gums," is a firm, resilient, pink tissue which covers the alveolar bone and through which the tooth's clinical crown protrudes. The gingiva may be divided into attached gingiva and free gingiva. The gingiva directly adjacent to the alveolar bone is referred to as attached gingiva. Gingiva which extends coronally (toward the crown) from the attached gingiva is called _____ gingiva.

The gingiva also attaches directly to the tooth. The attachment to the tooth is always slightly apical to the height of the visible tissue surrounding the tooth. There is, therefore, a space between the gingiva and the tooth, somewhat like a miniature trough, encircling the crown. We call this very narrow space the **gingival sulcus** (JIN juh vul, SULL kuss). In healthy mouths, the gingival sulcus ranges from almost non-existence to 3 mm in depth.

The free gingival groove is a shallow indentation or groove found in some areas of the mouth, paralleling the margin of the free gingiva and roughly corresponding to the deepest point of the gingival sulcus.

The surface of gingival tissue is covered with a cell tissue that is common to protective surface tissue throughout the body and it is called **epithelium** (e pith THEE lee um). The space located coronally from the connection of the epithelium to the tooth is called the gingival sulcus, which _____ (does/does not) completely surround each tooth.

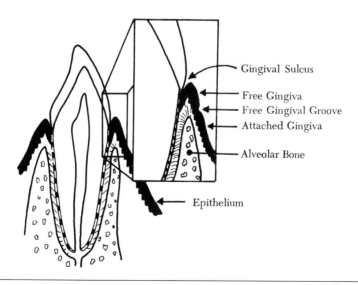

Gingival Sulcus

Free Gingiva

Free Gingival Groove

Attached Gingiva

Alveolar Bone

Epithelium

The free gingiva is further subdivided as **papillary** (PAP ill larry) and **mar- ginal** gingiva. The free papillary gingiva, or just papillary gingiva, occupies the space between the teeth. The marginal gingiva is free gingiva that is both facial and lingual, to each tooth. Therefore, the free gingiva that forms the boundary of each clinical crown is both papillary and marginal gingiva.

Permanent Mandibular Right
1. 1st Molar
2. 2nd Premolar
FACIAL

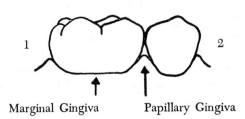

Marginal Gingiva   Papillary Gingiva

Papillary gingiva is located _____.

between teeth

Papillary and marginal gingiva collectively form the free gin- giva which extends coronally from the _____.

attached gingiva

The gingiva adjacent to the alveolar bone is called _____ gingiva.

attached

The free gingiva located facially and lingually to each tooth is called _____ gingiva.

marginal

Marginal gingiva is continuous with the free gingiva that ex- tends into the spaces between the teeth, that is the _____ gingiva.

Which of the schematic outlines shown below correctly diagrams the classification of
the gingiva?

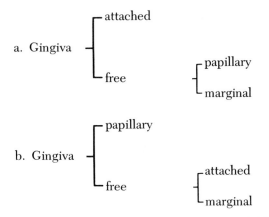

a. Gingiva ─┬─ attached
            │
            └─ free ─┬─ papillary
                     └─ marginal

b. Gingiva ─┬─ papillary
            │
            └─ free ─┬─ attached
                     └─ marginal

Classification a is correct

REVIEW TEST 5

1. Choose the *incorrect* statement.
   a. Cementum is classified as a supporting tissue.
   b. Papillary tissue is gingival tissue.
   c. The periodontal ligament is part of the marginal tissue.

2. Choose the *incorrect* statement.
   a. The cementodental junction is called the cervical line.
   b. The gingival sulcus is located between the tooth and the gingiva.
   c. Papillary gingiva occupies the space between the teeth.

3. Choose the *incorrect* statement.
   a. Pulpal stimulation causes the laying down of secondary dentin.
   b. Ameloblasts are bone producing cells.
   c. The dentin constitutes the major portion of the tooth.

MAKE A NOTE OF YOUR ANSWERS AND TURN TO PAGE 52

SECTION 6.0 LIFE HISTORY OF TEETH

All teeth initially develop from a <u>tooth germ—a small clump of cells capable of differentiating into the ameloblasts that form enamel, the odontoblasts that form dentin,</u> and the other specialized cells necessary to produce the complex structure we call a tooth. Both primary and permanent teeth form in this way. The cells differentiated from the tooth germ form the organic structure which is subsequently **calcified. Calcification** is the process through which tooth tissues become hardened by deposits of mineral salts, including calcium salts. The tooth tissues that are hardened by calcification are _____, _____, and, _____.

enamel, dentin, cementum

The <u>first tooth germs of the primary dentition</u> can be found <u>approximately at 5–7 weeks of fetal development</u>. The first tooth germs of the permanent dentition usually appear within 12 weeks after the first primary teeth begin to form—that is, they appear at approximately which point in fetal development? _____.

    a. at the first third
    b. at the midpoint
    c. at the last third

b. at the midpoint

<u>Dentin forms inwardly from the dentoenamel junction</u> and <u>enamel forms outwardly from the junction</u>. The development and calcification of tooth tissue is paralleled by development of the alveolar bone which will support the tooth. The bone forms a **crypt** <u>around the developing tooth.</u> The process of tooth and bone formation and eruption is time consuming. Are any teeth normally visible in the mouth at birth? _____.

No, not usually

The development of the hard tooth tissues in the crypt begins with the laying down of _____, then enamel, and, finally, cementum.

dentin

Which type of dentin is laid down in the crypt, *primary* or *secondary* dentin? _____.

67

The first primary teeth begin to calcify at about the midpoint of fetal development and calcification of <u>*all* primary teeth is normally completed at *three* to *four* years of age</u>. For permanent teeth, <u>calcification begins approximately at birth and is completed at eighteen</u> to twenty-five years of age. The development of a tooth begins with the formation of the <u>*crown*</u> and continues apically until the apex is formed. We could describe the stage of development of *permanent* teeth in a 12-year old child by saying:

"The hard tissues are not completely _____, and the _____ portion of some teeth have not completely formed."

SECTION 6.1   GROWTH CENTERS AND LOBES

Tooth development begins with increased cell activity in **growth centers** in the tooth germ. A growth center is an area of the tooth germ where the cells are particularly active. The active <u>cells create projections or mounds</u>. As the growth centers develop, <u>they unite with one another.</u> This union is called **coalescence**. The development of the tooth begins with the formation of the _____ (crown/root) and then continues in the direction of the _____ until the tooth is complete.

The initial formation of the crown is paralleled by growth of the alveolar bone, producing a _____ around the developing tooth.

Coalescence is a word you should know. It means "to fuse" or "to unite." Writing it once or twice may help you to remember it.

In the illustration, you see the occlusal view of a mandibular second molar. The growth centers have been marked with circles to indicate the center from which the tooth was formed.

How many growth centers make up the molar in this illustration? _____.

Permanent
Mandibular
Right
2nd Molar
OCCLUSAL

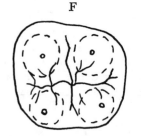

On the surface of crowns there may be grooves and/or cusps which mark significant anatomical divisions of the crown. In dental anatomy, we often use the term **lobes** to describe these divisions.

In molars, the number of growth centers and lobes are approximately the same. However, rather than describing teeth with reference to their growth centers, it is convenient to describe them in terms of the significant anatomical divisions, called _____.

lobes

Lobes are not the same as growth centers. For instance, incisors are believed to be formed initially from a single growth center, even though they are described as having four lobes. On a newly-erupted central incisor, the presence of three bulges on the incisal edge, called **mamelons and two facial grooves** appear to separate the facial and incisal portions of the incisor into three distinct areas. These three areas plus one area making up the lingual portion of the incisor crown, are called the _____ of the incisor.

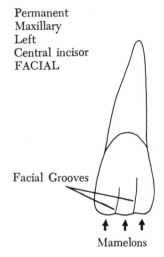

Permanent
Maxillary
Left
Central incisor
FACIAL

Facial Grooves

Mamelons

lobes

All anterior teeth show traces of four lobes, three facially and one lingually. The three facial lobes are visible as rounded eminences (mamelons) on newly-erupted incisors. The facial surface of incisors, especially central incisors, often show traces of the fusion of three lobes. This evidence of lobes is in the form of lines called _____ grooves.

Premolars usually have four lobes except the mandibular second premolar which frequently has five lobes (and two lingual cusps). Three lobes form the single facial cusp, and one or two lingually, depending upon the number of lingual cusps. Molars also have four or five lobes as a general rule. Each lobe of molar teeth is surmounted by a cusp. Fill in the table below by writing in the usual number of lobes and cusps for each tooth:

	NUMBER OF LOBES	NUMBER OF CUSPS
Molar	_____ or _____	_____ or _____
Premolar	_____ or _____	_____ or _____

	number of lobes	*number of cusps*
Molar	*4 or 5*	*4 or 5*
Premolar	*4 or 5*	*2 or 3*

The central lobe (No. 2) in each of the illustrations below is on which surface? _____.

Permanent
Mandibular
Right
1st Premolar
a. FACIAL
b. OCCLUSAL
c. LINGUAL

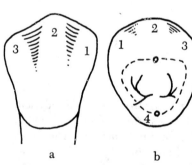
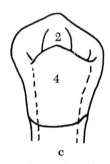

a   b   c

The incisors and canines are described as having how many lobes? _____.

The incisal edges of newly erupted incisors have three rounded bulges called _____. They suggest the location of *three lobes*.

What would be the location of the *fourth* lobe of these incisors? _____ (facial/lingual).

mamelons, lingual

SECTION 6.2 NAMES OF LOBES AND TOOTH SURFACES

Knowing the correct technical term for each of the tooth surfaces will be very important throughout the remainder of this course. Names of surfaces, often in combined terms, are constantly used to locate various anatomical features. If you prefer to review these surface identifications, see Section 2.2 on page 19.

All anteriors and premolars have three facial lobes and one lingual lobe with the exception of some mandibular second premolars which have two lingual lobes. All molars have two facial lobes and two lingual lobes with the exception of first molars which frequently have a fifth lobe.

For example, there are usually five lobes identified on the crown of the maxillary first molar, two to the facial, two to the lingual, and the fifth on the lingual side of the mesiolingual lobe. The facial lobes are known as the *mesiofacial* and *distofacial* lobes. The lingual lobes are known as the *mesiolingual* and *distolingual* lobes. The fifth lobe is a rudimentary lobe called the lobe of Carabelli, commonly called the **cusp of Carabelli**, deriving its name from the man who first described it. It is located _____ (facial/lingual/mesial/distal) to the mesiolingual lobe (see illustration).

Permanent Maxillary Right 1st Molar OCCLUSAL

Lobe (Cusp) of Carabelli

lingual

The cusp of Carabelli is found on the _____ molar.

Is the cusp of Carabelli found toward the mesial or distal surface of the tooth?

mesial ....GO TO BOTTOM OF THIS PAGE
distal ....GO TO NEXT FRAME

▶ From preceding frame   *distal is incorrect*

Distal is incorrect because the lobe of Carabelli is lingual to the mesiolingual lobe, placing it near the mesial and ligual surfaces.

Consider the illustration, *then carefully picture in your mind the arrangement of these lobes, and answer the question above again.*

Permanent
Maxillary
OCCLUSAL

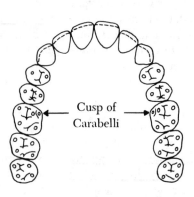

Cusp of
Carabelli

▶ From top of this page   *mesial is correct*

The mandibular first molar has five lobes also. The arrangement of the lobes differs from those of the maxillary first molar. There are two lingual lobes, mesiolingual and dis- tolingual; and two facial lobes, mesiofacial and distofacial. The fifth lobe is positioned distal to the distofacial lobe and is known as the distal lobe (*see diagram*).

Permanent
Mandibular
Right
1st Molar
OCCLUSAL

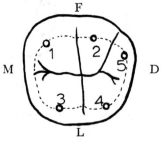

The locations of three of the four lobes making up an incisor are seen from the bumps along the incisal edge of young children's incisors. These bumps are called _____.

Both the <u>maxillary and mandibular second molars generally have four lobes,</u> two to the facial and two to the lingual. Except for the fifth lobe on each of the first molars, the arrangement of the other four lobes is similar to the second molars, and the same terms apply.

The two facial lobes are the _____ and _____ lobes.
The two lingual lobes are the _____ and _____ lobes.

Permanent
1. Maxillary
Left
2nd Molar
2. Mandibular
Right
2nd Molar
OCCLUSAL

Many variations occur in the lobe arrangement of the third molars. Either four or five lobes may be present. At times only three lobes may be seen, and sometimes more than five. Because of the wide variation in the third molars, it is impractical to establish a standard for them.

The variations which occur throughout human dentition are also partially caused by the relationship of one lobe to another. Therefore, variations occur resulting from (1) the number of lobes, (2) the shape of the lobe, and (3) the arrangement of the lobes. These variables together affect the shape of any one particular tooth. A tooth is actually a _____ (fusion) of several lobes which has developed into a tooth.

SECTION 6.3   DEVELOPMENT AND ERUPTION

The <u>*eruption*</u> of a tooth is most noticeable <u>when it penetrates the **oral mucosa**</u> (mew CO suh) and enters the oral cavity.

At the time the tooth begins to erupt, the crown is fully developed, but the _____ is not.

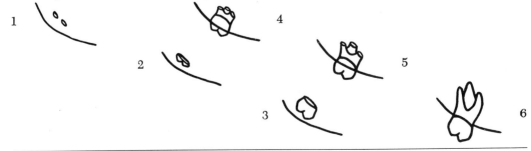

When the crown of the tooth is visible in the mouth, the process of enamel hardening, called _____, has been completed.

The tooth usually continues to erupt until it meets its __antagonist__ (opposing tooth) in the opposite jaw.

This complex process is called __active eruption__ and is the movement of teeth coronally through the oral mucosa. The active eruption of teeth in each dentition follows an **eruption sequence**, that is, an order of the progressive eruption of the teeth. The eruption sequence for the primary dentition is anterior to posterior except for the canines, which often lag behind the first molars. Which primary tooth can be expected to erupt first? _____.

Following is a table showing the most frequent eruption sequence and the range of eruption dates for primary teeth. The sequence, central incisor, lateral incisor, first molar, canine, second molar, is found in the majority of cases, with the first molar, and canine occasionally reversed. Study the table carefully.

✱ ERUPTION SEQUENCE AND DATES FOR __PRIMARY TEETH__

MAXILLARY AND MANDIBULAR	RANGE OF TYPICAL ERUPTION DATES
Central Incisors	6 months — 1 year
Lateral Incisors	9 month — 16 months
First Molars	1 year — 1½ years
Canines	1½ years — 2 years
Second Molars	2 years — 3 years

Which of the following series (A or B) of abbreviations represents the normal eruption sequence for primary teeth in each arch?

A: CI, LI, C, 1M, 2M
B: CI, LI, 1M, C, 2M

Although there is a great variability in eruption sequence when we consider whether or not a particular mandibular tooth preceeds a maxillary tooth, the most common sequence is shown below, where abbreviations again signify the teeth.

MOST COMMON ERUPTION SEQUENCE*

Maxillary:	CI LI	1M	C	2M	
Mandibular:	CI	LI	1M	C 2M	

*Adapted from Lunt, R. C. and Law, D. B. A review of the chronology of eruption of deciduous teeth. *JADA*, 89:872, Oct., 1974, with permission of Dr. Lunt.

There may be a considerable difference between the mandibular and maxillary eruption dates for any one patient, but these differences are not found in all patients. However, in general, the tooth that can be expected to erupt first is the primary _____ (maxillary/mandibular) central incisor.

mandibular

ERUPTION SEQUENCE AND DATES FOR PERMANENT TEETH

TYPICAL ERUPTION DATE IN YEARS	RANGE	ERUPTION SEQUENCE MAXILLARY	MANDIBULAR
6	6- 7		first molar
6	6- 7	first molar	
6	6- 7		central incisor
7	7- 8	central incisor	
7	7- 8		lateral incisor
8	8- 9	lateral incisor	
10	9-10		canine
10	10-12	first premolar	first premolar
11	10-12	second premolar	second premolar
11	11-12	canine	
12	11-13		second molar
12	12-13	second molar	
20	17-21	third molar	third molar

Now, study the table below of eruption sequence and dates for permanent teeth. The above eruption table for permanent teeth shows a major difference in the eruption time of mandibular and maxillary canines.

The mandibular canine usually erupts before the mandibular premolars. The maxillary canine usually erupts _____ (before/after) the maxillary premolars.

Also, as shown in the eruption table, the permanent mandibular teeth usually erupt before the maxillary teeth except for the premolars which have eruption dates very close together. For example, the mandibular central incisor usually erupts _____ (before/after) the maxillary central incisor.

---

before

An important difference between the eruption sequences for permanent and primary teeth is that the first molars erupt first in the permanent dentition. Recall that the permanent molars do not await the loss of any primary teeth in order to erupt— that is, the permanent molars are _____.

---

nonsuccedaneous

The first permanent teeth to erupt are an exception to the general rule of an anterior to posterior eruption sequence. These are the _____, sometimes called the six-year _____.

---

first molars, molars

The permanent maxillary canines also lag behind the first molars just as the primary _____ do.

---

canines

We learned before that the primary canines normally lag behind the primary _____.

---

first molars

Also, that the first *permanent* teeth to erupt are the _____.

---

first molars

When a tooth meets its antagonist, further active _____ is restrained and continues only as necessary to compensate for wear on the functional surfaces.

After the *primary* tooth has met its antagonist through active eruption, it functions to hold space while the child grows, helps with mastication, swallowing, speech, etc., until the permanent tooth begins movement towards the oral cavity. A permanent tooth that moves into a position formerly occupied by a primary tooth is called a ——————— tooth.

---

succedaneous

The succedaneous tooth continues its active eruption (root formation and movement) accompanied by the **resorbtion** of the roots of the primary tooth in its path.

Resorbtion of the primary tooth continues until the tooth has no root and no bone support and the epithelial attachment can no longer hold the tooth in place. The primary tooth then

———————.

---

falls out (or any synonym)

Soon after the primary tooth falls out, the erupting permanent tooth is in place to pierce the mucosa and move into view in the mouth.

The natural process whereby the primary teeth are lost is known as **exfoliation**. Remember this term from the fact that primary teeth are also called deciduous and that a deciduous tree loses its leaves through exfoliation. Only the ——————— dentition undergoes the process of exfoliation.

---

primary

The normal development of human dentition, therefore, consists of the active eruption, function, resorbtion of the root, and exfoliation of the primary teeth, followed by the appearance of the permanent teeth. The actual order of eruption for these teeth is known as the ———————.

---

eruption sequence

Before a succedaneous permanent tooth can enter the oral cavity, first the ——————— of the primary tooth root and finally the ——————— of that tooth must take place.

77

As the tooth actively erupts, an increasingly larger segment of the tooth is visible. The free gingiva determines the boundary of this visible segment, called the _____.

The process of active eruption is basically completed when the tooth assumes its position in the mouth and the root is fully formed. Some active eruption related to additional growth of cementum and alveolar bone near the apex continues throughout life to compensate for the wear of occluding surfaces of teeth. A process called **passive eruption** may begin once the tooth enters the oral cavity. Passive eruption is the migration of the soft tissue attachment near the cementoenamel junction to a more apical attachment exposing more clinical crown. This **recession** of the supporting tissues may be a very slow process and of little significance, but can become a critical factor in pathological condition (e.g., periodontal disease) by weakening the tooth's support or actually causing loss of the tooth.

The laying down of additional bone at the base of the alveolus would be associated with _____ (active/passive) eruption.

One other factor in the history of a normal tooth is **attrition**, the wearing away of the incisal or occlusal surfaces. Attrition is initially the wearing away of what tooth tissue? _____.

The enamel may show noticeable wear even though it is the _____ tissue in the body.

The most noticeable effect of attrition is the flattening of the occlusal cusp tips and incisal edges.

It is not uncommon for the incisal edges to have worn to such a extent through attrition that the dentin is exposed.

Teeth cannot all be expected to wear at the same rate as a result of attrition. Differences in rate of wear are common. For example, it is possible that the first teeth to erupt may experience the most wear. Can you remember which of the permanent teeth erupt first?

The central incisors ....GO TO BOTTOM OF PAGE 79
The first molar ....GO TO TOP OF PAGE 79
I'm tired ....GO TO MIDDLE OF PAGE 79

◆ From page 78   *first molar is correct*

It is a common misconception about the normal pattern of eruption for permanent teeth that the central incisors erupt first which, of course, is not generally true. It does happen in instances, but for the present time we will not consider variations.

There is typically a lag of about six years between the eruption of the first and second molars and another six years between the second and third molars. The lag occurs because the maxilla and mandible have not completed their development, and there is insufficient space for the remaining nonsuccedaneous teeth. Normally, therefore, the last of the permanent teeth to erupt are the _____.

third molars

The eruption sequence of the molars is important in considering attrition. Between the first and third permanent molars, there might be a considerable difference in wear from attrition because of a difference of how many years of use—6 years or 12 years? _____.

GO TO MIDDLE OF PAGE 80

◆ From page 78   *Tired?*

Place your left elbow on the circle below. Open your left hand and rest your chin in its palm for one minute.

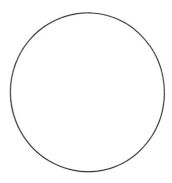

NOW RETURN TO THE QUESTION ON PAGE 78.

◆ From page 78   *central incisors is incorrect*

You may be thinking about the primary central incisors; they are usually the first primary teeth to erupt. The first permanent teeth to erupt are not normally the central incisors. The central incisors are succedaneous teeth and must wait for the exfoliation of the primary central incisors. The first, second, and third permanent molars are _____ and, therefore, do not follow any primary teeth.

All of the permanent molars cannot erupt early, however, for they must necessarily wait until the maxilla and mandible have reached the stage of development which allows enough room for them to erupt. Normally this means that the first permanent molars erupt about the sixth year, the second and third appearing later on at about six-year intervals.

TURN TO PAGE 75 AND REVIEW THE SECTION BEGINNING WITH THE ERUPTION SEQUENCE OF PERMANENT TEETH. WHEN YOU HAVE FINISHED, ANSWER THE LAST QUESTION ON PAGE 78 AGAIN.

12 years

The anterior teeth and premolars erupt at varying times within this interval of approximately twelve years. Therefore, we cannot expect these teeth to wear evenly.

Teeth, by meeting each of their antagonists through active eruption, form an imaginary **occlusal plane** along which each tooth makes contact with its antagonists. Is it correct to say that active eruption goes on throughout life, thereby maintaining the occlusal plane? ——————.

yes

The life history of a tooth consists, therefore, of its development from one or more growth centers, coalescence when multiple centers exist, active eruption with root formation, continued active eruption to compensate for incisal/occlusal wear, and, in some cases, passive eruption through apical recession of the gingival attachment. The primary teeth usually have much less passive eruption than permanent teeth since they are not retained in the mouth for as many years, but they do, of course, undergo resorbtion of their roots and exfoliation.

NOW, TAKE THE REVIEW TEST ON THE NEXT PAGE

REVIEW TEST 6

1. Choose the *incorrect* statement.
   a. Each tooth shows evidence of four or more lobes.
   b. Normally each tooth erupts after calcification of its crown is complete.
   c. Incisors develop from five growth centers.

2. Choose the *incorrect* statement.
   a. Grooves are visible lines which may separate the lobes.
   b. The fifth lobe normally found on the permanent mandibular first molars is known as the lobe of (cusp of) Carabelli.
   c. The lobe arrangement of most premolars is similar to that of the incisors.

3. Choose the *correct* statement:
   Normally, the first permanent teeth to erupt are . . .
   a. the central incisors
   b. the canines
   c. the first premolars
   d. the first molars

4. Choose the *incorrect* statement.
   a. The development of primary teeth is first evident in the crypt during the fifth to seventh week of fetal life.
   b. The primary eruption sequence is CI, LI, 1M, C, 2M.
   c. Active eruption of a tooth is completed when the tooth meets its antagonist.

MAKE A NOTE OF YOUR ANSWERS AND TURN TO PAGE 53

SECTION 7.0   OCCLUSION

Occlusion refers to movements of the mandible and to the contacting of the maxillary and mandibular teeth resulting from those movements. There is great variety in human occlusion. The study of occlusion is complex and demands far more attention than this volume could provide. We shall limit our discussion to some basic terminology and concepts.

Most commonly, the maxillary teeth overlap the mandibulars, and most teeth have two opposing teeth (antagonists). Which surface of the maxillary anterior teeth are touched by the mandibular anterior teeth—the incisal or lingual? _____.

PERMANENT LEFT QUADRANTS IN
OCCLUSION

SCHEMATIC DIAGRAM OF PERMANENT
LEFT QUADRANTS

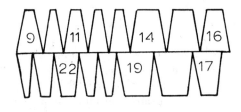

lingual

Which mandibular teeth commonly have one antagonist? _____.

SCHEMATIC DRAWING OF PERMANENT
MAXILLARY AND MANDIBULAR
LEFT QUADRANTS

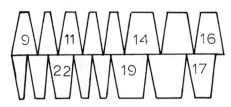

The maxillary teeth generally have two antagonists, except for the _____ molars, which have one antagonist.

SCHEMATIC DRAWING OF PERMANENT MAXILLARY AND MANDIBULAR LEFT QUADRANTS

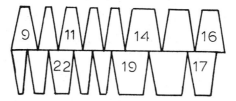

Teeth are like stone blocks in a gothic arch. In the most frequent occlusion, which arch is larger—maxillary or mandibular?_____

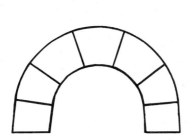 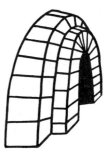

Tooth alignment usually involves a slight **horizontal overlap** and **vertical overlap**. Overlap is a term to describe the overlapping alignment seen when the two arches occlude. Horizontal overlap is also called **overjet** and vertical overlap is known as

Permanent
Maxillary
Mandibular
1. Incisors
   FACIAL (Occluded)
2. Central Incisors
   PROXIMAL (Occluded)

overbite. However, this text will use the simpler and more correct terms, horizontal overlap and vertical overlap. In Figure 2, identify the label (A or B) that represents horizontal overlap _____.

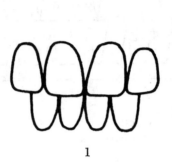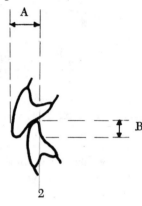

1   2

A, horizontal overlap

In 1899, Edward H. Angle developed a classification of human occlusion that is still basic and useful today. Angle described three classes of occlusion, **Class I, Class II, and** **Class III.** Class I is the most common (about 70% of the population), Class II less common (about 25%) and Class III least common (less than 5%).

Class I Occlusion

Permanent
Maxillary
Mandibular
1. First molars
   FACIAL
2. Central incisors
   PROXIMAL

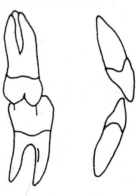

The classes can be defined in terms of the relationship between maxillary and mandibular first molars and incisors.

Angle felt, as many still do, that the first molars were good reference points because of their early eruption dates and significance in determining the space available for the succedaneous teeth. In Angle Class I occlusion, the **mesiofacial cusp** of the maxillary first molar lines up approximately with the facial groove of the mandibular first molar (see the illustration). The maxillary central incisors overlap the mandibulars. That is, the incisors show both _____ and _____.

In Angle Class II occlusion, the mesiofacial cusp of the maxillary first molar falls approximately between the mandibular first molar and second premolar. The lower jaw and chin may also appear small and withdrawn. The mandibular incisors occlude even more posterior to the maxillary incisors so that they may not touch at all. Compared to Class I, the maxillary incisors in Class II show more _____ (horizontal/vertical) overlap.

Class II Occlusion

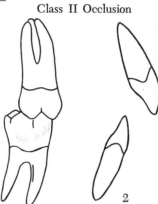

Permanent
Maxillary
Mandibular
1. 1st molars
   FACIAL
2. Central incisors
   PROXIMAL

horizontal

In Angle Class III occlusion, the mandibular teeth are in a more anterior position than in Class I. The chin may also protrude like a bulldog's does. The mandibular incisors overlap anterior to the maxillary incisors. The mesiofacial cusp of the maxillary first molar falls approximately between the mandibular first molar and the mandibular _____.

Class III Occlusion

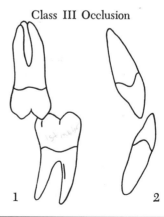

Permanent
Maxillary
Mandibular
1. 1st molars
   FACIAL
2. Central incisors
   PROXIMAL

second molar

The cusp of the maxillary first molar that serves as a reference point in identifying Class I, II, and III occlusion is the _____ cusp.

Viewed from the distal, the premolars and molars normally occlude so that the mandibular facial cusps strike the central portion of the occlusal surface of their antagonists. Where would the lingual cusps of the maxillary posteriors strike their mandibular antagonists? _____.

a. Central portion of the occlusal surface
b. Facial portion of the facial cusps

Permanent
Maxillary
Mandibular
First Premolars
DISTAL
Occluded

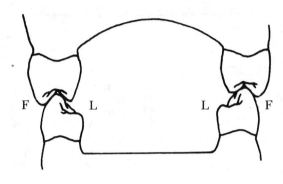

F   L   L   F

a, central portion

The facial cusps of mandibular posteriors and the lingual cusps of the maxillary posterior teeth are called <u>centric cusps</u>, because <u>they contact their antagonists and determine the position of the mandible in maximum opposing tooth contact</u> (**centric occlusion**). In contrast, <u>maxillary facial cusps and mandibular lingual cusps are called</u> **noncentric cusps**.

The form of teeth appears highly related to function in occlusion. For example, <u>the centric cusps seem more bulky and rounded</u> <u>than noncentric cusps.</u> Choose the letter (a or b) corresponding to the centric cusp shown on the right. _____

Permanent
Mandibular
Right
1st Premolar
MESIAL

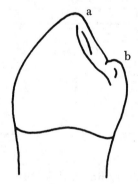

a
b

In some cases, you will see patients who have one or more <u>posterior teeth or an</u> entire quadrant which show a **cross-bite.** Study the drawing below of a left cross-bite, and compare it to the right side which is in normal relation.

Which cusp on the left maxillary premolar occludes in the central portion of the left mandibular premolar in this cross-bite case—facial or lingual? _____.

**Permanent
1st Premolars
DISTAL
Occluded
(Cross-bite)**

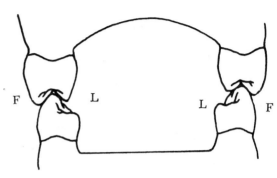

facial

The form of teeth is related to the way they occlude and function in the entire dentition. For example, the arch form of the upper and lower teeth determines to some extent the form of individual teeth.

1. Stone block arch
2. Permanent
   Maxillary
   OCCLUSAL

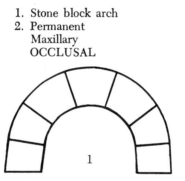

1

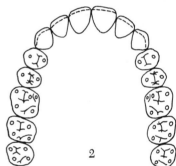

2

<u>Stone blocks used to form an arch are wider at their outer surface than at their inner surface.</u> When examining a dental arch, we can notice a similar relationship between the facial and lingual surfaces of the teeth, especially the anterior teeth. An incisal view of a maxillary central incisor (see right) demonstrates this concept.

Which surface of the incisor is narrower, the facial or lingual? _____

Permanent
Maxillary
Right
Central Incisor
INCISAL

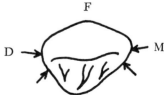

The study of the interrelationships of teeth in the arch should include an examination of the areas where adjacent teeth contact each other in the same arch. These **proximal contact areas** are described next.

 ## SECTION 7.1   PROXIMAL CONTACT AREAS

Each tooth contacts adjacent teeth on its proximal surfaces except the distal of third molars. The proximal surfaces are the _____ and _____ surfaces of a tooth.

Permanent
Maxillary
Left
1. Central Incisor
2. Lateral Incisor
FACIAL

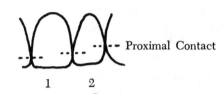

Proximal Contact

1   2

mesial, distal

Proximal surfaces usually have contact areas rather than contact points. Generally, newly erupted teeth will have small contact areas. As enamel wears over the years, these contact areas broaden into larger proximal contact _____ .

Permanent
Maxillary
Right
1. 2nd Premolar
2. 1st Premolar
3. Canine
OCCLUSAL

Contact Areas

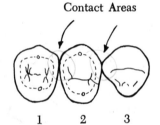

1   2   3

New Teeth

+

Age and Wear

areas

Most proximal contacts involve a mesial and a distal surface. The proximal contact that involves the mesial surface of both teeth is between the two _____ .

Permanent
Maxillary
OCCLUSAL

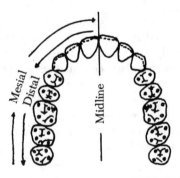

Mesial
Distal
Midline

Each tooth is supported, in part, through contact with its neighboring teeth. In turn, a tooth lends support to the entire dental arch through its two proximal _____.

Permanent
Maxillary
Right
1. Canine
2. Lateral Incisor
FACIAL

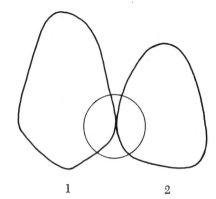

1   2

The only tooth surface that does not make proximal contact is the _____ of _____.

   (surface)   (teeth)

Just like stone blocks in an arch, teeth provide some of the stability of the human dental arch through contact with neighboring teeth.

All teeth have both mesial and distal contacts except the _____.

  a. central incisors
  b. last erupted molars

1. Stone block arch
2. Permanent Maxillary
OCCLUSAL

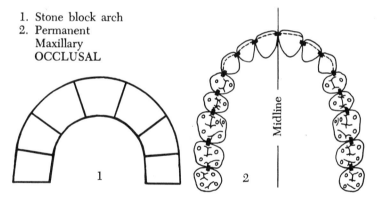

"Below" or cervical to each proximal contact and "between" adjacent teeth is the **interdental area**. The term that indicates the location "between" two teeth is _____.

Permanent
Mandibular
Right
1. 1st Molar
2. 2nd Premolar
3. 1st Premolar
FACIAL

Proximal Contact

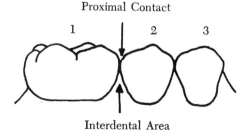

Interdental Area

Occupying much of the interdental area is a projection of the free gingival tissue called "**interdental papilla**" or simply, **papilla** (puh PILL luh). Viewed facially, the interdental area and the interdental papilla are generally _____ in shape.

Permanent
Mandibular
Right
1. 1st Molar
2. 2nd Premolar
3. 1st Premolar
FACIAL

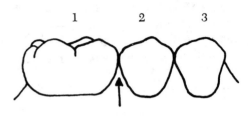

Interdental Papilla

The interdental area is often called the **interproximal area** or **interproximal space**. It is not really a space because tissue fills much of the area. Since that tissue is interdental papilla, it is convenient to call the area the interdental area. Recall that the free gingiva lying between teeth was called _____ gingiva. Now, another term for that tissue is interdental _____.

Permanent
Mandibular
Right
1. 1st Molar
2. 2nd Premolar
3. 1st Premolar
FACIAL

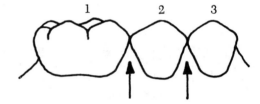

In healthy mouths, the tissue assumes much of the triangular shape of the interdental area from the facial view, but resembles a slightly sagging tent from the proximal view. The sagging area is the **coll** (CALL) of the papillary gingiva and is apical to the _____ area.

Permanent
Mandibular
Left
1st Premolar
MESIAL

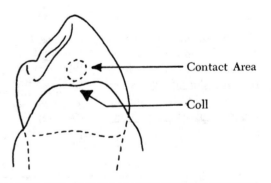

Contact Area

Coll

The cervical third of the proximal surfaces of all teeth are relatively flat or even slighly concave in some areas increasing the space for the free gingival tissue called the _____.

SECTION 7.2 EMBRASURES

The curved tooth surfaces that sweep away from the proximal contact areas form open spaces: the interdental area (gingival to the contact) and **embrasures** (elsewhere around the contact). There are *incisal* or *occlusal embrasures*, *lingual embrasures*, and *facial embrasures.* Thus, the proximal contact is surrounded by the interdental area and the spaces called _____.

Permanent
Mandibular
Right
1. 2nd Premolar
2. 1st Premolar
FACIAL
OCCLUSAL

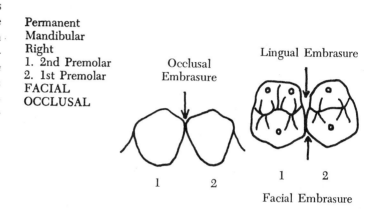

Occlusal
Embrasure

Lingual Embrasure

Facial Embrasure

1   2   1   2

These spaces allow chewed foods to escape from the occlusal surface. The best name for the spaces between teeth which allows food to escape from the occlusal surface is _____.

Permanent
Maxillary
Left
1. 2nd Premolar
2. 1st Molar
3. 2nd Molar
OCCLUSAL

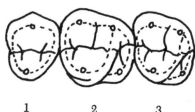

1   2   3

91

Embrasures make the natural hygienic factors in the mouth more effective by exposing tooth surfaces to oral fluids and the mechanical cleansing action of the tongue, lips, and cheeks. The curved surfaces discourage the impaction of food between the ——————.

Permanent
Maxillary
Left
1. 2nd Premolar
2. 1st Molar
3. 2nd Molar
OCCLUSAL

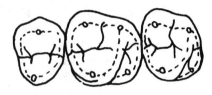

1   2   3

proximal surfaces

The embrasures also allow food to slide away from the chewing surfaces during mastication. This helps to protect the supporting structures from undue trauma by —————— (increasing/reducing) the forces exerted on the teeth during mastication.

reducing

The supporting structures are, therefore, protected from traumatic forces by the escape of food via the open —————— and by the transmission of occlusal forces to adjacent teeth through the solid ———

—————— ——————.

Permanent
Mandibular
Right
1. 1st Molar
2. 2nd Premolar
3. 1st Premolar
FACIAL

Proximal Contact   Embrasure

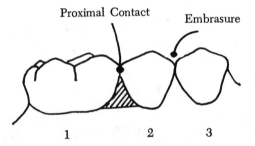

1   2   3

embrasures, proximal contact areas

The embrasures are named according to their location in relation to the contact. The embrasures located incisally or occlusally to the contact are called the incisal or occlusal embrasures. The embrasures located facially are called facial embrasures, and those located lingually are called lingual embrasures.

Facial and lingual embrasures are confluent with the interdental area; that is, their boundaries are indistinct and they blend together. The facial and lingual embrasures are also confluent with the space above the contact called the ——————.

incisal (occlusal) embrasure

DIRECTIONS FOR MATRIX TESTS

What we call *matrix tests* will appear from time to time in the remainder of the program. They will help you check your progress and review if necessary.

Examples of Completed MATRIX TESTS

MATCH ROWS AND COLUMNS WITH AN "X" IN THE CORRECT CELL.

	City	Country	Continent
France		X	
Paris	X		
Australia			X

ANSWER ALL NINE QUESTIONS (CELLS). USE ONE-WORD ANSWERS.

	Relative Size	Country	Seacoast
Our Town	Small	U.S.A.	Yes
Portland, Oregon	Medium	U.S.A.	No
London	Large	England	No

MATRIX TEST 1

Directions

    Place an X in the square that matches the left hand column with the top row. When you have completed the test, *turn to Page 96.*

	Interdental Area	Proximal Contact Area	Embrasure
Supports neighboring teeth . . .			
Allows for escape of resistant food . . .			
Contains the interdental papilla . . .			
Area between proximal tooth surfaces . . .			

94

REVIEW TEST 7

For each question, select the one most correct answer.
1. Cervical to the proximal contact area is the:
   a. occlusal table
   b. interdental area
   c. distal embrasure

2. What surrounds the proximal contact areas in facial, occlusal and lingual directions?
   a. papillary gingiva
   b. embrasures
   c. interdental area

3. What is located in the interdental area?
   a. alveolar bone
   b. attached gingiva
   c. interdental papilla

4. In the most common occlusion, which mandibular teeth have only one antagonist?
   a. third molars
   b. central incisors
   c. third molars and central incisors

5. In the most common occlusion, the facial cusp of a mandibular second premolar is a . . .
   a. centric cusp
   b. non-centric cusp
   c. cusp in cross-bite position

6. In reference to the position of the central incisors in occlusion, match the following:

   Tends toward

   a. mandibular incisors overlap anterior to maxillary incisors   I. Class I occlusion
   b. normal maxillary horizontal and vertical overlap   II. Class II occlusion
   c. extreme maxillary horizontal overlap   III. Class III occlusion

7. In reference to the position of the mesiofacial cusp of tooth number 14 (universal code) in occlusion, match the following:

   Tends toward

   a. cusp aligned between 18 and 19   I. Angle Class I
   b. cusp aligned between 19 and 20   II. Angle Class II
   c. cusp aligned with facial groove of 19   III. Angle Class III

MAKE A NOTE OF YOUR ANSWERS AND TURN TO PAGE 54

MATRIX TEST 1

Answers

If any items are missed, turn to the page indicated for review. Review, then retake the matrix test on page 94.

If all are correct, *turn to Page 95 and take Review Test 7.*

	Interdental Area	Proximal Contact Area	Embrasure
Supports neighboring teeth . . .		X (PP. 88–89)	
Allows for escape of resistant food . . .			X (P. 91)
Contains the interdental papilla . . .	X (PP. 89–90)		
Area between proximal tooth surfaces . . .	X (PP. 89–90)		

SECTION 8.0   LOCATION OF PROXIMAL CONTACTS AND EMBRASURES

Proximal contacts provide stability to the dental arch by helping support the individual tooth. These contact areas (located on the mesial and distal surfaces, excepting the third molars) are collectively called _____ surfaces.

Permanent
Maxillary
Anterior
FACIAL

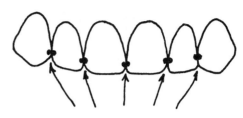

Contact Areas

proximal

Precisely locating a point (or area) on a surface requires two "coordinates." Locating contact areas between teeth requires describing two dimensions of the _____ surface.

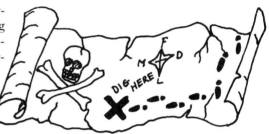

proximal

The proximal contact area is located in (1) the **incisocervical** or **occlusocervical dimension** and (2) the **faciolingual dimension.** In the diagram to the right, dimenson A is the _____ dimension, and B is the _____ dimension.

Permanent
Maxillary
Right
2nd Premolar
PROXIMAL

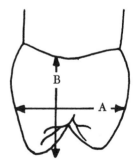

The contact location is determined by referring to thirds. Viewing the teeth from the facial aspect, the crowns are divided into three equal parts: the _____, _____, and _____ thirds.

Permanent
Maxillary
Right
1. Lateral Incisor
2. Central Incisor
FACIAL

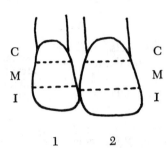

1   2

---

cervical, middle, incisal (occlusal)

Since a contact is between two teeth, two proximal surfaces are involved. For example, the contact between the lateral incisor and canine involves the distal surface of the _____ ____ and the _____ surface of the canine.

Permanent
Maxillary
Right
1. Canine
2. Lateral Incisor
FACIAL

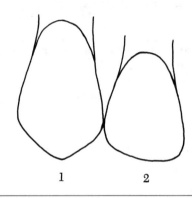

1   2

---

lateral incisor, mesial

The faciolingual location of the proximal contact and the configuration of two embrasures are seen from an occlusal or incisal view. The two embrasures outlined in an occlusal view are the _____ and _____ embrasures.

Permanent
Maxillary
Left
1. 2nd Premolar
2. 1st Molar
OCCLUSAL

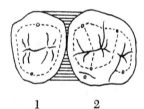

1   2

---

facial, lingual

The relative depth of the facial and lingual embrasures is determined by the location of the contact faciolingually. If the contact is located more facially, the embrasure with the greater depth is the _____ embrasure.

Permanent
Maxillary
Left
1. 2nd Premolar
2. 1st Molar
OCCLUSAL

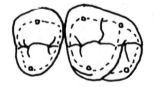

1   2

The drawings on the right and in the next frame show the proximal contacts of all teeth in both the incisocervical (occlusocervical) and faciolingual dimensions.

Permanent
1. Maxillary
2. Mandibular
Left Quadrants
FACIAL

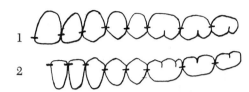

Study the drawing on the right and then answer the questions below and on the following page. Refer back to this drawing as necessary to answer the questions.

In the region of the anterior teeth, the facial and lingual embrasures have approximately equal depth. The proximal contacts between anterior teeth are _____ (centered/more to the facial) in the faciolingual dimension.

Permanent
Maxillary
Right Quadrant and
Left Central Incisor
OCCLUSAL

INCISO- OR OCCLUSOCERVICAL
LOCATION OF CONTACTS

FACIOLINGUAL
LOCATION OF
PROXIMAL CONTACTS
AND
EMBRASURES

In the region of the posterior teeth, the lingual embrasures are deeper than facial embrasures. This is because the proximal contacts between posterior teeth are toward the _____ (facial/lingual) surface in the faciolingual dimension.

Faciolingually, all proximal contacts are either displaced slightly toward the _____ or are _____ on the faciolingual axis of the crown.

The relative depth of facial and lingual embrasures is determined by the location of the contact in the _____ dimension.

The incisocervical or occlusocervical location of the proximal contacts may be seen by examining a _____ view of the teeth.

In the incisocervical or occlusocervical dimension, if you examine the location of the proximal contacts from the anterior teeth back to the posterior teeth, you will see that the contacts tend to be located in or near the incisal third between anteriors and in or near the middle third on the posteriors. Incisocervically, the central incisors of both arches have mesial contact areas well within the _____ thirds and incisal embrasures that are _____ (size).

It is possible to study the inciso/occlusocervical location of the proximal contacts of individual teeth and to summarize the location of the contacts of all teeth with two rules that apply in every case:

1. The more anterior the tooth, the more incisal/occlusal are the location of the proximal contacts.
2. For any tooth, the mesial contact area is more toward the incisal/occlusal than is the distal contact area.

Use the adjacent illustration to apply both of the rules concerning the location of the proximal contacts. The permanent maxillary central incisor has a mesial contact in the incisal (I) third, and the distal contact at the junction (J) of the incisal and middle thirds. The lateral incisors have their contacts more apical (Rule 1) than the centrals, with their mesial contact more incisal than their distal contact (Rule 2). Therefore, the permanent maxillary lateral incisor can be labeled J-M to indicate the location of its mesial contact (J—at the junction of the incisal and middle thirds) and distal contact (M—in the middle third). The maxillary canine can be labeled J-M also, which means that its mesial contact is at the _____ and its distal contact is in the _____.

Permanent
Maxillary
Left
1. Central Incisor
2. Lateral Incisor
3. Canine
FACIAL

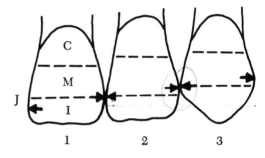

junction of incisal and middle thirds, middle third

All posterior teeth have proximal contacts in the middle third. The more posterior teeth—the molars—have contacts lower in the middle third than the premolars (Rule 1). Also, each posterior tooth has the mesial contact slightly more _____ (occlusal/apical) than the distal contact (Rule 2).

Both the mesial and distal contacts on each of the eight premolars are located occlusocervically, just cervical to the junction of the occlusal and middle thirds. Therefore, the contact areas on each of the premolars are in the _____ third of the crown.

Permanent
Maxillary
Left
1. Canine
2. 1st Premolar
3. 2nd Premolar
4. 1st Molar
Mandibular
5. Canine
6. 1st Premolar
7. 2nd Premolar
8. 1st Molar
FACIAL

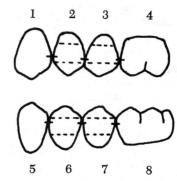

The first, second, and third molars of both arches have their mesial and distal contacts located approximately in the *center of the middle* third of the crown.

Both molars and premolars have contacts located in the middle third. However, the contacts on the premolars are located more _____ (cervically/occlusally) than those of the molars.

Permanent
Maxillary
Left
1. 2nd Premolar
2. 1st Molar
3. 2nd Molar
4. 3rd Molar
Mandibular
5. 2nd Premolar
6. 1st Molar
7. 2nd Molar
8. 3rd Molar
FACIAL

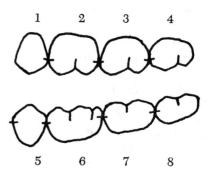

The inciso/occlusocervical locations of the proximal contacts of a maxillary quadrant can be labeled as follows:

Maxillary: IJ, JM, JM, MM, MM, MM, MM, MM

This labeling is a convenient means of remembering the locations of these proximal contacts, and it indicates that all of the premolars and molars have their mesial and distal contacts in the middle third (MM). The maxillary central incisor has its distal contact at the _____ thirds, which is labeled by the letter _____.

The permanent *mandibular* quadrants have the same rules as stated on page 100 for the location of their proximal contact areas. The difference between maxillary and mandibular proximal contact locations is that the mandibular incisors and canines have contacts all in the incisal third except the distal of the canine which is in the middle third. Thus, a mandibular quadrant can be labeled as follows:

Mandibular: II, II, IM, MM, MM, MM, MM, MM

Which are the letters that represent the mandibular canine's proximal contact locations? _____

The more anterior the location of a tooth in the dental arches, the more incisal or occlusal the location of the proximal contact areas. The distal contact areas are always slightly more _____ (occlusal/apical) in location than the mesial contact areas.

All posterior teeth, whether maxillary or mandibular, have proximal contacts in the _____ third.

Review the locations of the proximal contacts once more by using the labels below:

Maxillary: IJ, JM, JM, MM, MM, MM, MM, MM,
Mandibular: II, II, IM, MM, MM, MM, MM, MM,

List the four proximal surfaces that have differences in proximal contact location between the maxillary and mandibular arches:

_____ surface of the central incisors
_____ surface of the lateral incisors
_____ surface of the lateral incisors
_____ surface of the canines

SECTION 8.1   CONTOURS OF TOOTH CROWNS

It is important to study the curved **contours** of crowns because there are many occasions for the dentist to operate on these contours in restoring or replacing crown surfaces. There is clinical evidence that smooth and properly contoured (not too convex) crown surfaces promote tooth cleaning and gingival health.

Permanent
Mandibular
1st Premolar
FACIOLINGUAL
SECTION

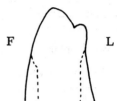

The curved contours of the crown are normally continuous with the gingiva, as shown in the drawing on the right. This form seems to help make the _____ (cervical/occlusal) areas of the teeth cleanable.

cervical

One of the best ways to study the contours of crowns is to focus on the **height of contour**.

The height of contour is an imaginary curved line encircling a tooth at its greatest bulge or circumference. One way to visualize this imaginary line is shown in the drawing on the right, where a light source is depicted as being directed toward the incisal edge of an incisor. The height of contour encircles the entire crown and would be incisal or occlusal to a real line that encircles the tooth, the _____ line or cementoenamel junction.

Maxillary
Right
Central Incisor
DISTOFACIAL VIEW

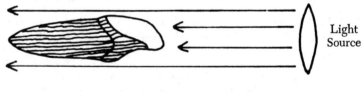

Light
Source

104

One can also see the location of the height of contour by moving a pencil around the crown at its greatest bulge or circumference, and marking the height of contour.

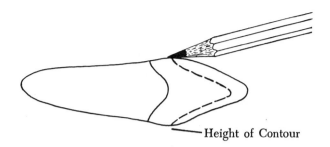

Height of Contour

The proximal contacts of a tooth lie _____ (along/above) the height of contour.

Permanent
Mandibular
Left
1st Premolar
MESIAL

Height of
Contour

Contact
Area

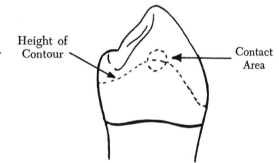

The facial and lingual heights of contour are seen when a tooth is drawn from a _____ view.

Permanent
1. Maxillary
   Right
   Central Incisor
   MESIAL
2. Mandibular
   Left
   1st Molar
   DISTAL

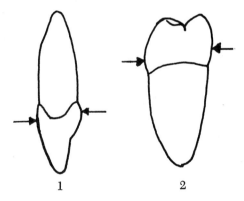

1   2

Anterior teeth have facial or lingual heights of contour in the cervical third of the crown.

Examine the drawings for height of contour. The height of contour occurs in the cervical third on both the facial and lingual surfaces for all maxillary and mandibular _____ (anterior/posterior) teeth.

Permanent
1. Maxillary
   Right
   Central Incisor
   MESIAL
2. Mandibular
   Left
   Central Incisor
   DISTAL

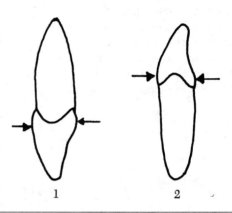

anterior

All maxillary and mandibular posterior teeth have the height of contour in the middle third on the _____ surface.

which side sticks out more?

Permanent
1. Maxillary
   Right
   2nd Molar
   MESIAL
2. Mandibular
   Right
   1st Molar
   MESIAL

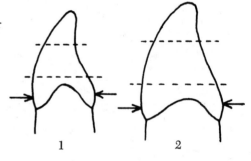

lingual

As with the maxillary incisors and canines, the mandibular anteriors have both the facial and lingual height of contour in the _____ third of the crown.

Permanent
Mandibular
Right
1. Central Incisor
2. Canine
MESIAL

Both maxillary posterior teeth and mandibular posterior teeth have the height of contour on the facial surface in the _____ third and the lingual height of contour in the _____ third.

Permanent
Mandibular
Right
1st Premolar
MESIAL

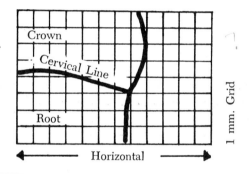

In addition to knowing the location of the height of contour, you should know the **amount of contour** in a horizontal direction from the cervical line.

One way to measure the amount of contour of a tooth surface is to place a grid over a drawing of a tooth, as is shown here. If the grid has lines that are 1 mm apart, what is the amount of contour shown? _____.

All maxillary teeth exhibit facial and *lingual* contours that measure approximately ½ mm horizontally. The *lingual* surface of the maxillary right canine has the height of contour in the _____ third that measures _____ mm.

The lingual surface of the maxillary left first molar has the height of contour in the _____ third that measures _____ mm.

Permanent
Maxillary
Right
1. Canine
2. 1st Molar
MESIAL

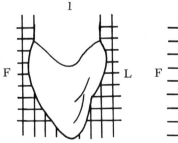
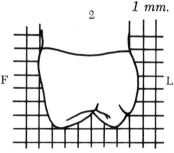

107

In proximal view, maxillary teeth give the impression that the amount of contour is greater on the facial than on the lingual surface (especially true for anterior teeth). However, careful examination will show that the contour, both facially and lingually, for all maxillary teeth measures approximately ——————— mm.

Permanent
Maxillary
Right
1. Central Incisor
2. 1st Premolar
MESIAL

1

2

1 mm.
Grid

½

You should know that ½ mm is a very small amount of contour. For example, one-half millimeter is only as thick as four sheets of paper from this text held tightly between the fingers. It is approximately equal to the thickness of a human fingernail.

The facial and lingual amounts of contour of the mandibular anteriors are very slight. Mandibular incisors and canines have facial and lingual amounts of contour that measure:

A. more than ½ mm
B. ½ mm
C. less than ½ mm

Permanent
Mandibular
Right
1. Central Incisor
2. Canine
MESIAL

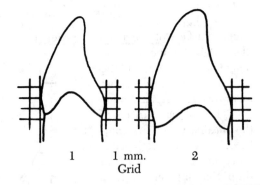

1

1 mm.
Grid

2

The amount of contour on the facial surfaces of *mandibular* posteriors are similar to those on the *facial* surfaces, of the *maxillary* posterior teeth, that is, they measure approximately ———— mm.

Permanent
Mandibular
Left
1. 1st Premolar
2. 1st Molar
DISTAL

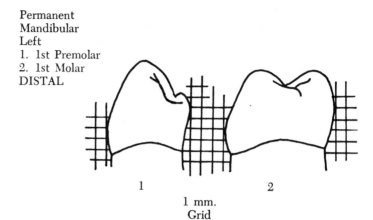

1   2

1 mm.
Grid

½

The <u>mandibular posterior teeth have *lingual* curvatures that measure nearly double those of the maxillaries.</u> The amount of contour on the *lingual* surface of *mandibular* posterior teeth approaches ———— mm in measurement.

Permanent
Mandibular
Right
1st Molar
MESIAL

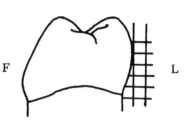

F   L

1

When examining teeth in the oral cavity, the location of the height of contour and the amount of contour may appear different than that of extracted teeth or drawings. The reason for this difference is shown in the drawing at the right of a permanent mandibular molar. Because teeth are often inclined (toward the lingual in the case of the mandibular molars), the <u>observed height of contour is noticeably different from the anatomical height of contour.</u> The observed height of contour is closer to the occlusal surface and the amount of contour appears greater than the anatomical contour would suggest.

Permanent
Mandibular
Right
1st Molar
MESIAL

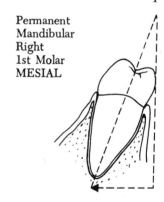

In preparation for the review test that follows, complete the following statements.

All permanent teeth have their height of contour in the cervical third on the ———— surface of the crown.

The height of contour is located in the cervical third on the lingual surface of all maxillary and mandibular _____ (anterior/posterior) teeth.

Both maxillary and mandibular premolars and molars have heights of contour approximately in the middle third on the _____ surface of the crown.

Which tooth surfaces have curvatures that measure less than ½ mm? _____
(indicate whether maxillary or mandibular, anterior or posterior, facial or lingual)
   Which tooth surfaces have curvatures that usually measure more than ½ mm? _____
(indicate whether maxillary or mandibular, anterior or posterior, facial or lingual)

In the discussion of facial and lingual contours, the *average* or most common tooth form was described. As with most anatomical features, individual deviations from the norm may occur on a specific tooth or a group of teeth.

Each of the following words is misspelled. Rewrite each word, spelling it correctly.

   1. Ginegiva   _____

   2. Facilingule   _____

   3. Maxallary   _____

   4. Procimal contracts   _____

   5. Cervacal   _____

   6. Embrazures   _____

GO TO THE NEXT PAGE AND TAKE MATRIX TEST 2

MATRIX TEST 2

Directions

Fill in each cell with the correct word, words or numbers.

When you have completed the test, *turn to Page 112 and check your answers.*

	Location (third) of facial height of contour	Location (third) of lingual height of contour	Amount of contour in mm.	
			Facial	Lingual
Maxillary Anteriors				
Maxillary Posteriors				
Mandibular Anteriors				
Mandibular Posteriors				

MATRIX TEST 2
(From Page 111)

Directions

If any items were missed, review the section on contours on the page indicated in the cell.

If all answers are correct, *take Review Test 8 on the next page.*

	Location (third) of facial height of contour	Location (third) of lingual height of contour	Facial	Amount of contour in mm. Lingual
Maxillary Anteriors	Cervical (P. 106)	Cervical (P. 106)	½ mm (P. 107)	½ mm (P. 107)
Maxillary Posteriors	Cervical (PP. 106–107)	Middle (PP. 106–107)	½ mm (P. 107)	½ mm (P. 109)
Mandibular Anteriors	Cervical (P. 106)	Cervical (P. 106)	less than ½ mm (P. 108)	less than ½ mm (P. 108)
Mandibular Posteriors	Cervical (PP. 106–107)	Middle (PP. 106–107)	½ mm (P. 108)	1 mm (P. 109)

REVIEW TEST 8

Choose the most correct answers and make a note of them. Turn to Page 55 to check your answers when you have finished.

1. In their position in the alveolar bone, the mandibular molars are . . .
   a. tipped toward the facial
   b. in an upright, vertical position
   c. tipped toward the lingual

2. The proximal contact is usually located
   a. at the mesial or distal height of contour
   b. in the cervical third of the crown
   c. in the middle third of the crown

3. Indicate the incisocervical or occlusocervical location of the following proximal contact areas. Write the name of the third (incisal, middle, etc.) and/or the junction of thirds where the area is located.
   a. mesial contact area of the maxillary central incisor _____
   b. distal contact area of the maxillary lateral incisor _____
   c. mesial contact area of the mandibular central incisor _____
   d. distal contact area of the mandibular canine _____
   e. mesial contact area of the maxillary second premolar _____
   f. distal contact area of the mandibular second molar _____

4. In the region of the anterior teeth, the facial embrasures are approximately
   a. as deep as the lingual embrasures
   b. deeper than the lingual embrasures
   c. not as deep as the lingual embrasures

5. Choose the correct statement:
   a. Contact areas between posterior teeth are displaced lingually from the center of the faciolingual axis.
   b. Contact areas between posterior teeth are displaced facially from the center of the faciolingual axis.

GO TO PAGE 55

2
PERMANENT ANTERIOR TEETH

SECTION 1.0   REVIEW OF TOOTH SURFACES

The crowns of posterior teeth can be described as cube-shaped, and the crowns of anterior teeth can be described as _____ -shaped.

Permanent
1. Mandibular Right 2nd Molar
2. Mandibular Right Central Incisor

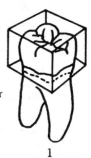 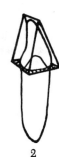

1   2

wedge

One side of the cube or wedge used to describe tooth crowns is taken up by the root, and, consequently, it is not classified or named as a tooth surface. This leaves four surfaces and the incisal edge which are named on anterior teeth, and _____ (number) surfaces on posterior teeth.

Permanent
1. Mandibular Right 2nd Molar
2. Mandibular Right Central Incisor

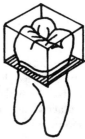 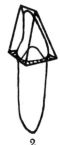

1   2

five

Each square surface has _____ edges or borders. A triangular surface has _____ (number) borders.

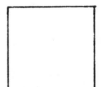 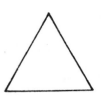

If the surface is more nearly trapezoidal in shape, there are _____ (number) borders to each surface. Any quadrilateral has _____ sides and angles.

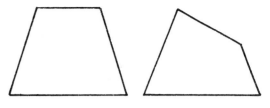

A rhombus is a modified square that has _____ sides.

If teeth were only square, rhomboidal, trapezoidal, or some other quadrilateral, they could be easily described, but they are complex in shape with numerous surface refinements. Each edge or border must be studied as well as the area within these borders, called a tooth _____.

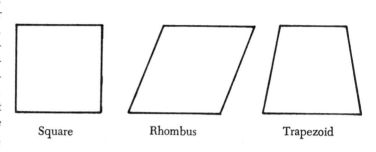

Square   Rhombus   Trapezoid

Using the analogy of the cube or wedge and considering the "top" of the cube (or wedge) to be the occlusal surface (or incisal edge) and the front the facial surface, the back side would then represent the _____ surface and the two sides the _____ and _____ surfaces.

Permanent
1. Mandibular Right 2nd Molar
2. Mandibular Right Central Incisor

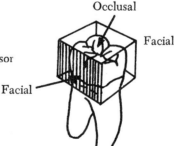

Viewed facially (from the "front" of the cube or wedge), one border is the **cervical border,** the side borders are referred to as mesial and distal, and the upper border is called _____ border.

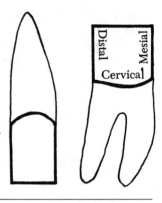

---

incisal (or occlusal)

From the lingual aspect, four borders are seen. One border is cervical; the other three borders are the _____, _____, and the _____ borders.

Permanent
Maxillary
Left
Central Incisor
LINGUAL

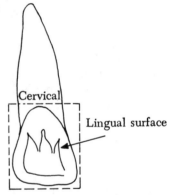

---

incisal (occlusal), mesial, distal

What surface on posterior teeth is designated by the shaded area? _____

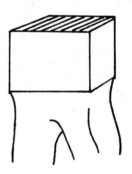

Three of the borders of the facial surface are also shared with other surfaces. For example, border (A) is a border of both the facial and the mesial surface. Often these borders are named by using a compound of two surfaces. In this case, the word would be _____.

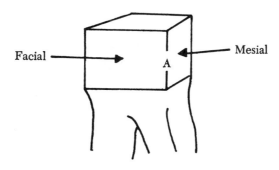

Facial ———→   A   ←——— Mesial

When two surfaces meet and share a border, the border is often called a **line angle.** The border formed by the intersection of the mesial and facial surfaces would be called the **mesiofacial line angle.** In a similar manner, the distal border of the facial surface may also be called the _____ line angle.

Each of the surfaces of anterior teeth can now be described. The edge of anterior teeth is called the _____ edge, and the four tooth surfaces labeled in the drawing above are the A. _____, B. _____, C. _____, and D. _____.

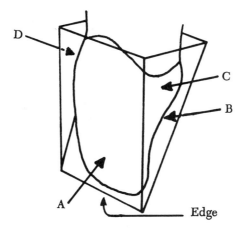

SECTION 1.1 MAXILLARY CENTRAL INCISOR: FACIAL VIEW

The first tooth to be described, the permanent maxillary central incisor, is one of the most prominent teeth in the dental arch. The universal code number for this tooth in the left quadrant is _____.

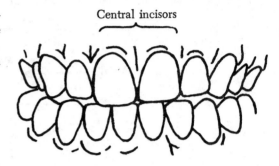

Central incisors

9

The maxillary central incisors contact one another across the midline on their _____ surfaces.

Permanent
Maxillary
Central Incisors
FACIAL

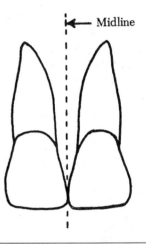

Midline

mesial

Viewed facially, the maxillary central incisor resembles a trapezoid. The four borders are called the _____, _____, _____, and _____ borders.

Permanent
Maxillary
Right
Central Incisor
FACIAL

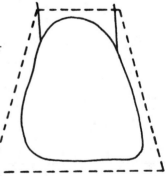

At eruption, the incisal surface has three mamelons which suggest three of the _____ (number) lobes of the central incisor.

Permanent
Maxillary
Right
Central Incisor
FACIAL

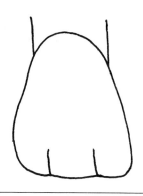

four

Three of the four lobes are revealed by the grooves seen on the _____ surface of the crown.

Permanent
Maxillary
Right
Central Incisor
FACIAL

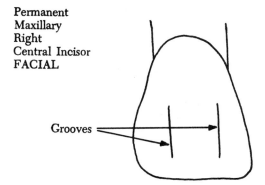

Grooves

facial

The junction of the mesial and facial surface is called the _____ line angle.

Permanent
Maxillary
Right
Central Incisor
MESIOFACIAL OBLIQUE

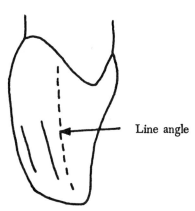

Line angle

Similarly, the junction of the distal and facial surfaces would form the _____ line angle.

Permanent
Maxillary
Right
Central Incisor
DISTOFACIAL OBLIQUE

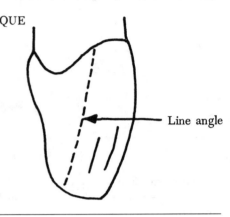

Line angle

Of these two line angles or edges, the mesiofacial is slightly longer. Thus, the distance between the incisal edge of the tooth and the cervical line is greater at the _____ (mesial/distal) border of the facial surface.

The facial surface of the central incisor is convex at both the mesial and distal borders. The mesiofacial line angle is said to be very slightly convex with the distofacial line angle somewhat _____ (more/less) convex.

    The shorter line angle of the two is the _____ line angle.

Permanent
Maxillary
Right
Central Incisor
FACIAL

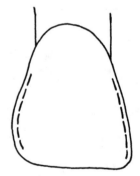

The angle formed at the intersection of the mesial and incisal surfaces is called the **mesioincisal angle.** As illustrated, the mesioincisal angle is a (an) (obtuse, acute) _____.

Permanent
Maxillary
Left
Central Incisor
FACIAL (INCISAL THIRD)

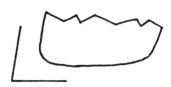

Obtuse angle is incorrect
Acute angle is correct

An obtuse angle is an angle that measures more than 90°. The illustration in the frame above indicates an angle of less than 90°. The mesioincisal angle of a maxillary central incisor is less than 90° and, therefore, is an acute angle.

Permanent
Maxillary
Left
Central Incisor
FACIAL

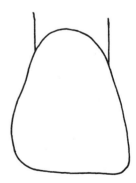

The distoincisal angle of the central incisor is _____ (more/less) rounded then the mesioincisal angle.

Permanent
Maxillary
Right
Central Incisor
FACIAL

Of the two proximal line angles of the facial surface, the _____ is the longer, and the _____ is more curved.

Permanent
Maxillary
Right
Central Incisor
FACIAL

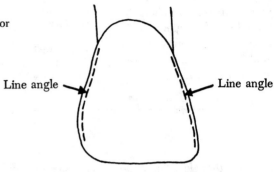

Line angle ⟶   ⟵ Line angle

The cervical line forms the fourth border of the facial or lingual surface, its curve blending into the mesial and distal borders. The illustration shows that the convexity is directed toward the root. The **crest of convexity** is slightly _____ (mesial/distal) to the longitudinal axis of the tooth as seen from a facial view.

Permanent
Maxillary
Left
Central Incisor
FACIAL

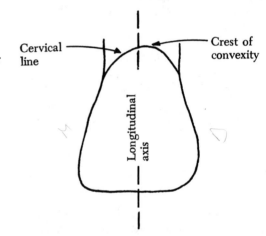

Cervical line   Crest of convexity

Longitudinal axis

In Figure 1, the mesial surface is toward _____ (A/B). In Figure 2, the mesial surface is toward _____ (A/B).

Permanent
Maxillary
Central Incisor
FACIAL

B   A

Fig. 1

A   B

Fig. 2

To which maxillary quadrant does this tooth belong? _____ (right/left)

Permanent
Maxillary
Central Incisor
FACIAL

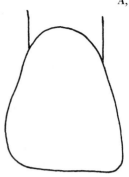

right

Within its four borders, the facial surface of the maxillary central incisor is very slightly convex horizontally (from mesial edge to distal edge, or mesiodistally) and vertically (incisocervically). In other words, the facial surface is curved in _____ (one/two) dimensions.

Permanent
Maxillary
Right
Central Incisor
MESIOFACIAL OBLIQUE

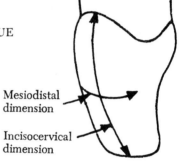

Mesiodistal dimension

Incisocervical dimension

two

Each of the following words is misspelled. Rewrite each, spelling it correctly.

distil _____
oclusal _____
labiul _____
mesiel _____
maxilarry _____

distal, occlusal, labial, mesial, maxillary

MATRIX TEST 1

Directions . . .

Place an X in the square matching the left hand column with the top row.

When you have completed the test, remove the sheet and turn to Page 185 *to check your answers.*

MAXILLARY CENTRAL INCISOR Facial View	MESIAL	DISTAL	NEITHER
More rounded incisal angle on the maxillary central incisor.			
Displacement of crest of convexity of cervical line of facial surface.			
Line angle that is shorter in facial view.			
Line angle that is more nearly straight.			

CHECK YOUR ANSWERS ON PAGE 185. GO TO PAGE 125 AFTER COMPLETING THIS TEST.

SECTION 1.2   MAXILLARY CENTRAL INCISOR: LINGUAL VIEW

The outline of a maxillary central incisor is the same when viewed from either the facial or lingual aspect. However, the lingual surface is slightly smaller than the facial surface. (true/false) _____.

true

Recall that stone blocks used to form an arch are wider at their outer surface than at their inner surface. When examining a dental arch, we can notice a similar relationship between the facial and lingual surfaces of the teeth. The three views shown below of a maxillary central incisor demonstrate this concept.

1. Stone Arch
2. Permanent Maxillary Arch OCCLUSAL

Permanent Maxillary Central Incisor
3. INCISAL
4. LINGUAL
5. FACIAL

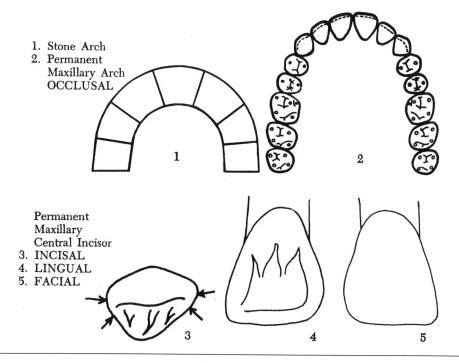

Similar to the facial surface, the lingual surface at the cervical line is convex toward the root and its crest of convexity is displaced toward the _____ (mesial/distal).

Permanent
Maxillary
Left
Central Incisor
LINGUAL

Crest of convexity
of cervical line

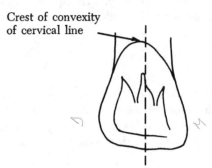

distal

Along the mesial and distal margins, rounded ridges of enamel unite in a sweeping curve along the cervical line. Cervically, the ridge is called the **linguocervical ridge.** The two lateral ridges are called the _____ **marginal ridge** and the _____ **marginal ridge.**

Permanent
Maxillary
Left
Central Incisor
LINGUAL

Marginal
ridge

Marginal
ridge

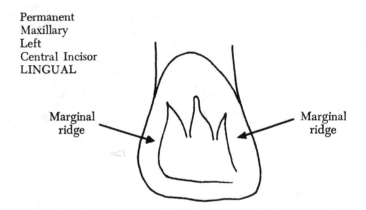

mesial, distal

Identify the lettered areas using the correct nomenclature. A. _____ B. _____ C. _____.

Permanent
Maxillary
Left
Central Incisor
LINGUAL

A

B

C

A. *distal marginal ridge; B. mesial marginal ridge; C. linguocervical ridge*

On the lingual surface, the pronounced convexity can be referred to in two ways. The bulge in the cervical third that follows the curve of the cervical line can be called the linguocervical ridge. When referring to the entire convexity, which represents the fourth or lingual lobe, we use the term **cingulum** (SING gue lum).

Which of the labels (A or B) in the drawing on the right indicates the cingulum? _____ Which indicates the linguocervical ridge? _____.

Permanent
Maxillary
Left
Central Incisor
LINGUAL

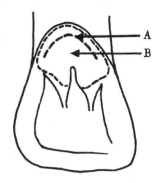

B. cingulum; A. linguocervical ridge

In contrast to the convexity of the cingulum and marginal ridges, the remaining lingual surface is concave. This concavity, called a fossa, is named for the surface on which it occurs. It is, therefore, called the _____ fossa.

Permanent
Maxillary
Left
Central Incisor
LINGUAL

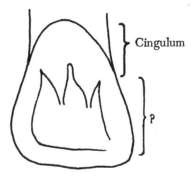

Cingulum

?

lingual

In some individuals there is a shallow pit called the **lingual pit.** This pit is in the cervical portion of the _____ fossa.

Permanent
Maxillary
Right
Central Incisor
LINGUAL

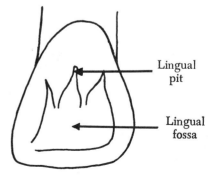

Lingual
pit

Lingual
fossa

127

The lingual fossa is concave in both dimensions and may have a small cervical extension called the _____.

Permanent
Maxillary
Right
Central Incisor
LINGUAL

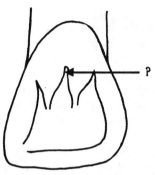

lingual

In contrast to the facial surface of this incisor tooth, which is slightly _____ (concave/convex), the lingual surface is both _____ and _____ when viewed from a proximal aspect.

Permanent
Maxillary
Right
Central Incisor
DISTAL

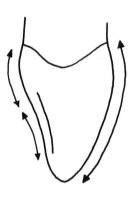

lingual pit

---

convex, concave, convex

The three major ridges of the lingual surface are the _____, the _____, and the _____.

Permanent
Maxillary
Right
Central Incisor
LINGUAL

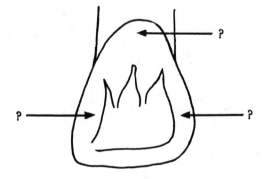

The major convexity on the lingual surface in the cervical and middle thirds is the _____.

The major concavity is the _____ which occasionally has a slight cervical extension called the _____.

Permanent
Maxillary
Left
Central Incisor
LINGUAL

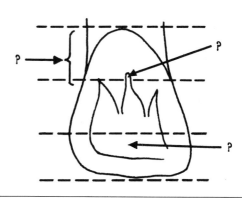

REVIEW TEST 1

MAKE A NOTE OF YOUR ANSWERS AND TURN TO PAGE 186 TO CHECK THEM.

1. The more convex line angle on the surface of the maxillary central incisor is the . . .
   a. mesiofacial
   b. distofacial

2. The longer of the two line angles on the maxillary central incisor is the . . .
   a. mesiofacial
   b. distofacial

3. The maxillary central incisor at eruption has how many mamelons?
   a. one
   b. three
   c. five
   d. four

4. The maxillary central incisor has how many lobes?
   a. three
   b. four
   c. five

5. Where are the following anatomical characteristics located on the lingual surface of the maxillary central incisor—in the cervical, middle or incisal thirds?
   (Hint: Some of these are located in more than one of the thirds)
   Draw a circle around the correct locations:

   a. cingulum: *cervical middle incisal*
   b. linguocervical ridge: *cervical middle incisal*
   c. lingual fossa: *cervical middle incisal*

ANSWERS ON PAGE 186

SECTION 2.0   MAXILLARY CENTRAL INCISOR: PROXIMAL VIEW

Viewing the maxillary central incisor from the mesial side reveals a triangular profile with the apex at the _____.

The base corresponds roughly to the _____.

Permanent
Maxillary
Left
Central Incisor
MESIAL

Cervical line

Incisal Edge

incisal edge, cervical line

The most _prominent feature_ of the lingual profile is the _____.

Permanent
Maxillary
Left
Central Incisor
MESIAL

cingulum

In mesial profile, the cingulum appears _____ (convex/concave), but the remaining sweep of the lingual surface is gently _____ (convex/concave).

Permanent
Maxillary
Left
Central Incisor
MESIAL

Cingulum →

convex, concave

As shown, the cingulum occurs in both the _____ and _____ thirds of the anatomical crown.

Permanent
Maxillary
Right
Central Incisor
DISTAL

Examine the diagrams. The incisal edge occurs in the incisal third of the crown; the
height of contour of the facial and lingual
surfaces occurs in the _____ third, and
the lingual fossa is in the _____ and
_____ thirds.

Permanent
Maxillary
Right
Central Incisor
1. LINGUAL
2. DISTAL

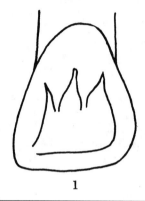
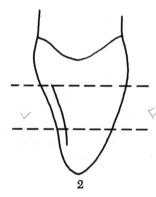

1   2

As seen in a proximal view, the cervical line
appears as a rounded "U" shape with the
"bottom" of the "U" projecting toward the
_____ surface.

Permanent
Maxillary
Right
Central Incisor
DISTAL

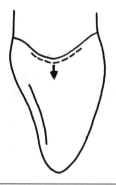

cervical line → ÷ b/t enamel + cementum

From a proximal view of the maxillary central incisor, you will observe that the tooth
axis that bisects the root apex and the incisal
edge, also crosses through the crest of convexity of the _____ (cervical line/lin-
guocervical ridge).

Permanent
Maxillary
Right
Central Incisor
DISTAL

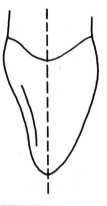

132

From a mesial view, the outline of the central incisor is roughly similar to what geometric shape? _____ .

Permanent
Maxillary
Right
Central Incisor
MESIAL

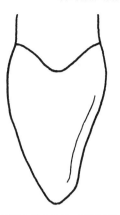

cingulum - convexity

The mesial view is very similar to the distal. Again, on the lingual surface one observes the large _____ (cingulum/lingual pit) occurring in the cervical and middle thirds.

Permanent
Maxillary
Right
Central Incisor
MESIAL

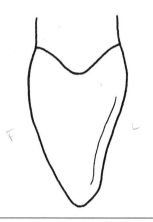

On the facial surface, the convexity is smooth with its height of contour occurring in the _____ third.

Permanent
Maxillary
Right
Central Incisor
DISTAL

Height of contour →

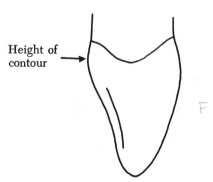

133

To review briefly, on both facial and lingual aspects, these heights of contour occur in the ———— of the crown.

Permanent
Maxillary
Right
Central Incisor
DISTAL

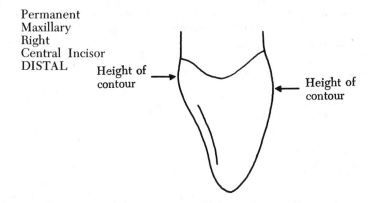

Height of contour →

← Height of contour

The curvature of the cementoenamel junction (or cervical line) on the distal surface is similar to that of the mesial surface, the exception being the amount of curvature. For example, if the cervical line has a curvature that measures 3.5 mm on the mesial surface, the distal curvature will measure 2.5 mm. Although the amount of difference may vary, the amount of curvature of the cervical line on all teeth is greater on the ———— surface.

Permanent
Maxillary
Right
Central Incisor
1. MESIAL
2. DISTAL

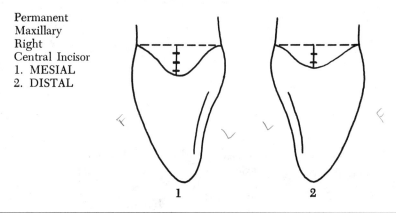

1   2

How many of the following terms are spelled correctly?

mesial-distel
cervikal
lingual fose
mesiodistally

SECTION 2.1 MAXILLARY CENTRAL INCISOR: INCISAL VIEW

Viewing the maxillary central incisor from the incisal surface reveals the narrowness of the incisal surface. Much of facial surface can be seen. On the lingual surface, the most striking prominence is the large _____.

Permanent
Maxillary
Right
Central Incisor
1. DISTAL
2. INCISAL

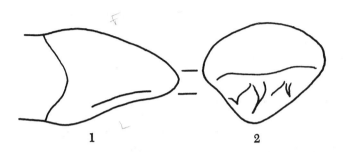

cingulum

When examining a specimen tooth (maxillary central incisor) from an incisal view, how much of the root can be seen?

    A. The root is completely obscured
       in an incisal view.............GO TO NEXT FRAME
    B. Only a small portion of the root
       is visible in an incisal view .....GO TO NEXT FRAME

Incisal to the cingulum is the large lingual concavity, the _____.

Permanent
Maxillary
Central Incisor
PROXIMAL

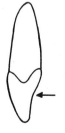

The incisal edge of a central incisor is centered over the root in the faciolingual direction. Thus, the plane that bisects the incisal edge and the cervical line on the proximal surfaces also bisects the _____.

Permanent
Maxillary
Central Incisor
PROXIMAL

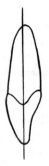

Examining a maxillary central incisor from the incisal view reveals three evident features of crown anatomy. First, the proximal surfaces taper in toward the cingulum. Second, very slight grooves are present on the facial surface. Third, the incisal view shows a geometric outline that is roughly _____ in shape.

Permanent
Maxillary
Right
Central Incisor
INCISAL

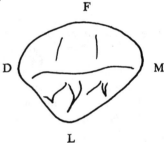

As we examine the facial surface progressively toward the incisal, the mesiodistal arc of convexity becomes less convex, until near the incisal border the curve of convexity is almost _____.

Permanent
Maxillary
Right
Central Incisor

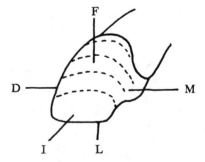

136

SECTION 2.2 MAXILLARY LATERAL INCISOR

The maxillary lateral incisor closely resembles its neighbor, the central incisor. Facially, the geometric shape of the lateral incisor is the same; that is, _____ in shape.

Permanent
Maxillary
Right
Lateral Incisor
FACIAL

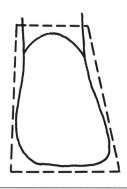

trapezoidal or quadrilateral

The lateral incisor is smaller than the central incisor in all dimensions. Mesiodistally (horizontally), it is _____ (narrower/wider); incisocervically (vertically), it is _____ (longer/shorter).

Permanent
Maxillary
Right
1. Lateral Incisor
2. Central Incisor
FACIAL

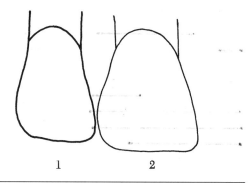

narrower, shorter

A maxillary lateral incisor is <u>more rounded</u> from a facial view than its adjacent central incisor. The angles formed by the intersection of the incisal with the two proximal surfaces are definitely rounded. Of the two incisal angles, the more rounded is the _____ angle.

Permanent
Maxillary
Right
Lateral Incisor
FACIAL

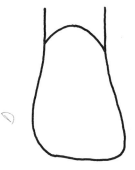

137

Keeping in mind the over-all comparison in curvature between a maxillary lateral and central incisor, which tooth has the more rounded distofacial line angle? _____ .

Permanent
Maxillary
Right
1. Lateral Incisor
2. Central Incisor
FACIAL

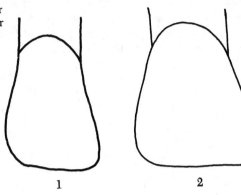

1   2

Although the lateral incisor is more curved than the central incisor, there is one feature that is an exception. The mesiofacial line angles of the two maxillary incisors closely resemble each other. The maxillary lateral incisors will deviate from the norm more often than any other tooth, with the exception of the third molars. At times, the general trend of a more rounded form for the lateral incisor is reversed, so that the mesial border of a lateral incisor appears to be _____ than that of the central incisor.

Permanent
Maxillary
Right
1. Lateral Incisor
2. Central Incisor
FACIAL

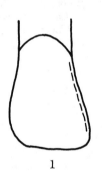 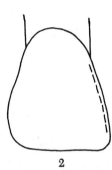

1   2

Lingually, the features of a maxillary lateral incisor are more prominent than those of a central incisor. Each of the four convexities that form the borders of the lingual surface is well developed. By comparison to the central incisor, these well-developed ridges create a lingual fossa that is slightly _____ (deeper/shallower).

Permanent
Maxillary
Right
1. Central Incisor
2. Lateral Incisor
LINGUAL

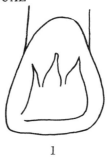 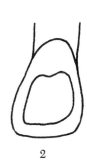

1   2

The mesial and distal marginal ridges unite, cervically, with the major lingual convexity, the _____.

Permanent
Maxillary
Right
Lateral Incisor
LINGUAL

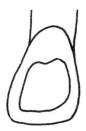

Incisally, a well developed **linguoincisal ridge** completes the marginal convexity of the lingual surface. Which of the following statements describes the effect the well-developed linguoincisal ridge has on the incisal surface of the lateral incisor?

The faciolingual measurement of the incisal edge of the maxillary central and maxillary lateral incisor would be . . .

a.   the same on both incisors
b.   relatively thicker on the lateral incisor

Permanent
Maxillary
Right
Lateral Incisor
1. LINGUAL
2. MESIAL
Central Incisor
3. MESIAL

  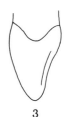

1   2   3

139

A maxillary central incisor is larger than a maxillary lateral incisor, but the well developed linguoincisal ridge on a lateral incisor gives the <u>lateral incisor added thickness at the incisal.</u>

The lingual surface of a maxillary lateral incisor has mesial and distal marginal ridges that are _____ (more/less) prominent than a maxillary central incisor.

---

more

The term used to identify area (A) is _____ _____ _____.

Permanent
Maxillary
Right
Central Incisor
LINGUAL

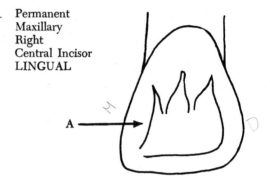

A ⟶

---

mesial marginal ridge

The term used to identify area (B) (right) is _____ ridge.

Permanent
Maxillary
Right
Central Incisor
LINGUAL

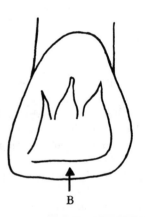

B

Area (B) is called _____ (lingual fossa/ lingual pit).

Permanent
Maxillary
Right
Central Incisor
LINGUAL

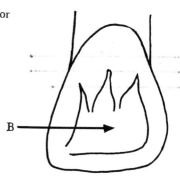

B

The cingulum is indicated by arrow (A,B, or C). _____.

Permanent
Maxillary
Left
Central Incisor
LINGUAL

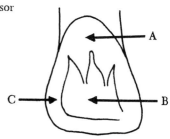

A

C   B

A is correct; (B is the lingual fossa; C is the distal marginal ridge)

From a facial view, which tooth is larger: a maxillary central incisor or a maxillary lateral incisor? _____.

maxillary central incisor

From a proximal view, which tooth appears relatively thicker at the incisal: a maxillary central incisor or a maxillary lateral incisor? _____.

141

Both proximal surfaces of a maxillary lateral incisor are generally similar to the proximal surfaces of a central incisor. The actual amount of curvature of the cervical line is slightly less on the proximal surfaces of a _____ incisor.

Permanent
Maxillary
Right
1. Lateral Incisor
2. Central Incisor
MESIAL

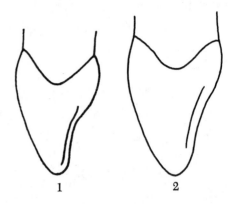

lateral

As on a maxillary central incisor, the cervical line on the proximal surface of a maxillary lateral incisor appears as a rounded "U" shape. The cervical line is convex toward the _____ edge.

Permanent
Maxillary
Right
Lateral Incisor
MESIAL

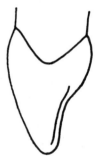

incisal

As with all teeth, the lateral incisors are relatively flat on the proximal surfaces, gingival to the interproximal contact area. This relatively flat contour allows room for the gingival tissue called the _____.

Permanent
Maxillary
Right
Lateral Incisor
1. FACIAL
2. MESIAL

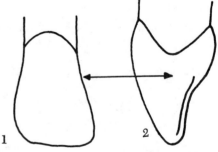

On which proximal surface of any given tooth does the cervical line have the greater amount of curvature? _____.

Although a maxillary central incisor is larger than a <u>lateral incisor,</u> the lateral incisor appears to be <u>more rounded from an incisal view.</u> Because a lateral incisor is narrower mesiodistally, the <u>curvature on the facial surface is proportionately greater than that of a</u> <u>central incisor.</u> Lingually, the major convexities (the mesial and distal marginal ridges, the linguoincisal ridge, and cingulum) are more fully developed on a lateral incisor.

Of the two drawings below, which is the lateral incisor (incisal view), 1 or 2?

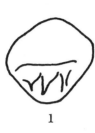 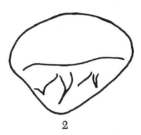

1   2

Identify each of the four teeth by arch (maxillary/mandibular), quadrant (right/left), and tooth name.

A. Permanent   _____   _____   _____
B. Permanent   _____   _____   _____
C. Permanent   _____   _____   _____
D. Permanent   _____   _____   _____

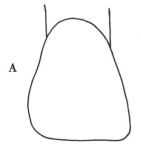 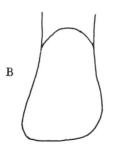 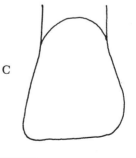 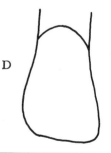

A   B   C   D

A. Permanent maxillary right central incisor; B.
Permanent maxillary left lateral incisor; C.
Permanent maxillary left central incisor; D.
Permanent maxillary right lateral incisor

Each of the following terms is spelled incorrectly. Revise each.

1. cervecol   1. _____

2. fosse   2. _____

3. conkave   3. _____

4. meseodistol   4. _____

1. cervical; 2. fossa; 3. concave; 4. mesiodistal

GO TO THE NEXT PAGE AND TAKE THE MATRIX TEST.

MATRIX TEST 2

Directions . . .

Place an X in the square matching the left hand column with the top row. When you have completed the test, *turn to Page 187 to check your answers.*

	MAXILLARY CENTRAL INCISOR	MAXILLARY LATERAL INCISOR	BOTH INCISORS
Quadrilateral shape (facial view)			
Longer incisocervically			
Relatively thicker (at incisal edge)			
More distinct lingual features			

ANSWERS ON PAGE 187

REVIEW TEST 2

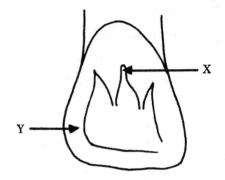

1. The correct name for the structure labeled "X" is:
   a. Lingual fossa
   b. Lingual pit
   c. Linguocervical ridge

2. In the drawing, "Y" represents the:
   a. Mesial marginal ridge
   b. Distal marginal ridge

3. Choose the **correct** statement:
   a. The lateral incisor usually has a straighter distofacial line angle than the central incisor.
   b. The lateral incisor has a rounder distofacial line angle than the central incisor.

4. Choose the **correct** statement:
   a. The lateral incisor has more curvature to the cervical line on the mesial and distal surface than does the central incisor.
   b. The cervical line of the lateral incisor has less curvature on the mesial and distal surfaces than does the cervical line on the corresponding surfaces of the central incisor.

5. Which of the following descriptions of the maxillary central incisor is correct in all aspects (a, b, or neither)?
   a. The height of contour on the facial and lingual surfaces occurs in the cervical third. On the proximal surfaces the cervical line is "U" shaped, with the "U" centered on the tooth axis. The cervical line has more curvature on the distal surface than on the mesial.
   b. The height of contour on the facial and lingual surfaces occurs in the cervical third. On the proximal surfaces the cervical line is "U" shaped, with the "U" displaced toward the facial. The cervical line has more curvature on the mesial surface than on the distal.

6. Choose the **incorrect** statement:
   a. The distoincisal angle of the maxillary lateral incisor is more rounded than the mesioincisal angle.
   b. The maxillary central incisor has more distinct mesial and distal marginal ridges than the maxillary lateral incisor.

c. The anatomy of the maxillary lateral incisor shows great variation among different individuals—more variation than any other tooth, except the third molar.

7. If someone said, "The maxillary incisors are relatively flat on their proximal surfaces, gingival to the proximal contact areas," which of the following responses would be the most complete and accurate reply you could make:
a. "This is false because they are convex."
b. "That is false, because the line angles of these teeth are curved."
c. "That is true, because the enamel is thin."
d. "That is true, because this flatness provides space for the interdental papilla."

MAKE A NOTE OF YOUR ANSWERS AND TURN TO PAGE 188 TO CHECK THEM.

147

SECTION 3.0 MANDIBULAR CENTRAL INCISORS

The mandibular incisors are the <u>smallest teeth of the human dentition</u>. In normal occlusion, the maxillary central incisor occludes with the central and lateral incisors of the mandibular arch. Which incisor normally has only one antagonist? _____

_____ _____

Permanent
1. Maxillary Incisors
2. Mandibular Incisors
FACIAL

1

2

mandibular central incisor

The form of a mandibular incisor is distinctly different from that of a maxillary incisor. Despite the differences in tooth form, the maxillary and mandibular incisors have general similarities that place them in the classification of incisors. Each of the crowns of the incisors has a _____ shape.

wedge

As with maxillary anteriors, the mandibular incisors have _____ (number) lobes.

four

Similar to maxillary incisors, the incisal edges of newly erupted mandibular incisors have three rounded bumps. These bumps, which suggest three of the four lobes, are called _____.

Permanent Mandibular Incisors FACIAL

mamelons

The four lobes are called the **distofacial, central-facial, mesiofacial, and lingual lobes.** Which three lobes represent that part of the tooth seen in a facial view? _____ _____

_____.

The fourth lobe is represented on the lingual surface of the crown by the prominent convexity called the _____.

Permanent
1. Maxillary
2. Mandibular
Central Incisor
PROXIMAL

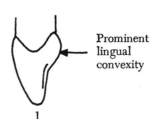 Prominent lingual convexity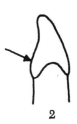

1

2

cingulum

As seen from a facial view, the geometric outline of a mandibular incisor is roughly quadrilateral. From a proximal view, each of the eight incisors has a geometric outline that is roughly _____.

Permanent
Maxillary
Right
Central Incisor
1. FACIAL
2. DISTAL
Mandibular
Right
Central Incisor
3. FACIAL
4. DISTAL

1 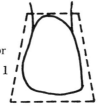 2

3 4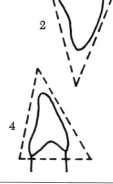

triangular

The nomenclature established for the maxillary incisors applies to the corresponding features of mandibular incisors. The prominent features are located in similar positions on the crowns of all eight incisors.

For example, the intersection of the facial and mesial surfaces forms the mesiofacial line angle, and the concavity of the lingual surface is termed the lingual _____.

149

The facial surface of a mandibular central incisor is <u>curved in the incisocervical and mesiodistal dimensions</u>. In both dimensions, the facial surface is slightly _____ (convex/concave).

Permanent
Mandibular
Right
Central Incisor
1. INCISAL
2. DISTAL

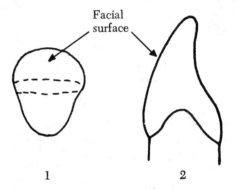

Facial surface

1   2

convex

Incisocervically, the imaginary line encircling the tooth and <u>defining the peak or height of curvature</u> is called the _____ __ _____.

Permanent
Mandibular
Right
Central Incisor
1. FACIAL
2. MESIAL

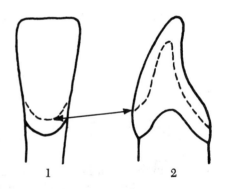

1   2

height of contour

The **height of contour** is an imaginary curved line that completely surrounds the crown. On the facial and lingual surfaces of a mandibular incisor, the height of contour occurs in the _____ third of the crown.

Permanent
Mandibular
Right
Central Incisor
DISTOFACIAL

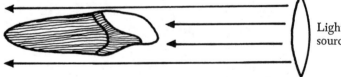

Light source

Recall that the **amount of contour** is a horizontal measurement. On the facial and lingual surfaces of a mandibular incisor, the amount of contour is _____.

**Permanent
Mandibular
Right
Lateral Incisor
DISTAL**

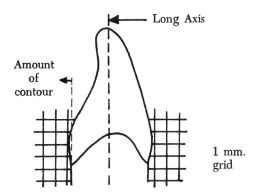

more than ½ mm ....GO TO NEXT FRAME
less than ½ mm ....GO TO TOP OF PAGE 152

From top of this page

More than ½ mm is incorrect

Let us review some material presented earlier. For the majority of the teeth in the human dentition, the facial and lingual amount of contour measures approximately ½ mm. There are, however, several exceptions, the mandibular incisors being one. The amount of contour on the mandibular incisors is very slight, at times nearly indistinguishable. Therefore, on mandibular incisors, the facial and lingual amount of contour measures less than ½ mm.

**Permanent
Mandibular
Right
Central Incisor
MESIAL (CERVICAL THIRD)**

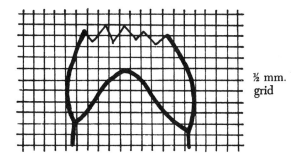

½ mm. grid

The reduction of curvature on the facial surface is typical of the contours of the entire crown of a mandibular incisor. Facially, the slight mesiodistal convexity of a mandibular central incisor is most pronounced in the cervical third of the crown. The degree of convexity of the facial surface decreases progressively from the narrow cervical third toward the wider, nearly flat _____ edge.

Permanent
Mandibular
Right
Central Incisor
1. FACIAL
2. INCISAL

L

D

M

F

1

2

---

incisal

As the facial surface becomes less convex, it becomes wider, so the broadest portion of a mandibular central incisor is found near the _____.

Permanent
Mandibular
Right
Central Incisor
FACIAL

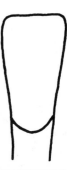

When one examines a mandibular central incisor from a facial view, it is difficult to identify characteristics that distinguish the mesial from the distal surface. The distinguishing features are very slight.

Permanent
Mandibular
Right
Central Incisor
FACIAL

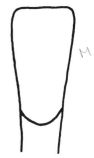

From the facial view
1. The distofacial line angle is slightly more convex.
2. The cervical line has its crest slightly toward the distal.
3. The straight line distance between the end-points of the distofacial line angle is slightly less than the straight-line distance between the end-points of the mesiofacial line angle. That is, the incisal edge is inclined slightly toward the gingival at the distal.
4. The distoinciscal angle is slightly greater than the mesioincisal angle.

Permanent
Mandibular
Central Incisor
FACIAL

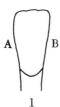

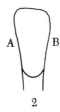

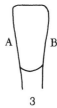

The drawings above represent three mandibular central incisors. In each drawing, which letter—"A" or "B"—is toward the distal?

_____   _____   _____.

(Figure 1)   (Figure 2)   (Figure 3)

Fig. 1-A; Fig. 2-B; Fig. 3-B

Both the mesioincisal and the distoincisal angles of a mandibu- lar central incisor are acute. Of the two angles, which is more acute? _____

---

mesioincisal

From a facial view, the cervical line is convex toward the _____ of the tooth. The crest of this convexity is slightly _____ (distal/mesial) to the midline of the facial surface.

---

root, distal

Let the geometric shape shown represent the outline of the facial surface on a model of a mandibular central incisor that has been dropped on a tray. Which of the line segments (A, B, C, D) represents the incisal and cervical borders? Incisal ___ Cervical _____.

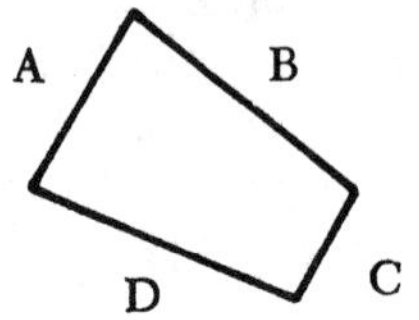

---

incisal, A; cervical, C

The faint facial grooves seen on the facial surfaces of the maxillary incisors are absent on the mandibular central incisors except when they are newly erupted. Compared to maxillary centrals, the mandibular centrals have a facial surface that is quite _____ and straight.

---

smooth

The geometric outlines of the facial and lingual surfaces of the mandibular central incisor are similar. How many borders or edges does the outline have? _____.

Permanent
Mandibular
Right
Central Incisor
1. FACIAL
2. LINGUAL

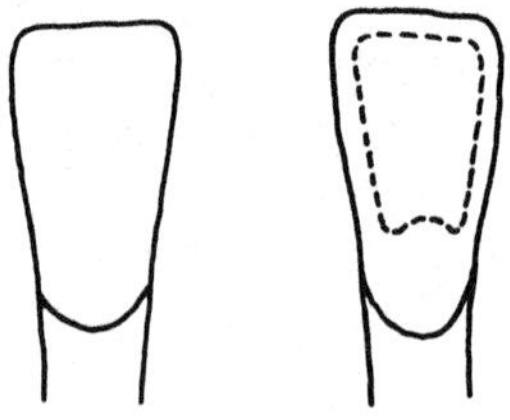

---

four

As with maxillary incisors, the lingual surface is somewhat _____ (smaller/larger) than the area within the facial sur- face.

As seen from an incisal view, the smaller lingual outline is a result of the convergence toward the _____ surface.

Permanent Mandibular Right Central Incisor INCISAL

In contrast to what is observed on the maxillary incisors, the mesial and distal marginal ridges of the mandibular central incisor are quite _____ (size).

Permanent Mandibular Right Central Incisor LINGUAL

Comparing the lingual convexity of the maxillary and mandibular central incisors, the cingulum on the lingual surface of a mandibular central incisor is _____ (less/more) pronounced.

Permanent Mandibular Right Central Incisor MESIAL

The lingual surface of a mandibular central incisor is concave in both the incisocervical and mesiodistal dimensions. The small cingulum and indistinct marginal ridges result in a shallow and generally less distinct lingual _____.

The resulting lingual surface of a mandibular central incisor forms a smooth area that flows in a concave, then convex curve from the incisal edge to the cervical line. The less pronounced lingual anatomy results in the absence of small extensions of the fossa into the cingulum. A mandibular central incisor, therefore, has no lingual _____ .

**Permanent
Mandibular
Right
Central Incisor
1. MESIAL
2. LINGUAL
3. INCISAL**

1   2   3

Although the lingual fossa of a mandibular central incisor is small or less distinct, the lingual surface is concave in two dimensions: the incisocervical dimension and very slightly concave in the _____ dimension.

Contributing to the smooth lingual surface of a mandibular central incisor are the reduced marginal ridges and cingulum and the absence of a lingual _____ (pit/fossa).

Permanent
Mandibular
Right
Central Incisor
LINGUAL

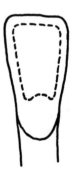

Like the crowns of the maxillary incisors, the mandibular central incisor crown (mesial view) is approximately _____ in shape.

Permanent
Mandibular
Right
Central Incisor
MESIAL

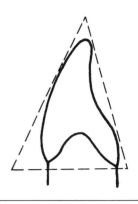

triangular

The apex of this triangle represents the _____ edge of the tooth; the base of the triangle corresponds roughly to the

_____.

incisal, cervical line

The vertical axis of the tooth that bisects the cervical line on the mesial surface shows the incisal edge displaced slightly toward the _____ surface.

Permanent
Mandibular
Right
Central Incisor
MESIAL

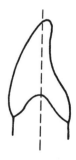

lingual

As seen from a mesial view, the facial surface of a mandibular central incisor is _____ (convex/concave).

Permanent
Mandibular
Right
Central Incisor
MESIAL

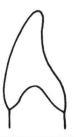

The bulk of the convexity of the lingual surface occurs in the _____ third of the crown and forms the _____.

Permanent
Mandibular
Right
Central Incisor
MESIAL

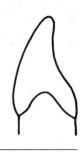

The mesial view also shows a concavity of the lingual surface from the small _____ to the _____ edge.

Permanent
Mandibular
Right
Central Incisor
MESIAL

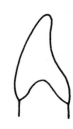

Identify the lettered areas.
    A. _____
    B. _____
    C. _____

Permanent
Mandibular
Right
Central Incisor
LINGUAL

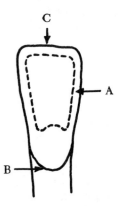

There is a difference in the amount of curvature of the cervical line on the two proximal surfaces. The cementoenamel junction curves slightly more toward the incisal on the mesial. <u>On which of the two proximal surfaces is the cervical line *less* convex toward the incisal?</u> _____.

Permanent
Mandibular
Right
Central Incisor
1. MESIAL
2. DISTAL

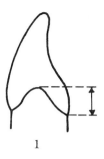 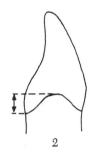

1   2

distal

The crest of convexity of the cervical line is more incisally located on the _____ (mesial/distal) surface (Fig. 1 and Fig. 3).

The incisal edge slopes slightly downward (Fig. 2) toward the distal surface and the distofacial line angle is slightly _____ (shorter/longer) than the mesiofacial.

Permanent
Mandibular
Right
Central Incisor
1. DISTAL
2. FACIAL
3. MESIAL

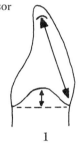 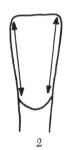 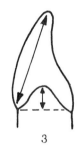

1   2   3

mesial, shorter

The mesial surface is slightly _____ (longer/shorter) than the distal, and the incisal edge slopes down towards the _____.

Permanent
Mandibular
Right
Central Incisor
FACIAL

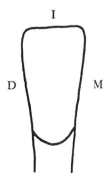

From the incisal view, we see the proximal surfaces taper in toward the _____ (facial/lingual) surface.

like skull shape

Permanent
Mandibular
Right
Central Incisor
INCISAL

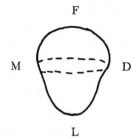

With normal occlusion, the mamelons on mandibular incisors are eventually worn away. Maxillary and mandibular incisors do <u>not usually occlude end to end</u>, but <u>occlude so that the mandibular incisors strike the incisolingual surfaces of the maxillary incisors</u> (Fig. 2). Under normal conditions, which portion of the incisal edge on a mandibular incisor receives more wear?

Permanent
1. Incisors
FACIAL (OCCLUDED)
2. Central Incisors
PROXIMAL (OCCLUDED)

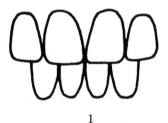 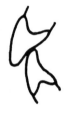

1   2

linguoincisal ....GO TO
NEXT FRAME

facioincisal .GO TO TOP OF
PAGE 161

◆ From preceding frame

linguoincisal is incorrect

Try the following experiment. Slide your lower jaw back and forth in a faciolingual direction. You, like most people, will probably feel the mandibular incisors slide over the lingual surface of the maxillary incisors. Does the abrasion on the mandibular incisors involve a portion more toward the facial or the lingual? _____.

facial

PLEASE RETURN TO THE MIDDLE OF THIS PAGE AND ANSWER AGAIN.

With increased wear at the facioincisal, the incisal edge tends to incline. In some individuals, the incisal edge of a mandibular incisor has an obvious slope downward toward the _____ (facial/lingual) surface.

Permanent
Central Incisors
PROXIMAL

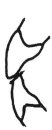

facial

Attrition also influences the incisal edge of maxillary incisors. On a maxillary incisor, which area (facioincisal/linguoincisal) receives more wear? _____

Permanent
Central Incisors
PROXIMAL

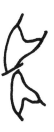

linguoincisal

With added wear at the linguoincisal portion, the incisal edge of a maxillary incisor tends to slope upward toward the lingual. The worn edges of maxillary and mandibular incisors tend to be:

Parallel . . . . GO TO TOP OF PAGE 162

Perpendicular . . . . GO TO NEXT FRAME

Suppose a pencil is placed in the mouth and the incisors closed on two opposite parallel surfaces. The slope of the pencil represents the incline of the worn incisal edges of both maxillary and mandibular incisors. The slope is upward toward the lingual and downward toward the facial. With wear, the incisal edges of maxillary and mandibular incisors tend to become parallel surfaces.

Permanent
1. Maxillary
2. Mandibular
Central Incisors
PROXIMAL

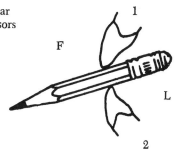

CONTINUE ON PAGE 162

When describing the slope of worn incisal edges of the maxillary and mandibular incisors, we say that the incisal edge of a maxillary incisor is inclined toward the lingual, and the incisal edge of a mandibular incisor is inclined toward the _____ surface.

Permanent
1. Maxillary
2. Mandibular
Central Incisor
PROXIMAL

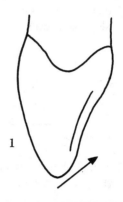

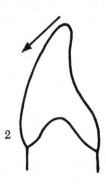

1

2

facial

TURN TO PAGE 163 AND TAKE THE MATRIX TEST.

MATRIX TEST 3

Directions . . .

Place an X in the square that matches the left hand column with the top row. Turn to Page 184, and check your answers.

	MESIAL	DISTAL
Which border is longer in facial view?		
Which border is more convex in facial view?		
More acute angle with the incisal . . .		
Crest of convexity of the cervical line is displaced to which side on facial view?		
Incisal edge sloped down toward . . .		
Cervical line on this profile more convex towards the incisal . . .		

ANSWERS ON PAGE 189

REVIEW TEST 3

Make a note of your answers, and turn to Page 190 to check them.

1. Choose the CORRECT statement:
   a. The mandibular central incisor has a less prominent lingual fossa than the maxillary central incisor and the marginal ridges are less distinct.
   b. A lingual pit is occasionally found on the mandibular central incisor.

2. Mandibular incisors have an amount of contour on the facial and lingual surfaces that measures:
   a. between 1 mm and ½ mm
   b. approximately ½ mm
   c. less than ½ mm

3. What is the word that describes the process that causes adult mandibular incisors to show no signs of the mamelons that were present at eruption (in cases where the adult has had the most common type of occlusion)?

4. Which one of the following teeth has only one antagonist in the normal (most frequent) occlusion?
   a. maxillary central incisor
   b. maxillary lateral incisor
   c. mandibular central incisor
   d. mandibular lateral incisor

ANSWERS ON PAGE 190

SECTION 4.0   MANDIBULAR LATERAL INCISORS

The mandibular lateral incisors are very similar to central incisors, but a few minor distinctions should be emphasized. Which of the two mandibular incisors shown is wider mesiodistally? _____

Permanent
Mandibular
Right
1. Lateral Incisor
2. Central Incisor
FACIAL

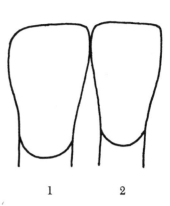

(1) lateral incisor

Does the same relationship hold for the maxillary incisors? _____ (yes/no)

Which maxillary incisor is wider mesiodistally? _____

Permanent
1. Maxillary
2. Mandibular
Right
Incisors
FACIAL

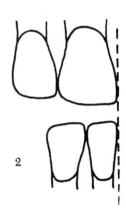

no; maxillary central incisor

The lingual fossa on a mandibular lateral incisor is slightly more evident than that on a mandibular central incisor because of the somewhat more evident mesial and distal _____ ridges.

Permanent
Mandibular
Right
1. Central Incisor
2. Lateral Incisor
LINGUAL

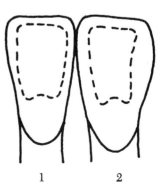

The mandibular lateral incisor also has more curvature on the distal surface than the central incisor. Which of the two diagrams represents a mandibular lateral incisor? _____ (Figure 1/Figure 2)

Permanent
Mandibular
Right
Incisors
FACIAL

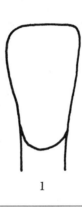
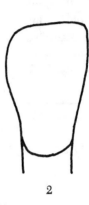

1   2

Figure 2

In general, which mandibular incisor has the more evident convexities and concavities? _____

The greater prominence of the lingual fossa on the lateral incisor is _____ (like/unlike) the relationship between the maxillary incisors.

The mesial surface of a mandibular lateral incisor tends to be slightly _____ (shorter/longer) than the distal.

Permanent
Mandibular
Right
Lateral Incisor
1. LINGUAL
2. FACIAL

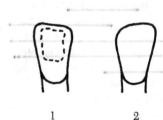

1   2

Although these general distinctions exist, they are very slight. The best method for distinguishing a mandibular lateral from a central incisor is to examine the functioning surface, that is, the _____ edge.

The <u>chief identification of a mandibular lateral incisor is made from an incisal view.</u> You will notice a <u>slight rotation of the distal end of the incisal surface</u> toward the _____ surface, due to the location of the tooth in the arch.

Permanent
Mandibular
1. Right
Lateral Incisor
INCISAL
2. Mandibular
   arch
OCCLUSAL

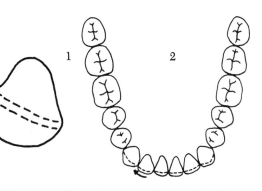

The two diagrams represent a mandibular right and left lateral incisor. Which diagram represents a mandibular right lateral incisor? _____ (Fig. 1/ Fig. 2)

Permanent
Mandibular
Lateral Incisors
INCISAL

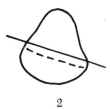

1   2

Figure 2

In the rotation on the incisal edge, which end is rotated lingually? _____

For review, identify the lettered areas on the lingual surface of the anterior tooth. Use complete dental terminology.

Permanent
Maxillary
Right
Central Incisor
LINGUAL

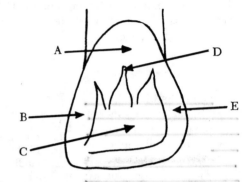

A. _____
B. _____
C. _____
D. _____
E. _____

A. cingulum; B. mesial marginal ridge; C. lingual fossa; D. lingual pit; E. distal marginal ridge

Which of the following words are spelled correctly:

1. mandibalar
2. inciser
3. mamilons
4. cervical
5. mesiel

6. incisaly
7. mesiodistal
8. cingalum
9. mesioincisel
10. facial

cervical, mesiodistal, facial

GO TO NEXT PAGE AND TAKE THE MATRIX TEST.

MATRIX TEST 4

Directions . . .

Supply a one-word answer to each box in the two columns indicated.
Turn to Page 191 and check your answers.

	Mandibular Central Incisor	Mandibular Lateral Incisor
Relative size (larger/smaller)		
Relative prominence of the lingual fossa (more/less)		
Relative amount of curvature of the distal surface (more/less)		
Is the incisal edge rotated slightly on the root? (yes/no)		
If yes (above), is the mesial or the distal rotated to the lingual?		

ANSWERS ON PAGE 191

REVIEW TEST 4

NOTE: This is a review of both Sections 3 and 4. Make a note of your answers and then turn to Page 192 to check them.

1. Choose the correct statement.
   a. On the mandibular central incisor, the distofacial line angle is more curved than the mesiofacial line angle.
   b. On the mandibular central incisor, the cervical line is curved more toward the incisal on the distal surface than on the mesial surface.

2. Which of the following anatomical characteristics are found on all incisors? (choose as many as are correct)
   a. lingual fossa
   b. lingual pit
   c. distoincisal angle
   d. mamelons
   e. height of contour in the cervical third on the facial and lingual surfaces of the crown.
   f. four lobes

3. The best way to tell the difference between a mandibular lateral incisor and a mandibular central incisor is to inspect which surface?
   a. mesial
   b. lingual
   c. incisal
   d. distal

ANSWERS ON PAGE 192

SECTION 5.0   MAXILLARY CANINE: FACIAL VIEW

The <u>maxillary canines are the longest, most stable teeth in the mouth (considering crown and root together)</u>. The teeth are sometimes referred to as "<u>cuspids;</u>" however, they are more correctly designated the maxillary _____.

**Permanent
Maxillary
Left
Canine
FACIAL**

canines

The geometric form of the crown is irregular. Unlike the other anterior teeth, the crown presents _____ (number) facial borders.

**Permanent
Maxillary
Left
Canine
FACIAL**

five

The facial surface of the maxillary canine has five borders. Two of these form the incisal edge and are <u>called the mesial and distal **cusp ridges;**</u> the other three are the _____, _____, and _____ borders.

This is the first tooth encountered having a cusp as the prominent crown feature. Cusps always have four ridges, but how many ridges can be seen from a facial view? _____

Permanent
Maxillary
Right
Canine
FACIAL

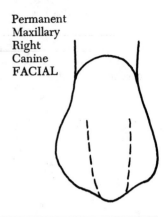

three (mesial, facial, distal)

The cusp tip divides the incisal edge into two parts. These two features are often referred to as the mesial cusp _____ and the distal cusp _____.

Permanent
Maxillary
Right
Canine
FACIAL

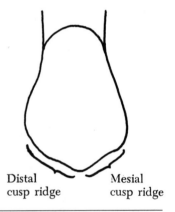

Distal
cusp ridge

Mesial
cusp ridge

ridge, ridge

The crowns of all anterior teeth have five surfaces. One surface of a canine is divided into two parts by the cusp tip. Both of these parts combine to make up the one _____ surface.

The facial surface is bounded by five borders, the incisal edge providing two of them. The five are the _____, _____, and _____ borders and the _____ and _____ cusp ridges.

Permanent
Maxillary
Right
Canine
FACIAL

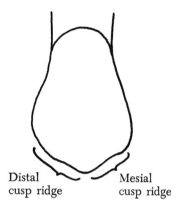

Distal cusp ridge   Mesial cusp ridge

---

mesial, distal, cervical; mesial, distal

The four surfaces and the edge numbered above are called the:

1. _____
2. _____
3. _____
4. _____
5. _____

Permanent
Maxillary
Right
Canine
a. FACIAL
b. MESIAL

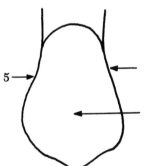
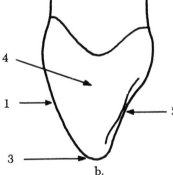

a.   b.

From the facial view, the cervical line is convex toward the root. Unlike the incisors, the cervical line has its crest of convexity slightly toward the mesial. In the diagram, which is toward the mesial (A/B)? _____

Permanent
Maxillary
Right
Canine
FACIAL

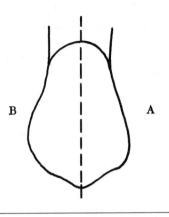

B   A

A

The mesioincisal angle of the maxillary incisors approaches a right angle, especially the central incisors. The mesioincisal angle of the canine, however, is not so well defined. From the facial aspect, the mesioincisal angle is more of a _____ than an angle.

Permanent
Maxillary
Right
Canine
FACIAL

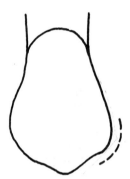

concavity......GO TO MIDDLE OF PAGE 175
convexity ....GO TO NEXT FRAME

◗ From preceding frame

convexity is correct

Both the mesial and distal borders are first concave, then convex, from the cervical line to the cusp tip. Which border has the less distinct "S-shape" curvature, the mesial or distal? _____.

Permanent
Maxillary
Right
Canine
FACIAL

D   M

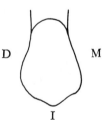

I

The distal border has a pronounced convexity at the distoincisal angle that tends to accentuate the degree of concavity found in the _____ (cervical/incisal) third of the distal border.

Permanent
Maxillary
Right
Canine
FACIAL

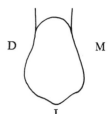

The mesial border has less overall convexity than the distal border which makes the cervical concavity on the mesial appear less pronounced, often approaching a _____ (straight/convex) outline in the cervical third.

◆ From page 174

"Concave" means having a hollow or recess. The mesioincisal angle of a maxillary canine appears as a convexity.

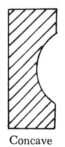
Concave

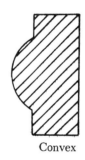
Convex

The crest of the cervical line is slightly mesial to the long axis of the tooth (facial view). However, the cusp tip of the incisal edge is _____ (mesial/distal/centered).

Permanent
Maxillary
Right
Canine
FACIAL

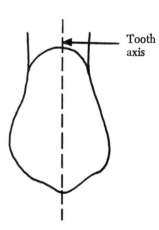
Tooth axis

The widest portion of the crown, mesiodistally, is located at the proximal contact areas. As is true of all teeth, which proximal contact area is located more cervically? _____ _____

Permanent
Maxillary
Right
Canine
FACIAL

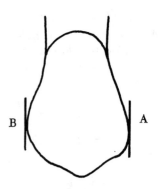

B   A

The mesial contact area of a maxillary canine is located approximately at the junction of the incisal and middle thirds of the crown. The distal contact area is located in the _____ third of the crown.

Permanent
Maxillary
Right
Canine
FACIAL

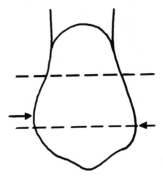

Keeping in mind that the cusp tip is centered mesiodistally, which cusp ridge is longer? _____ _____ (mesial cusp ridge/distal cusp ridge)

The distal ridge of the canine cusp is _____ (shorter/longer) than the mesial ridge of the cusp.

Permanent
Maxillary
Right
Canine
FACIAL

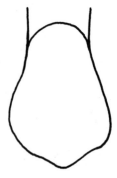

Which is the distal cusp ridge? _____
(A/B)

Permanent
Maxillary
Canine
FACIAL (Incisal Third)

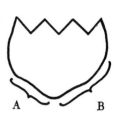

A   B

The <u>facial surface of the maxillary canine is marked by a prominent facial ridge.</u> The facial ridge is not centered on this surface but is located toward the _____ surface.

Permanent
Maxillary
Right
Canine
FACIAL

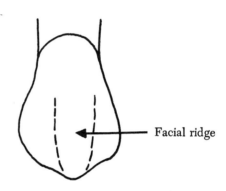

Facial ridge

The shape of the facial surface of the maxillary canine is pentagonal. This is explained by the incisal edge being divided into two ridges by the _____ (cusp tip/facial ridge).

Permanent
Maxillary
Right
Canine
FACIAL

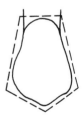

SECTION 5.1   MAXILLARY CANINE: LINGUAL VIEW

Because of the crown form, there are features on the lingual surface of a canine that are generally not present on incisors; i.e., lingual ridge, mesiolingual fossa, and distolingual fossa. Similar to the incisors, however, area (A) is termed the _____.

Permanent
Maxillary
Right
Canine
LINGUAL

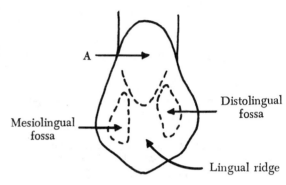

A

Distolingual fossa

Mesiolingual fossa

Lingual ridge

Typical of most teeth, the lingual surface of a canine is narrower than the facial surface. The lingual surface is marked by a prominent ridge extending from the cusp tip to the cingulum. This ridge is called the _____.

Cervically, the lingual ridge blends into the well developed _____.

Permanent
Maxillary
Right
Canine
LINGUAL

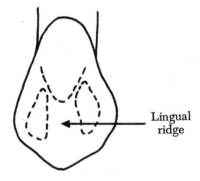

Lingual ridge

The concavities and convexities (fossae and ridges) on the lingual surface are more prominent than the topographical features of the facial surface. Which of the two surfaces is narrower mesiodistally? _____

Between the lingual ridge and distal marginal ridge is the

_____.

lingual pit . . . . .GO TO NEXT FRAME
distolingual fossa . . . . .GO TO BOTTOM OF THIS PAGE

◗ From preceding frame

lingual pit is incorrect

Unlike the lingual surface of the incisor teeth, the maxillary canine has two distinct fossae, the disto- and mesiolingual fossae.

**Permanent
Maxillary
Right
Canine
LINGUAL**

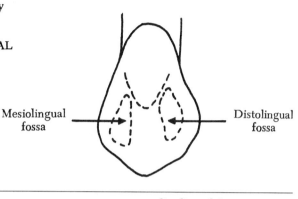

Mesiolingual fossa ——— Distolingual fossa

◗ From top of this page

distolingual fossa is correct

Incisal to the cementoenamel junction, the cingulum is convex both mesiodistally and incisocervically. The cervical portion of the cingulum is sometimes called the linguocervical _____.

**Permanent
Maxillary
Right
Canine
LINGUAL**

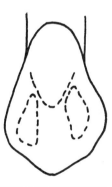

Match each of the terms below with one of the lettered areas in the diagram.

_____ lingual ridge

_____ distolingual fossa

_____ cervical line

_____ cingulum

_____ mesial marginal ridge

_____ mesiolingual fossa

Permanent
Maxillary
Right
Canine
LINGUAL

E, lingual ridge; B, cingulum; F, distolingual fossa; C, mesial marginal ridge; A, cervical line; D, mesiolingual fossa

SECTION 5.2 MAXILLARY CANINE: PROXIMAL VIEW

The proximal views of a maxillary canine have several features in common with the incisors. The overall geometric shape is roughly triangular with the cusp tip representing the apex of the triangle. The facial surface appears boldly convex. The lingual surfaces of incisors and canines are "S-shaped" in that they are concave in approximately the middle third and convex in the cervical third. The canine has more bulk, however, especially in the faciolingual dimension, than do the incisors.

The following refer to proximal views of a maxillary canine.

The lingual surface is both concave and convex from the _____ to the incisal edge.

A continuous convexity extends from the cervical line to the incisal edge on the _____ surface.

Permanent
Maxillary
Right
1. Canine
2. Central Incisor
MESIAL

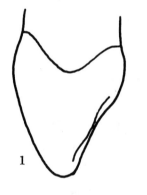
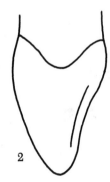

On which proximal surface does the cervical line show the least amount of curvature? _____

Compared to the incisors, <u>the canine has a greater measurement from the height of contour on the facial surface to the height of contour on the lingual surface.</u> Thus, the crown of a canine has a greater _____ measurement than the crown of an incisor.

SECTION 5.3   MAXILLARY CANINE: INCISAL VIEW

In the incisal view, the canine tooth shows the marked _____ (convexity/concavity) of the cingulum.

Permanent
Maxillary
Right
Canine
INCISAL

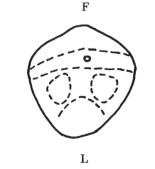

Evidence of the four lobes can be seen from the incisal view of a canine. Which of the three lobes of the facial surface is most prominent? _____

Permanent
Maxillary
Right
Canine
INCISAL

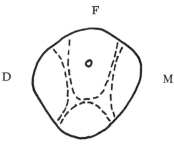

From the facial view, the cusp tip is formed by the junction of the mesial and distal ————— ridges.

Permanent
Maxillary
Canine
FACIAL (Incisal ⅓)

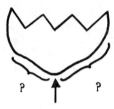

The cervical line marks the boundary between the anatomical crown and the anatomical root. It consists of a series of arcs that curve either incisally or apically. On which surfaces of the maxillary anterior teeth does the cervical line curve toward the root? —————

GO TO THE NEXT PAGE FOR MATRIX TEST 5

MATRIX TEST 5

Directions . . .

Place an X in the square that matches the left hand column with the top row. Turn to Page 193 and check your answers.

MAXILLARY CANINE	MESIAL	CENTRAL	DISTAL
Location or placement of cusp tip.			
Location or placement of crest of convexity of the cervical line (facial view)			
Border (facial view) with less pronounced convexity and concavity			
Cervical line on this surface has a crest that is more incisally located.			
Cusp ridge (longer/shorter)			

ANSWERS ON PAGE 193

183

REVIEW TEST 5

Make a note of your answers so you can check them on Page 194.

In each pair of statements about the maxillary canine, choose the one that is **correct.**

The Maxillary Canine

1.
    a. The lingual ridge of the cusp blends into the mesial marginal ridge.
    b. The lingual ridge of the cusp separates two lingual fossae.

2.
    a. The distal contact area is more toward the incisal than the mesial contact area is.
    b. The mesial contact area is at the junction of the incisal and middle thirds.

3.
    a. The facial surface is wider mesiodistally than the lingual.
    b. The cervical line has a crest that is more incisally located on the distal than on the mesial surface.

4.
    a. The facial ridge is displaced toward the distal from the center of the facial surface.
    b. The facial ridge represents the central-facial lobe.

ANSWERS ON PAGE 194

CONTINUE ON PAGE 203 AFTER THIS TEST

TEST ANSWER SECTION

MATRIX TEST 1
(From Page 124)

If any questions were missed, *turn to the page indicated and review.*
If all answers were correct, *turn to Page 125 and continue.*

MAXILLARY CENTAL INCISOR Facial View	MESIAL	DISTAL	NEITHER
More rounded incisal angle on the maxillary central incisor.		X (P. 121)	
Displacement of crest of convexity of cervical line on facial surface.		X (P. 122)	
Line angle that is shorter in facial view.		X (P. 122 or P. 120)	
Line angle that is more nearly straight.	X (P. 122 or P. 120)		

REVIEW TEST 1

(From Page 130)

CORRECT ANSWERS: 1. b. distofacial, 2. a. mesiofacial, 3. b. three, 4. b. four, 5. a. cervical and middle, b. cervical, c. middle and incisal.

IF YOU GOT ALL QUESTIONS CORRECT, congratulations, you have completed Section 1. Take a break now and do something that will reward your study progress. You might eat or drink something, go somewhere or talk to someone, or whatever interests you at the moment. If you do this immediately and consistently after finishing sections of this program it will make your studying more pleasant and it will help you learn. *When you return, go to Page 131.*

IF YOU MISSED ONE OF THE QUESTIONS, read the instructions for that question below. Review and then retake the review test.

1. IF YOU MISSED QUESTION 1, review the convexity of the mesiofacial and distofacial line angles on Pages 120–122.

2. IF YOU MISSED QUESTION 2, review the length of the line angles on Page 122.

3. IF YOU MISSED QUESTION 3, review the number of mamelons (3) on Page 119.

4. IF YOU MISSED QUESTION 4, review the number of lobes on Page 119.

5. IF YOU MISSED QUESTION 5, review the location of the anatomical characteristics by reading Pages 126 and 127 which explains the difference between cingulum and linguocervical ridge. Also, look at Pages 128–129 where the lingual surface is divided into thirds.

IF YOU MISSED TWO OR MORE QUESTIONS, it would be to your benefit to review this section again, starting on Page 114. Do not be discouraged at this. It is easier the second time! Retake the Review Test also.

MATRIX TEST 2
(From Page 145)

If any questions were missed, *turn to Page indicated for review.*
If all answers were correct, *turn to Page 146 and take Review Test 2.*

	MAXILLARY CENTRAL INCISOR	MAXILLARY LATERAL INCISOR	BOTH INCISORS
Quadrilateral shape (facial view)			X (P. 137)
Longer incisocervically	X (P. 137)		
Relatively thicker (at incisal edge)		X (P. 139)	
More distinct lingual features		X (PP. 138–139)	

REVIEW TEST 2
(From Pages 146–147)

CORRECT ANSWERS: 1. b. lingual pit, 2. b. distal marginal ridge, 3. b. is more correct, 4. b. is correct, 5. neither statement is correct in all respects, 6. b. is incorrect, 7.d. is most complete.

IF YOU GOT ALL QUESTIONS CORRECT, congratulations! Take a break—you deserve to reward yourself for your study progress. Do this immediately, before you continue, and it should help your learning. *When you return, start on Page 148.*

IF YOU MISSED ONE OF THE QUESTIONS, read the instructions for that question below. Review and then retake the review test for Section 2.

1. IF YOU MISSED QUESTION 1, review on Pages 128–129.

2. IF YOU MISSED QUESTION 2, see Pages 140–141.

3. IF YOU MISSED QUESTION 3, read Pages 137–138 carefully.

4. IF YOU MISSED QUESTION 4, see Page 142.

5. IF YOU MISSED QUESTION 5, review each of the separate facts on Pages 132–134.

6. IF YOU MISSED QUESTION 6, check statement "a" on Pages 137–138, statement "b" on Pages 137–138 or statement "c" on Pages 138–139.

7. IF YOU MISSED QUESTION 7, see Pages 142–143 which explains not only that the proximal surfaces are flat in this location, but why.

IF YOU MISSED TWO OR MORE QUESTIONS, it would be important for you to review this section again, starting on Page 131. It will be important for much of your future study for you to be able, for example, to tell the differences between lateral and central incisors. Retake the review test for Section 2 after you have reviewed.

MATRIX TEST 3

(From Page 163)

If any questions were missed, *turn to the Page indicated for review.*
If all answers were correct, *turn to Page 164 and take Review Test 3.*

	MESIAL	DISTAL
Which border is longer in facial view?	X (P. 153)	
Which border is more convex in facial view?		X (P. 153)
More acute angle with the incisal . . .	(mesioincisal angle) X (PP. 153–154)	
Crest of convexity of the cervical line is displaced to which side on facial view?		X (P. 153)
Incisal edge sloped down toward . . .		X (PP. 159–160)
Cervical line on this surface more convex towards the incisal . . .	X (P. 159)	

REVIEW TEST 3
(From Page 164)

CORRECT ANSWERS: 1. a 2. c 3. attrition 4. c

IF YOU GOT ALL QUESTIONS CORRECT, you deserve a break. Stop now and take a break to reward yourself for study progress. Do something that is interesting to you right now, such as getting something to eat or drink, taking a walk, exercising, or your favorite pastime. Try to match the time you spend on your break with the time you spent completing this section, if you can. *When you return, continue on Page 165.*

1. IF YOU MISSED QUESTION 1, review the correctness of statement "a" on Pages 155–156, or the incorrectness of statement "b" on Page 156.

2. IF YOU MISSED QUESTION 2, review the amount of contour on Pages 150–151.

3. IF YOU MISSED QUESTION 3, review attrition on Pages 161–162.

4. IF YOU MISSED QUESTION 4, review the occlusion of the incisors on Page 148.

IF YOU MISSED TWO OR MORE QUESTIONS, return to Page 148 and do a quick review of this section. The section that follows relies on your mastery of this section, in order to enable you to compare the mandibular central and lateral incisors. *Review and then take this review test again.*

MATRIX TEST 4
(From Page 169)

If any questions were missed, *turn to the page indicated for review.*
If all answers were correct, *turn to Page 170 for Review Test 4.*

	Mandibular Central Incisor	Mandibular Lateral Incisor
Relative size (larger/smaller)	SMALLER	LARGER (P. 165)
Relative prominence of the lingual fossa (more/less)	LESS	MORE (PP. 165–166)
Relative amount of curvature of the distal surface (more/less)	LESS	MORE (PP. 165–166)
Is the incisal edge rotated slightly on the root? (yes/no)	NO	YES (P. 167)
If yes (above), is the mesial or the distal rotated to the lingual?		DISTAL (P. 167)

REVIEW TEST 4
(From Page 170)

CORRECT ANSWERS: 1. a 2. a, c, d, e, f (all but the pit) 3. c

IF YOU GOT ALL QUESTIONS CORRECT, congratulations—give yourself a short break and then resume study on Page 171.

IF YOU MISSED ANY ONE OF THE QUESTIONS, read the directions for review below. Review and then retake the Review test for Section 4.

1. IF YOU MISSED QUESTION 1, review the facial line angles of the central incisor in Section 3, Page 153, or the curvature of the cervical line on Page 159.

2. IF YOU MISSED QUESTION 2, review the lingual surface on Page 156 of Section 3 (central incisors) and Pages 165–166 (lateral), Section 4. It should be clear from the fact that all incisors have distal and incisal surfaces (edges) that all have a distoincisal angle. Review mamelons on Page 148, Section 3. Review the location of the height of contour on Page 150, Section 3, where all incisors are included. Review the number of lobes on Pages 148–149.

3. IF YOU MISSED QUESTION 3, review Pages 166–167, Section 4.

IF YOU MISSED MORE THAN ONE QUESTION, review both Sections 3 and 4, starting on Page 148. Your future patients will want you to be able to identify the distinguishing features of mandibular incisors! Review and then retake the review test for Section 4 again.

MATRIX TEST 5
(From Page 183)

If any questions were missed, *turn to the page indicated for review.*
If all answers were correct, *turn to Page 184 and take the Review Test.*

MAXILLARY CANINE	MESIAL	CENTRAL	DISTAL
Location or placement of cusp tip.		X (PP. 175–176)	
Location or placement of crest of convexity of the cervical line (facial view)	X (P. 174)		
Border (facial view) with less pronounced convexity and concavity.	X (PP. 174–175)		
Cervical line on this surface has a crest that is more incisally located.	X (P. 181)		
Cusp ridge (longer/shorter)	shorter (P. 176)		longer (P. 176)

REVIEW TEST 5
(From Page 184)

CORRECT ANSWERS: 1. b. 2. b. 3. a. 4. b

IF YOU GOT ALL QUESTIONS CORRECT, very good. Take a break now and do something interesting to reinforce your effective study effort. When you return, *continue on Page 203, the beginning of Section 6.*

IF YOU MISSED ONE QUESTION, read the directions for reviewing the question below. After reviewing, retake the review test for Section 5.

1. IF YOU MISSED QUESTION 1, review on Pages 178–179.

2. IF YOU MISSED QUESTION 2, review contact locations on Pages 175–176.

3. IF YOU MISSED QUESTION 3, review facial width on Pages 178–179, or the cervical line in Page 181.

4. IF YOU MISSED QUESTION 4, review the location of the facial ridge on Page 177 or the lobes on Pages 181–182.

IF YOU MISSED TWO OR MORE QUESTIONS, go to Page 171, the beginning of Section 5 and review this section. Since the maxillary canine is the most stable tooth in the mouth, it won't be upset that you had to review its anatomy again.

If any questions were missed, *turn to the Page indicated for review.*
If all answers were correct, *turn to Page 211 and take the Review Test.*

	Maxillary Canine	Mandibular Canine
Compare the crown width (mesiodistal dimension). (More/less/same)	MORE (P. 203)	LESS
Compare the crown length (incisocervical dimension). (More/less/same)	LESS (P. 203)	MORE
Compare the convexity of the cervical line. (Proximal view). (More/less/same)	LESS (P. 208)	MORE
Compare the line formed by the mesial edge of the crown and root (Facial view). (Curved/straight)	CURVED (P. 203)	STRAIGHT

REVIEW TEST 6
(From Page 211)

CORRECT ANSWERS: 1. b 2. a 3. a 4. a

IF YOU GOT ALL QUESTIONS CORRECT, you deserve some self-reinforcement. Take a break right now and do something that interests you. This will help to make your studying a more effective and pleasant experience. When you return, *continue on Page 212, the beginning of Section 7.*

IF YOU MISSED ONE OF THE QUESTIONS, *read the directions for review below. Review and then retake test for Section 6, Page 211.*

1. IF YOU MISSED QUESTION 1, review the cingulum on Pages 203, 205, and 207. Review the incisal edge on Page 208.

2. IF YOU MISSED QUESTION 2, review the inclination of the cusp tip of the mandibular on Page 208. Review the incisal anatomy of the maxillary canine on Page 181, Section 5.

3. IF YOU MISSED QUESTION 3, review the curvature of the cervical line on Page 205, or the lingual features on Page 203.

4. IF YOU MISSED QUESTION 4, review the distal on Page 204.

IF YOU MISSED TWO OR MORE QUESTIONS, *return to Page 203*, the beginning of Section 6, and go over the material again. If a patient in the future should happen to bite you with a canine, you'll want to know if it's mandibular or maxillary.

MATRIX TEST 7
(From Page 219)

If any items were missed, *review the section by referring to the page in the cell.* You may also want to use the capital letters (I, J, M), shown below, as an aid to review. If all answers are correct, *turn to Page 220 and take Review Test 7.*

TOOTH		INCISOCERVICAL LOCATION OF . . .	
		MESIAL CONTACT AREA	DISTAL CONTACT AREA
MAXIL-LARY	CENTRAL INCISOR	incisal third (P. 213 to 214), *I*	junction of incisal and middle thirds (P. 214), *J*
	LATERAL INCISOR	junction of incisal and middle thirds (P. 214), *J*	middle third (P. 215), *M*
	CANINE	junction of incisal and middle thirds (P. 215), *J*	middle third (P. 215), *M*
MANDI-BULAR	CENTRAL INCISOR	incisal third (P. 214), *I*	incisal third (P. 216), *I*
	LATERAL INCISOR	incisal third (P. 216), *I*	incisal third (P. 216), *I*
	CANINE	incisal third (P. 216), *I*	middle third (just cervical to junction) (P. 216), *M*

197

REVIEW TEST 7
(From Page 220)

CORRECT ANSWERS: 1. a 2. b 3. c

IF YOU GOT ALL QUESTIONS CORRECT, congratulations—take a short break and then resume studying on Page 221, Section 8 (the second to last section in this chapter).

IF YOU MISSED ONE OF THE QUESTIONS, read the directions for reviewing that question, below. Review and then retake Review Test 7, Page 220.

1. IF YOU MISSED QUESTION 1, review the amounts of contour on Pages 212–213.

2. IF YOU MISSED QUESTION 2, compare the size of the incisal embrasure between the lateral and central on Page 214 to the size of the occlusal embrasure between canine and premolar on Pages 216–217.

3. IF YOU MISSED QUESTION 3, review Pages 212–213.

IF YOU MISSED TWO OR MORE QUESTIONS, start on Page 212 and review all of Section 7. The proximal contacts, embrasures, and the heights of contour will be important in your studies of restorative dentistry and you should master them now while fresh in your mind. *Retake the Review Test 7, Page 220, after you complete your review.*

MATRIX TEST 8
(From Page 234)

If any questions were missed, *turn to the page indicated for review.*
If all answers are correct, *turn to Page 235 and take Review Test 8.*

	Maxillary			Mandibular		
	C.I.	L.I.	C	C.I.	L.I.	C
Facial and lingual surface of horizontal section convex in mesiodistal direction.	X (P. 221)	X (P. 225)	X (P. 230)	X (PP. 226 –227)	X (PP. 226 –227)	X (PP. 232 –233)
Deviation of the apex is most often toward the mesial.	(PP. 228 –229)	(P. 226)		(P. 227)	(PP. 228 –229)	X (PP. 231 –232)
Occasionally bifurcated.						X (P. 233)
Longest root in the dental arch.			X (P. 229)			
Lingual surface more narrow than facial surface in the mesiodistal direction.	X (P. 221)	X (P. 221)	X (P. 221)	X (P. 221)	X (P. 221)	X (P. 221)

199

REVIEW TEST 8
(From Page 235)

CORRECT ANSWERS: 1. b 2. c 3. distal, mandibular 4. b

IF YOU GOT ALL QUESTIONS CORRECT, you have learned a good deal about the roots of anterior teeth. Take a break now before continuing on the last section in this chapter. When you return, begin on Page 236.

IF YOU MISSED ONE OF THE QUESTIONS, read the directions for review below. Go to the page indicated and search for the correct answer to the question. After reviewing, retake the Review Test 8, Page 235.

1. IF YOU MISSED QUESTION 1, review the pointedness of the apex of the mandibular canine on Page 232.

2. IF YOU MISSED QUESTION 2, review the longitudinal grooves on one or more of the following pages: Pages 228, 230, 233.

3. IF YOU MISSED QUESTION 3, review the distal deviation of root apexes on one of the following pages: Page 226 (maxillary lateral incisor), Page 227 (mandibular central incisor), Page 229 (all incisors). Review the opposite deviation of the mandibular canine on Page 232.

4. IF YOU MISSED QUESTION 4, review Page 228.

IF YOU MISSED TWO OR MORE OF THE QUESTIONS review Section 8, Pages 221–233. Knowledge of root anatomy will be important in clinical tasks such as extractions and root surface cleaning. *Restudy this section and then retake the Review Test 8, Page 235.*

If any items were missed, *turn to the page indicated for review.*
If all were correct, *turn to Page 244 and take Review Test 9.*

Pulp of Anterior teeth	Max. Central Incisor	Mand. Central Incisor	Max. Canine
In which direction is the pulp chamber widest at the roof?	Mesio-distal (P. 236)	Mesio-distal (P. 238)	Neither— Roof pointed (P. 240)
Of these three teeth, which has accessory canals most frequently?	(P. 239)	(P. 239)	X (P. 241)
Of these three teeth, which is most likely to have a divided root canal?	(P. 236)	X (P. 239)	(PP. 241–242)
Approximate shape of the root canal as seen in a horizontal section taken at the mid-root.	Round (circular) (P. 237)	Ellip-tical (P. 238)	Round (circular) (P. 241)

REVIEW TEST 9
(From Page 244)

CORRECT ANSWERS: 1. Mandibular central and lateral incisors, mandibular canine 2. b 3. a-1, b-2, c-3

IF YOU GOT ALL QUESTIONS CORRECT, congratulations, you have completed Chapter 2 of *Dental Anatomy*. This means that you have completed over 40% (2 out of 5 chapters, with Chapter 5 a short one) of the *Dental Anatomy* series. Give yourself a reward equal to the effort you invested in studying this chapter—you have earned it.

IF YOU MISSED ONE OF THE QUESTIONS, read the directions for review below for that question. Review on the pages indicated and then retake the review test on Page 244.

1. IF YOU MISSED QUESTION 1, review the double root canals of mandibular incisors (Page 239) and/or mandibular canines (Page 241).

2. IF YOU MISSED QUESTION 2, review the number of apical foramina on Page 239 (mandibular incisors) or Page 241 (mandibular canine).

3. IF YOU MISSED QUESTION 3, review the number of pulp horns on Page 236 (maxillary central incisor), Page 237 (maxillary lateral incisor) or Page 240 (maxillary canine—examine the illustrations which show a single pointed horn at the roof of the pulp chamber).

IF YOU MISSED TWO OR MORE QUESTIONS, review this section again, Pages 236–242. There will be many occasions in the dental office in which knowledge of pulp anatomy will be important. Your future patients will appreciate your knowledge because of nerves embedded in their pulp! *Review and then retake the review test in Page 244.*

SECTION 6.0 MANDIBULAR CANINE

The form and outline of the maxillary and mandibular canines are practically alike. Although the crown lengths of the two teeth are nearly the same (the mandibular canine is slightly longer than the maxillary), the mandibular canine is _____ (narrower/wider) mesiodistally than the maxillary canine.

Permanent
1. Maxillary
2. Mandibular
Right
Canine
FACIAL

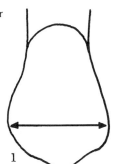
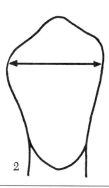

1   2

narrower

The lingual surface of the mandibular canine is smoother, the cingulum less developed, and the lingual and marginal ridges are less prominent than those of the maxillary canine. The cingulum is area _____ (A/B/C.)

Permanent
Mandibular
Right
Canine
LINGUAL

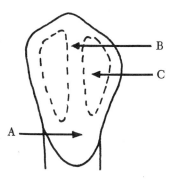

B

C

A

A

From the facial aspect, the line formed by the mesial outline of the crown and root of a maxillary canine is definitely curved. On a mandibular canine this line has less curvature; in fact it is nearly _____.

Permanent
1. Maxillary
2. Mandibular
Right
Canine
FACIAL

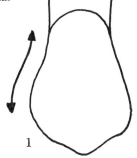
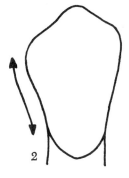

1   2

When compared with a maxillary canine, a mandibular canine has a distal contact area that is more toward the _____ (cervical/incisal).

Permanent
1. Maxillary Left
2. Mandibular Right
Canine
FACIAL

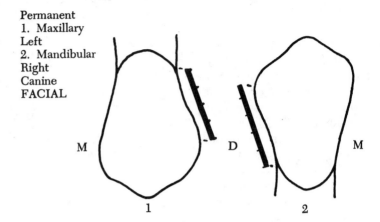

1   2

Because the distal contact is more cervical than the mesial, the incisocervical length of the distal surface is _____ (longer/ shorter) than the mesial.

Permanent
Mandibular
Right
Canine
FACIAL

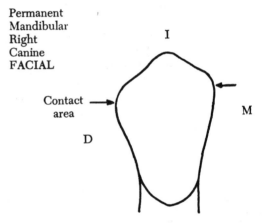

Contact → area

I

M

D

Running cervically from the cusp tip in the center of the facial surface is the _____ ridge.

Permanent
Mandibular
Right
Canine
FACIAL

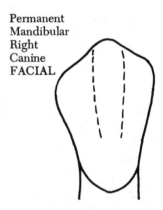

Facially, the cervical line of the mandibular canine has a semicircular curvature. Which of the two canines (maxillary/mandibular) has the more symmetrically contoured cervical line? _____

Permanent
1. Maxillary
2. Mandibular
Right
Canine
FACIAL

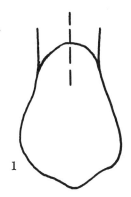
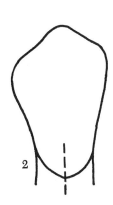

1

2

On which canine is the crest of curvature of the cervical line displaced toward the mesial on the facial surface? _____ (maxillary/mandibular)

SECTION 6.1   MANDIBULAR CANINE: LINGUAL VIEW

The lingual features of a mandibular canine are less prominent than those of a maxillary canine. The cingulum is relatively smooth, and the marginal ridges are less distinct. Are the comparisons between the lingual surfaces of a maxillary and mandibular canine similar to or the opposite of the comparisons between the lingual surfaces of the maxillary and mandibular incisors? _____

Permanent
Mandibular
Right
Canine
LINGUAL

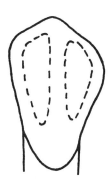

Running from the cusp tip to the cervical line and dividing the lingual surface to form two shallow fossae is a prominence called the _____.

mesial marginal ridge . . . . GO TO MIDDLE OF PAGE 207
lingual ridge . . . . GO TO TOP OF PAGE 206

◗ From page 205 or 207   *lingual ridge is correct*

Mesial and distal to the lingual ridge are the
_____ and _____.

Permanent
Mandibular
Right
Canine
LINGUAL

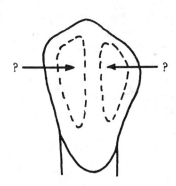

mesiolingual fossa, distolingual fossa

Area (A) is called the _____; area (B) is
the _____.

Permanent
Mandibular
Right
Canine
LINGUAL

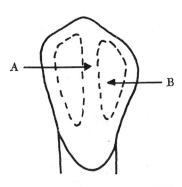

lingual ridge, distolingual fossa

The areas marked (A) and (B) are the _____
and _____ respectively.

Permanent
Mandibular
Right
Canine
LINGUAL

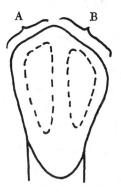

Compared with the features of the maxillary canine (lingual surface), those of the mandibular canine are _____ (more/less) prominent.

GO TO BOTTOM OF THIS PAGE

◗ From page 205   *mesial marginal ridge is incorrect*

The mesial marginal ridge runs from the mesioincisal angle to the linguocervical ridge, but it does not divide the lingual surface to form the mesial and distal lingual fossa.

Permanent
Mandibular
Right
Canine
LINGUAL

mesial marginal ridge

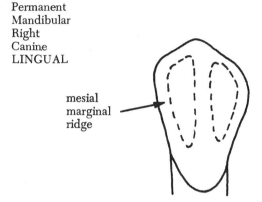

GO TO TOP OF PAGE 206 AND CONTINUE

◗ From top of this page   *less*

SECTION 6.2   MANDIBULAR CANINE: PROXIMAL VIEW

The cingulum on the mandibular canine appears _____ (more/less) prominent than on the maxillary canine.

Permanent
1. Maxillary
2. Mandibular
Right
Canine
MESIAL

Cingulum

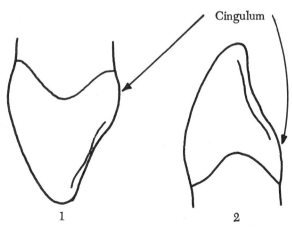

1   2

The incisal portion of the crown of a mandibular canine is
_____ (thinner/thicker) faciolingually than that of the
maxillary canine.

Comparing proximal views, one sees that the cusp tip of the mandibular canine is displaced toward the _____ (facial/lingual) from the long axis of the tooth.

Permanent
1. Maxillary
2. Mandibular
Right
Canine
MESIAL

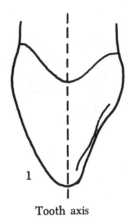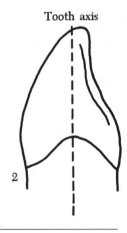

Tooth axis

Tooth axis

lingual

The cervical lines (mandibular canine, mesial and distal surfaces) are more convex incisally than those on the maxillary canine. On both canines, the cervical line is more convex on the _____ (mesial/distal) surface.

Permanent
1, 2 Mandibular
3, 4 Maxillary
Right
Canine
PROXIMAL (Cervical Third)

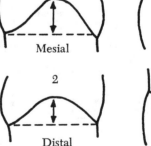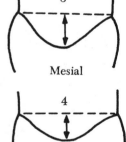

Mesial

Mesial

Distal

Distal

mesial

The cusp tip divides the mesial and distal cusp ridges. Which
is slightly longer? _____

From an incisal view, the incisal edge of a mandibular canine appears to slant toward the lingual. Which end of the incisal edge is located more lingually? _____

Permanent
Mandibular
Right
Canine
INCISAL

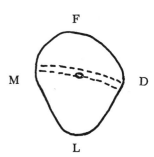

In the diagram, A is the _____ cusp ridge, and B is the _____ cusp ridge.

Permanent
Mandibular
Right
Canine
INCISAL

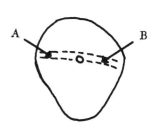

From a facial view, the incisal edge on a newly erupted mandibular canine has a cusp tip that is more pointed than that of a maxillary canine. With wear, the cusp tip on a mandibular canine flattens. Which of the two drawings represents a newly erupted mandibular canine? _____

Permanent
Mandibular
Right
Canine
FACIAL

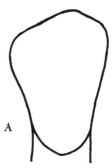

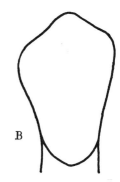

A   B

On which two surfaces of anterior teeth does the cervical line curve toward the root? _____ and _____

MATRIX TEST 6

Directions . . .

Supply the correct word for each empty cell, matching the left hand column with the top row.

When you have completed the test, turn to Page 195 to check your answers.

	Maxillary Canine	Mandibular Canine
Compare the crown width (mesiodistal dimension). (More/less/same)		
Compare the crown length (incisicervical dimension). (More/less/same)		
Compare the convexity of the cervical line. (Proximal view). (More/less/same)		
Compare the line formed by the mesial edge of the crown and root (Facial view). (curved/straight)		

ANSWERS ON PAGE 195

REVIEW TEST 6

Make a note of your answers so you can check them on Page 196.

Below are four sets of statements concerning the canine teeth. Choose the correct one from each pair.

1.
    a. The mandibular canine has a more prominent cingulum than does the maxillary canine.
    b. The incisal edge (proximal view) of the mandibular canine is thinner than that of the maxillary canine.

2.
    a. The cusp tip of the mandibular canine is displaced slightly to the lingual.
    b. The cusp tip of the maxillary canine is displaced slightly to the lingual.

3.
    a. On its facial surface, the mandibular canine has a more smooth, semicircular cervical line.
    b. The mandibular canine has the more prominent lingual features.

4.
    a. The mandibular canine has a longer distofacial line angle (distal border) than the maxillary canine.
    b. The maxillary canine has a distal contact area that is closer to the incisal edge.

ANSWERS ON PAGE 196

SECTION 7.0   HEIGHT OF CONTOUR OF ANTERIOR TEETH

Anterior teeth have facial or lingual heights of contours in the _____ third of the crown.

Permanent
1. Maxillary
Right
Central Incisor
MESIAL
2. Mandibular
Left
Central Incisor
DISTAL

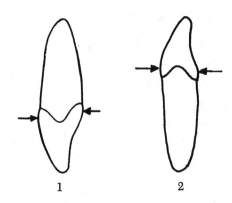

1   2

cervical

Examine the diagrams for height of contour. The height of contour occurs in the cervical third on both the facial and lingual surfaces for maxillary _____ teeth.

Permanent
1. Maxillary
Right
Lateral Incisor
MESIAL
2. Maxillary
Right
Canine
MESIAL

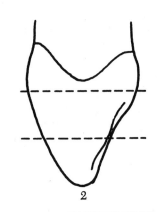

1   2

anterior

In proximal view, maxillary teeth give the impression that the amount of contour is greater on the facial than on the lingual surface (especially true for anterior teeth). However, careful examination will show that the contour, both facially and lingually, for all maxillary teeth measures approximately _____ mm.

Permanent
Maxillary
Right
1. Central Incisor
2. 1st Premolar
MESIAL

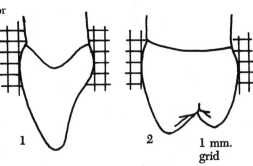

1   2   1 mm.
grid

As with the maxillary incisors and canines, the mandibular anteriors have both the facial and lingual height of contour in the _____ third of the crown.

Permanent
Mandibular
Right
1. Central Incisor
2. Canine
MESIAL

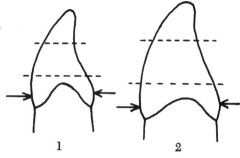

1   2

cervical

The facial and lingual contours of the mandibular anteriors are slight. Mandibular incisors and canines have facial and lingual contours that measure

A. more than ½ mm
B. ½ mm
C. less than ½ mm

Permanent
Mandibular
Right
1. Central Incisor
2. Canine
MESIAL

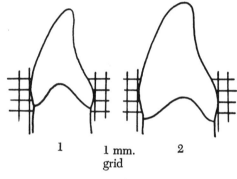

1   1 mm.   2
           grid

C. less than ½ mm

SECTION 7.1 PROXIMAL CONTACTS OF ANTERIOR TEETH

The incisocervical or occlusocervical location of the proximal contacts may be seen by examining a _____ view of the teeth.

Permanent
Maxillary
Incisors
1. FACIAL
2. INCISAL

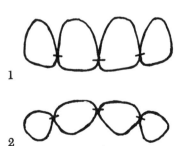

1

2

Notice the small incisal embrasure between the two maxillary central incisors. This is because of the nearly right-angled mesioincisal angles of the incisors and the incisocervical location of their mesial contact areas in the _____ third of the crown.

Permanent
Maxillary
Incisors
FACIAL

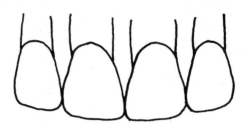

In the mandibular arch, the central incisors have contact areas located in the _____ third, forming a small incisal embrasure. This embrasure may be obliterated by wear of the incisal edges. No embrasure means that the contact area extends "up" to the _____.

Permanent
Mandibular
Central Incisors
FACIAL

Slight or absent
incisal embrasure

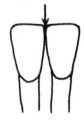

incisal, incisal edge (or mesioincisal angle)

Incisocervically, the central incisors of both arches have mesial contact areas well within the incisal thirds (which can be described by the letter "I"), and the incisal embrasures are _____ (size).

small

Incisocervically, the contact between a maxillary central and lateral incisor occurs approximately at the junction of the incisal and middle thirds. Therefore, "the junction of the incisal and middle third," or simply "J," describes the location of the mesial contact area for a maxillary _____ incisor and the distal contact area for a maxillary _____ incisor.

Permanent
Maxillary
Left
1. Central Incisor
2. Lateral Incisor
FACIAL

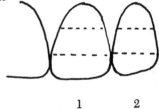

1   2

In the mandibular arch, the contact between the incisors is located near the incisal edge. Because of wear at the incisal edge, the incisal embrasures may become very _____ (small/large).

Permanent
Mandibular
Right
1. Lateral Incisor
2. Central Incisor
FACIAL

Contact area

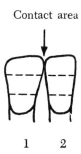

1   2

small

The proximal contact involving the maxillary canine and lateral incisor is located incisocervically so that the distal contact area of the lateral incisor is in the middle third ("M") of the crown. The mesial contact area of the canine is located at the junction ("J") of the incisal and middle thirds of the canine crown. The long distal ridge of the canine cusp locates the distal contact area in the middle third ("M").

Review the locations of the proximal contacts of anterior teeth with the aide of the pairs of letters given below. For example, "IJ" means that the mesial contact is located in the incisal third (I) and the distal contact is located at the junction (J) of the incisal and middle thirds.

	CENTRAL INCISOR	LATERAL INCISOR	CANINE
MAXILLARY	IJ	JM	JM
MANDIBULAR	II	II	IM

Which two anterior teeth can be described as having a "JM" pattern of proximal contact locations? _____ and _____.

215

Which of the following statements is the most correct?

    A. Incisocervically, each maxillary anterior tooth has a distal contact area that is located more cervically than its mesial contact area. . . GO TO NEXT FRAME

    B. Some of the maxillary anterior teeth have mesial contact areas that are located more cervically than their distal contact areas. . . GO TO MIDDLE OF PAGE 217

◗ From preceding frame or page 218

statement A is correct

The mandibular incisors (central and lateral) have both mesial and distal contacts in the _____ third.	Permanent Mandibular Central Incisors FACIAL	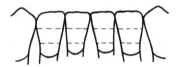

---

incisal

Because of the location of the contacts and wear at the incisal edges, the incisal embrasures between the mandibular incisors are _____ (size).

---

small (slight, etc.)

As with mandibular incisors, mandibular canines have mesial contacts incisocervically in the _____ third of their crowns.

---

incisal

Mandibular canines have distal contacts that are located slightly cervical to the junction of the incisal and middle thirds. The contact, therefore, is located in the _____ third of the crown.	Permanent Mandibular Right 1. 1st Premolar 2. Canine FACIAL	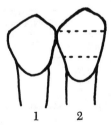

The distal ridge of the canine cusp contributes to the size of the occlusal embrasure between the canine and first premolar. The occlusal embrasure between the canine and first premolar is _____ (smaller/larger) than the embrasures between the incisors.

Permanent
Mandibular
Right
1. 1st Premolar
2. Canine
FACIAL

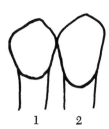

1   2

larger

The distal contact of mandibular canines is located _____ (cervical/incisal) to the junction of the incisal and middle thirds.

cervical

GO TO PAGE 219 AND TAKE THE MATRIX TEST

◆ From page 216

The term "cervically" means toward the cervical line. Which is more cervically located, the middle third or the incisal third of a crown? _____

Which is located more cervically: (A) a contact in the incisal third or (B) a contact at the junction of the incisal and middle thirds? _____

217

Let's clarify the location of the mesial and distal contact areas. Study the drawings below. The dots correspond to the location of the proximal contact.

Which teeth have their mesial contact areas in the incisal third? _____

Which teeth have their mesial contact areas at the junction of the incisal and middle thirds? _____

MAXILLARY ANTERIOR TEETH

	CENTRAL INCISOR	LATERAL INCISOR	CANINE
MESIAL	I	J	J
DISTAL	J	M	M
FACIAL	IJ	JM	JM

central incisors, lateral incisors and canines

Which maxillary anterior teeth have their distal contacts in the middle third? _____

Which maxillary anterior teeth have their distal contacts at the junction of the middle and incisal thirds? _____

canines and lateral incisors, central incisors

If one part of a tooth is located more toward the cervical line than another part, it is said to be located more cervically. Which one of the following statements is correct?

    A. Maxillary incisors and canines have proximal contacts that are located more cervically on the distal surface than on the mesial surface.

    B. All of the maxillary incisors and canines have distal contacts in the middle third of their crowns.

A is correct

NOW GO TO MIDDLE OF PAGE 216 AND CONTINUE

MATRIX TEST 7

Directions . . .

Fill in each cell with the correct letter, word or words.

When you have completed the test, *turn to Page 197 and check your answers.*

TOOTH		INCISOCERVICAL LOCATION OF	
		MESIAL CONTACT AREA	DISTAL CONTACT AREA
MAXIL-LARY	CENTRAL INCISOR		
	LATERAL INCISOR		
	CANINE		
MANDI-BULAR	CENTRAL INCISOR		
	LATERAL INCISOR		
	CANINE		

ANSWERS ON PAGE 197

REVIEW TEST 7

Make a note of your answers so that you can check them on Page 198.

1. In which arch(es) do the anterior teeth have facial and lingual amounts of contour that measure less than ½ mm?
   a. mandibular
   b. maxillary
   c. both arches

2. Choose the CORRECT statement:
   a. The incisal embrasure between the maxillary lateral incisor and maxillary central incisor is larger than the occlusal embrasure between the mandibular canine and first premolar.
   b. The process of attrition can completely eliminate the incisal embrasures between the mandibular central incisors.

3. In which arch(es) do the facial and lingual heights of contour occur in the cervical third of the crowns of all anterior teeth:
   a. mandibular
   b. maxillary
   c. both arches

ANSWERS ON PAGE 198.

SECTION 8.0 ROOTS OF ANTERIOR TEETH:
MAXILLARY CENTRAL INCISOR

The root of the maxillary central incisor is roughly cone shaped. A horizontal section (cross-section) of the root is sometimes described as having a triangular form with rounded edges but the exact shape varies depending on the part of the root from which the horizontal section is drawn. Similar to the crown, the <u>mesial and distal root surfaces converge toward the lingual,</u> slightly distorting the conical form. The lingual convergence reduces the lingual measurement of the root in the _____ (mesiodistal/faciolingual) direction.

Permanent
Maxillary
Right
Central Incisor
1. FACIAL
2. HORIZONTAL
   SECTION

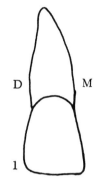
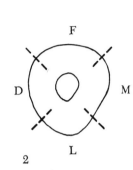

mesiodistal

The roots of all single-rooted teeth (incisors, canines, and most premolars) show a lingual convergence similar to the maxillary central incisor. As illustrated by a horizontal section taken in the cervical portion of the maxillary central incisor, which root surface is the narrowest? _____.

Permanent
Maxillary
Right
Central Incisor
HORIZONTAL SECTION

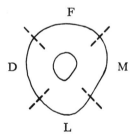

The definition of <u>cervix</u> is "the neck" or "any constricted part." Barring extreme variations, <u>every tooth is constricted in the region of the cementoenamel junction or cervical line</u>. Constrictions of this type occur whenever two convex forms (Fig. 1) or one convex and one straight form (Fig. 2) are united.

If the total form of a tooth is examined (Fig. 3, 4), the cervical constriction would be called a _____ (convex/concave) region.

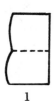 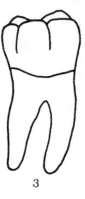 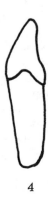

| 1 | 2 | 3 | 4 |

Because of the higher degree of variability in form at the apical portion of a root, our discussion of root anatomy will concentrate on the more consistent form exhibited by the _____ portion of the root.

Permanent
Maxillary
Right
Central Incisor
FACIAL

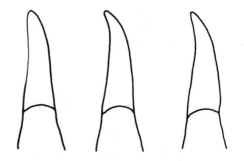

Viewed from the mesial, which root surface of the maxillary central incisor is more convex in the longitudinal direction? _____ (facial/lingual)

Permanent
Maxillary
Right
Central Incisor
MESIAL

F   L

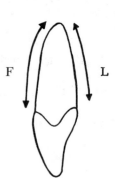

As seen in the horizontal section (Fig. 2), the faciolingual curvature of the mesial root surface of the maxillary central incisor has a convex portion and a portion that tends to be straight or flat. The convex portion is toward the _____ (facial/lingual), the straight portion toward the _____ (facial/lingual).

Permanent
Maxillary
Right
Central Incisor
1. FACIAL
2. HORIZONTAL
   SECTION

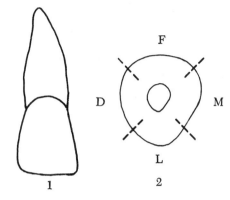

The faciolingual curvature of the distal surface is entirely _____.

Permanent
Maxillary
Right
Central Incisor
1. FACIAL
2. HORIZONTAL
   SECTION

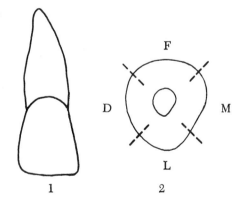

SECTION 8.1 ROOTS OF ANTERIOR TEETH:
MAXILLARY LATERAL INCISOR

The root form of the maxillary lateral incisor is highly variable. Typically, it is different from that of the central incisor. The roots of the two incisors are nearly equal in length; but in proportion to crown length, the maxillary lateral incisor has a root that is proportionally _____ (shorter/longer) than the central incisor.

Permanent
Maxillary
Right
1. Lateral Incisor
2. Central Incisor
FACIAL

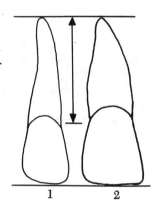

In the mesiodistal direction, which maxillary incisor has a thicker root? _____

Permanent
Maxillary
Right
1. Lateral Incisor
2. Central Incisor
FACIAL

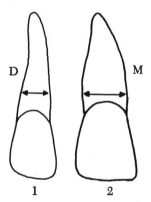

Which maxillary incisor has the thicker root in the faciolingual direction? _____

Permanent
Maxillary
Right
1. Central Incisor
2. Lateral Incisor
MESIAL

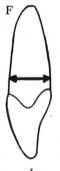 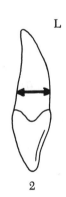

The mesial and distal surfaces of the maxillary lateral incisor sometimes have a broad groove running in the longitudinal direction. Named for the direction they run, these grooves are called _____ grooves.

Permanent
Maxillary
Right
Lateral Incisor

1. MESIAL
2. DISTAL
3. HORIZONTAL

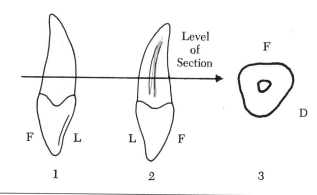

Level of Section

1   2   3

When present, a longitudinal groove is sometimes distinct, sometimes faint. The <u>presence of a longitudinal groove causes the mesial and distal root surfaces to have a faciolingual curvature that varies from</u> nearly flat to _____ (concave/convex).

Permanent
Maxillary
Right
Lateral Incisor
MID-ROOT
　HORIZONTAL SECTIONS

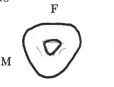

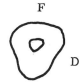

Because the root form of the lateral incisor is highly variable, the shape of the horizontal section varies. Longitudinal grooves may or may not be present on the mesial and distal root surfaces of the maxillary lateral incisor. On which of these two root surfaces does a longitudinal groove appear more often? _____

Permanent
Maxillary
Right
Lateral Incisors
MID-ROOT
　HORIZONTAL SECTIONS

225

Of the two maxillary incisors, <u>one has a blunt apex, the other a pointed one.</u> The apex of the maxillary lateral incisor is _____.

Permanent
Maxillary
Right
1. Lateral Incisor
2. Central Incisor
FACIAL

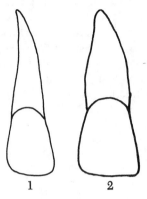

1 2

The apical portion of the root of different specimens of maxillary lateral incisors may be found to show deflections or deviations in any direction. Examine the drawings on the right, which show the most common deviations. The facial view shows a deviation toward the _____ (mesial/distal) and the proximal view shows a deviation toward the _____ (facial/lingual).

but max.c.incisors root - more lingual

Permanent
Maxillary
Right
Lateral Incisor
1. FACIAL
2. MESIAL

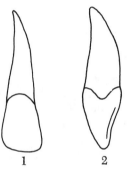

1 2

SECTION 8.2 ROOTS OF ANTERIOR TEETH: MANDIBULAR INCISOR

The <u>roots of the mandibular incisors are flattened or pinched from the mesial and distal directions.</u> In which of the two horizontal directions do the roots of the mandibular incisors have the greater measure?

_____

Permanent
Mandibular
Right
Central Incisor
1. FACIAL
2. MESIAL
3. HORIZONTAL
   SECTION

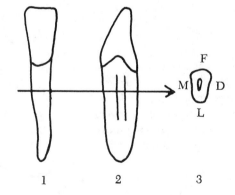

1 2 3

Viewed from the facial, the root of the mandibular central incisor is symmetrical and straight; that is, the mesial and distal surfaces tend to be relatively straight in the _____ direction.

Permanent
Mandibular
Right
Central Incisor
FACIAL

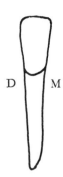

D   M

The apical portion of the root on the mandibular central incisor may deviate toward the _____.

Permanent
Mandibular
Right
Central Incisor
FACIAL

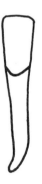

Longitudinal grooves may or may not be present on the mesial and distal root surfaces of the mandibular central incisor. When present, these grooves are broad and run most of the root length, causing the faciolingual curvature to vary from nearly flat to _____.

Permanent
Mandibular
Central Incisor
PROXIMAL

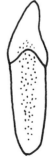
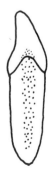

227

In form, the root of the mandibular lateral incisor resembles that of the mandibular central incisor, the chief distinction being the size of the two roots. In all directions, the root of the mandibular lateral incisor is _____ (larger/smaller) than that of the mandibular central incisor.

Permanent
Mandibular
Right
1. Lateral Incisor
2. Central Incisor
FACIAL

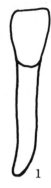
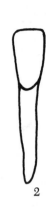

1   2

larger

The root of which mandibular incisor has the greater circumference? _____

lateral

Of the maxillary and mandibular incisors, which one is least likely to have longitudinal grooves on the mesial and distal root surfaces?

_____ _____ _____
   (arch)   (tooth)   (name)

maxillary central incisor

Study the drawings on the right. All the teeth have been drawn with their crowns toward the top of the page even though they may be maxillary. Identify each of the incisors shown above by writing their names below.

A._____
B._____
C._____
D._____

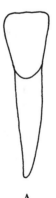
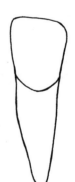
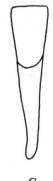
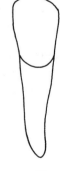

A   B   C   D

(IF YOU MISSED ANY PART OF THIS QUESTION, REVIEW ON PAGES 226–228 BEFORE CONTINUING)

Is this statement true or false?

"Each of the four types of teeth in the class incisors has a root apex that may deviate toward the distal." _____

true

SECTION 8.3   ROOTS OF ANTERIOR TEETH: MAXILLARY CANINE

The root of the maxillary canine is the longest in the dental arch. Does the maxillary canine also have the longest crown in the dental arch? _____ (yes/no)

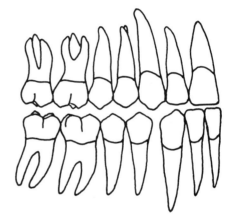

no

In the faciolingual direction, the mesial and distal surfaces of the maxillary canine are broad and generally flattened in the middle portion. At the facial and lingual borders of the mesial and distal surfaces, the curvature is more _____.

Permanent
Maxillary
Right
Canine
1. MESIAL
2. HORIZONTAL SECTION

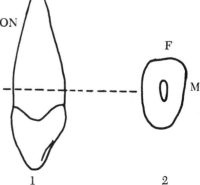

The crown of the mandibular canine is as long or longer than the crown of the maxillary canine. Generally, the tooth with the longest root in the central arch is the _____
(arch)

_____
(tooth)

The mesial and distal surfaces may be concave in the faciolingual direction. A concavity exists whenever a _____ _____ is present.

Permanent
Maxillary
Right
Canine
1. MESIAL
2. HORIZONTAL SECTION

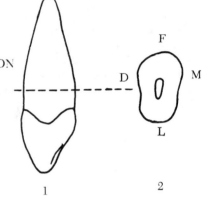

As is true for the maxillary lateral incisor, the maxillary canine has a longitudinal groove more often on which surface, mesial or distal? _____

The apical portion of the root on the maxillary canine tapers to form a bluntly pointed apex. Because of the relative width of the root in the faciolingual and mesiodistal directions, this tapering is more marked on the _____ and _____ surfaces (facial and lingual or mesial and distal).

Permanent
Maxillary
Right
Canine
1. FACIAL
2. MESIAL

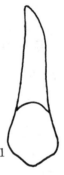 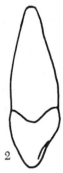

facial and lingual

SECTION 8.4 ROOTS OF ANTERIOR TEETH: MANDIBULAR CANINE

The permanent mandibular canine has the longest root of any tooth in the _____.

permanent dentition . . . . .GO TO NEXT FRAME
mandibular arch . . . . .GO TO BOTTOM OF THIS PAGE

Permanent
Mandibular
Right
Canine
FACIAL

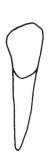

♦ From preceding frame

permanent dentition is incorrect

The maxillary canine has the longest root of any tooth in the dental arch. It is true, however, that the mandibular canine has the longest root of any tooth in the _____ arch.

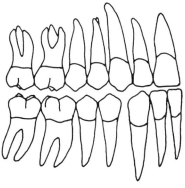

♦ From top of this page

mandibular arch is correct

The mesiodistal width of the root of the mandibular canine is less than that of the maxillary canine and greater than that of the mandibular incisor.

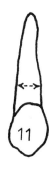

Similar to the root of the maxillary canine, the apical portion of the root of the mandibular canine tapers toward the apex. Which of the two canines has the more pointed apex?
_____

Permanent
1. Mandibular
Left
2. Maxillary
Right
Canine
FACIAL

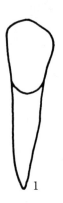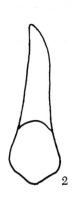

mandibular

When the apex of the mandibular canine shows a deviation from the tooth axis, it is often toward the incisors or in a _____ direction.

Permanent
Mandibular
Left
Canine
FACIAL

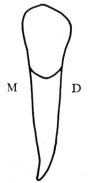

mesial

As concerns the mesial or distal deviations of the apical portions of the roots of anterior teeth, the mesial deviation of the mandibular canine is _____.
    a.   unique
    b.   the same as other anterior teeth

Longitudinal grooves are generally present on the mesial and distal root surfaces of the mandibular canine. Because of these grooves, the mesial and distal root surfaces are concave in the _____ direction.

Permanent
Mandibular
Left
Canine
1. MESIAL
2. HORIZONTAL
   SECTION

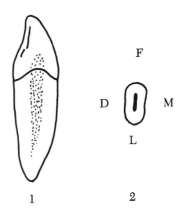

1   2

faciolingual (horizontal)

Occasionally, the root of the mandibular canine will be bifurcated. As suggested by the longitudinal grooves, whenever a bifurcation exists, the two terminal roots are called the _____ and _____ roots.

Permanent
Mandibular
Right
Canine
MESIAL

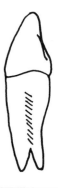

facial, lingual

Of the anterior teeth, which is most likely to have longitudinal grooves? Which is least likely to have longitudinal grooves?

most likely   _____   _____
                     (arch)   (tooth name)

least likely   _____   _____
                     (arch)   (tooth name)

mandibular canine, maxillary central incisor

GO TO THE NEXT PAGE AND TAKE THE MATRIX TEST

MATRIX TEST 8

Directions . . .

Place an X in the space matching the left hand column with the top row. When you have completed the test turn to Page 199.

Root Form	Maxillary			Mandibular		
	C.I.	L.I.	C	C.I.	L.I.	C
Facial and lingual sur-face of horizontal section convex in mesiodistal direction.						
Deviation of the apex is most often toward the mesial.						
Occasionally bifurcated.						
Longest root in the dental arch.						
Lingual surface more narrow than facial surface in the mesio-distal direc-tion.						

ANSWERS ON PAGE 199.

REVIEW TEST 8

Make a note of your answers so you can check them on Page 200.

1. The canine with the more pointed apex is the . . .
   a. maxillary canine
   b. mandibular canine

2. The roots of all but one anterior tooth are likely to have longitudinal grooves on the mesial and distal surfaces. The tooth that is not likely to have longitudinal grooves is the . . .
   a. mandibular lateral incisor
   b. maxillary canine
   c. maxillary central incisor

3. Which of the following pairs of terms best completes the statements?
   When the apex of a root shows a deviation, it is generally toward the ———— (mesial/distal).
   Whenever a deviation in the opposite direction occurs, the tooth is generally a ———— (maxillary/mandibular) canine.

4. Of the two mandibular incisors, which has a root that is larger in all dimensions?
   a. mandibular central incisor
   b. mandibular lateral incisor

ANSWERS ON PAGE 200

SECTION 9.0 PULP ANATOMY OF ANTERIOR TEETH: MAXILLARY INCISORS

The description of the pulp cavity of a permanent tooth indicates the average form after the root is formed. If the root of a tooth in the mouth of a young person is not completely formed, the average description will not be applicable.

In older people, secondary dentin may occupy part of the original pulp cavity. The progressive change in the pulp cavity that begins with the early formation of a tooth in the crypt takes place as the pulp performs its primary function of laying down _____.

dentin

The maxillary central incisor has a large, simple pulp cavity. Near the roof, the pulp chamber is widest in the _____ direction.

Permanent
Maxillary
Right
Central Incisor
LONGITUDINAL SECTIONS
1. MESIAL
2. FACIAL

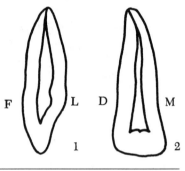

mesiodistal

In a mesiodistal longitudinal section, three pulp horns may be seen at the roof of the pulp chamber. These horns roughly correspond to the three facial _____.

Permanent
Maxillary
Right
Central Incisor
LONGITUDINAL SECTION
FACIAL

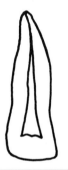

lobes

A faciolingual longitudinal section of the maxillary central incisor shows the pulp cavity tapering toward the incisal and apical. The gradual taper of the pulp cavity is interrupted by a slight faciolingual constriction at the level of the _____.

Permanent
Maxillary
Right
Central Incisor
LONGITUDINAL SECTION
MESIAL

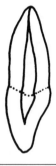

A series of horizontal sections show that the pulp cavity of the maxillary central incisor gradually changes from an elliptical to a circular shape. Near the roof of the pulp chamber, the shape is elliptical. This elliptical form is widest in the _____ direction.

Permanent
Maxillary
Right
Central Incisor
1. LONGITUDINAL SECTION
2. HORIZONTAL SECTIONS

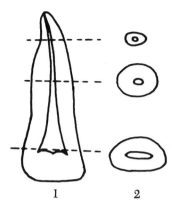

1   2

mesiodistal

The pulp cavity of the maxillary lateral incisor is similar in shape to that of the maxillary central incisor except that the lateral usually has _____ (two/three) pulp horns. Because of the relative sizes of the two teeth, the measurements of the pulp cavity of the lateral incisor are slightly _____ (larger/smaller) than those of the maxillary central incisor.

Permanent
Maxillary
Right
1. Central Incisor
2. Lateral Incisor
LONGITUDINAL SECTIONS

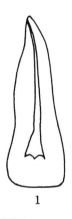 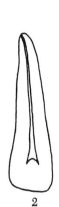

1   2

two, smaller

The pulp cavity of either maxillary incisor may have fine, irregular constrictions along the incisoapical path and accessory canals. Which maxillary incisor is more likely to have accessory canals?

Permanent
Maxillary
Right
1. Central Incisor
2. Lateral Incisor
LONGITUDINAL SECTIONS
FACIAL

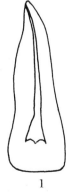 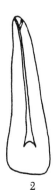

1   2

SECTION 9.1 PULP ANATOMY OF ANTERIOR TEETH: MANDIBULAR INCISORS

In the mandibular arch, the pulp canals of the two incisors are similar. For most of its incisoapical length, the pulp cavity of a mandibular incisor is wider in the _____ direction.

Permanent
Mandibular
Right
1. Central Incisor
2. Lateral Incisor
LONGITUDINAL
   SECTIONS
a. MESIAL
b. FACIAL

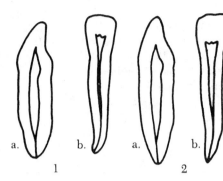

faciolingual

Examine the series of horizontal sections. Near the roof of the pulp chamber, the elliptical form of the pulp cavity is widest in the _____ direction.

Permanent
Mandibular
Right
Lateral Incisor
1. LONGITUDINAL SECTION
FACIAL
2. HORIZONTAL SECTIONS

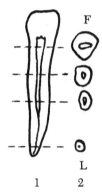

mesiodistal

Near mid-root of a mandibular incisor, the elliptical form is widest in the _____ direction.

Permanent
Mandibular
Right
Lateral Incisor
1. LONGITUDINAL SECTION
FACIAL
2. HORIZONTAL SECTIONS

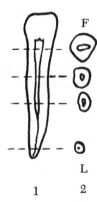

Near the apex of a mandibular incisor, the horizontal form of the pulp cavity is _____.

Permanent
Mandibular
Right
Lateral Incisor
1. LONGITUDINAL SECTION FACIAL
2. HORIZONTAL SECTIONS

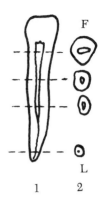

circular (round or synonym)

Sometimes, a thin wall of dentin divides the flattened root canal of the mandibular incisor. These two root canals are called the _____ and _____ root canals.

Permanent
Mandibular
Right
Central Incisor
LONGITUDINAL SECTIONS
MESIAL

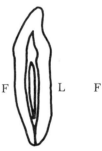 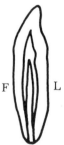

facial, lingual

If two root canals are present, they either have separate apical foramina or converge apically to form a single canal. Mandibular incisors have few accessory canals, relative to maxillary incisors. The incisor with the most variable root and most frequent accessory canals is the _____.

Permanent
Mandibular
Right
Central Incisor
LONGITUDINAL
  SECTIONS
MESIAL

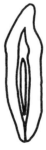 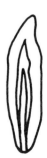

SECTION 9.2   PULP ANATOMY OF ANTERIOR TEETH: CANINES

As is true of all teeth, the pulp cavity pattern of the maxillary canine is that of the general form of the tooth. Which longitudinal section (sections) shows the roof of the pulp chamber to be pointed? _____ (mesiodistal/faciolingual/both)

Permanent
Maxillary
Right
Canine
LONGITUDINAL SECTIONS
1. MESIAL
2. FACIAL

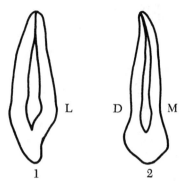

both

Similar to the horizontal measurements of the root, the cervical portion of the root canal of the maxillary canine is widest in the _____ direction.

Permanent
Maxillary
Right
Canine
LONGITUDINAL
    SECTIONS
1. MESIAL
2. FACIAL

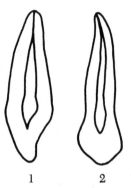

faciolingual

A series of horizontal sections through the root of the maxillary canine show the form of the root canal gradually changing from elliptical to nearly circular. The elliptical form is most evident in the _____ (cervical/apical) portion of the root, and is widest in the _____ direction.

Permanent
Maxillary
Right
Canine
1. LONGITUDINAL SECTION
2. HORIZONTAL SECTIONS

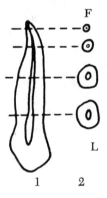

In the cervical portion of the root of the maxillary canine, a horizontal section shows the root canal to have an _____ form; but a horizontal section in the apical portion shows the root canal form to be nearly _____.

Permanent
Maxillary
Right
Canine
1. LONGITUDINAL
   SECTION
2. HORIZONTAL SECTIONS

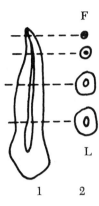

F

L

1   2

If the drawings illustrate a representative sample, about _____% of the maxillary canines will have accessory canals which usually run in a _____ direction.

Permanent
Maxillary
Right
Canine
LONGITUDINAL
   SECTIONS

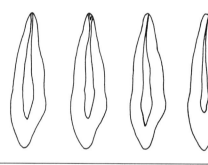

In the mandibular canine, the form of the pulp chamber and root canal is very similar to that of the maxillary canine. The chief exception is related to the relative frequency of a bifurcated canine root in the mandibular arch. Of all anterior teeth, the mandibular canine is the most likely to have _____ (number) root canals.

Permanent
Mandibular
Right
Canine
LONGITUDINAL
   SECTIONS
MESIAL

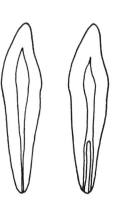

241

In the mandibular canine, a bifurcated root canal is more common than a bifurcated root. If two canals are present through most of the root length on single-rooted mandibular canines, there may be either a common or separate ——————.

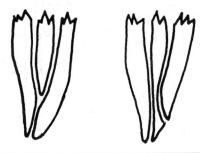

apical foramen (foramina)

MATRIX TEST 9

Directions . . .

Write your response (usually one word or an "X") in the square that matches the left hand column with the top row. *Turn to Page 201 to check your answers.*

Pulp of Anterior teeth	Max. Central Incisor	Mand. Central Incisor	Max. Canine
In which direction is the pulp chamber widest at the roof?			
Of these three teeth, which has accessory canals most frequently?			
Of these three teeth, which is most likely to have a divided root canal?			
Approximate shape of the root canal as seen in a horizontal section taken at the mid-root.			

ANSWERS ON PAGE 201

REVIEW TEST 9

Make a note of your answers so you can check them on Page 202.

1. If you were involved in clinical operations on several patients' root canals, you would have to be alert to the possibility of double root canals on which anterior teeth?

_____   _____

_____   _____

_____   _____
           (arch)   (tooth name)

2. Choose the CORRECT statement:
   a. When anterior teeth have two root canals they have two apical foramina.
   b. When anterior teeth have two root canals they have either one or two apical foramina.

3. For each of the anterior teeth listed below, write down the number of pulp horns typically found on the roof of their pulp chambers.
   a. maxillary canine _____
   b. maxillary lateral incisor _____
   c. maxillary central incisor _____

ANSWERS ON PAGE 202

3

THE PERMANENT PREMOLARS

SECTION 1.0 MAXILLARY PREMOLARS

Although the surfaces of posterior crowns are actually smoothly contoured, we can imagine the crown as a cube sitting on its root. The five visible sides of the cube are the facial, lingual, mesial, distal and occlusal surfaces. The sides intersect at right angles and form the edges (or lines) of the cube.

In correct dental terminology, these edges are called line _____.

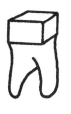 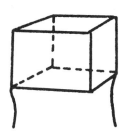

angles

Although **line angles** do not appear as distinct lines on the tooth crown, these lines provide a useful reference in describing the crown. How many line angles are present on a posterior tooth? _____

eight

The eight line angles of a posterior tooth are _____.

mesiofacial   mesiocclusal
distofacial   distocclusal
mesiolingual   faciocclusal
distolingual   linguocclusal

Which line angle is indicated by label **a**? _____

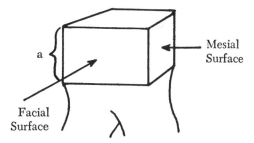

Another term in dental anatomy is **point angle.** A point angle is formed by the intersection of three surfaces, similar to the point that is formed by the intersection of three surfaces on a cube (point **B** is formed by the intersection of surfaces **a, b, c**).

Although the crown of a tooth does not exhibit distinct points, the concept of a crown as a modified cube with point angles at the "corners" is used for descriptive purposes.

The crown of a posterior tooth has four point angles. One point angle is located at each of the four "corners" of the _____ surface.

The four point angles of a posterior tooth are named by the three surfaces that intersect to form the "point." The names are _____

mesiofaciocclusal   mesiolinguoocclusal
distofaciocclusal   distolinguoocclusal

Which point angle is indicated by label **a**?

_____

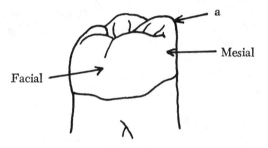

Before describing each posterior tooth, let's clarify the term **marginal ridge.**

The two marginal ridges of an anterior tooth can be viewed from a lingual aspect, but the marginal ridges of a posterior tooth are viewed from an occlusal aspect. Just as the marginal ridges form the mesial and distal borders of the lingual surface for an incisor, the mesial and distal marginal ridges of a posterior tooth form the mesial and distal borders of the _____ surface.

Permanent
1. Maxillary
Right
Central Incisor
LINGUAL
2. Mandibular
Right
1st Molar
OCCLUSAL

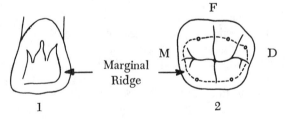

Similar to the cusp of the canines, each cusp of a posterior tooth has <u>four ridges.</u> Using the cusp tip as the starting point, the ridges are named for <u>the direction they run as seen from the occlusal view</u>. The ridge labeled **a** is a facial ridge; the ridge labeled **b** is a _____ ridge.

Permanent
Maxillary
Right
1st Premolar
OCCLUSAL

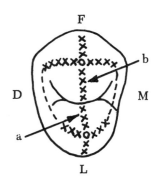

The cusp labeled **X** is located on the mesial portion of the crown. The cusp labeled **Y** is on the distal portion of the crown. Ridge **a** is the distal ridge of cusp **X**; ridge **b** is the _____ ridge of cusp **Y**.

Permanent
Maxillary
Right
1st Molar
OCCLUSAL

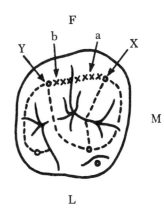

Of the two ridges labeled, which is a mesial ridge?
_____ (a/b)

Permanent
Maxillary
Right
1st Molar
OCCLUSAL

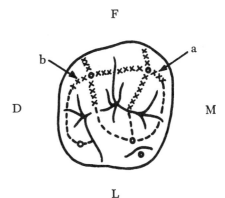

On posterior teeth, the occlusal surface, bounded by the mesial and distal ridges of the cusps and the two marginal ridges is often referred to as the **occlusal table.** Although the two terms name the same part of the tooth, they are not used interchangeably. "Occlusal table" is used when discussing the functional aspects of the crown, as in occlusion. "Occlusal surface" is used in more general discussions, such as anatomical descriptions of the tooth.

What is the appropriate term for the following discussion?

"Since the lingual cusp of the mandibular first premolar is nonfunctional, the lingual portion of the facial cusp contributes more significantly to the occlusal _____."

table

A maxillary first premolar has two cusps. How many ridges form the boundary of its occlusal table? _____ (four/six).

Permanent
Maxillary
Right
1st Premolar
OCCLUSAL

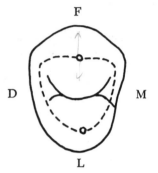

six

The boundary of the occlusal table is formed by the two marginal ridges, the two ridges of the facial cusp, and the two ridges of the lingual cusp for a total of six.

There are eight permanent premolar teeth, two in each quadrant. They lie behind the canines and in front of the permanent _____.

Permanent
Maxillary
Left Quadrant
FACIAL

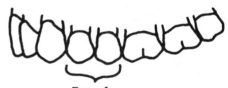

Premolars

The permanent premolars assume the positions formerly occupied by the deciduous molars. The permanent premolars and all permanent anterior teeth are called **succedaneous teeth.** A succedaneous tooth is a permanent tooth that assumes a position previously occupied by a _____ tooth.

1. Permanent
2. Primary
Maxillary
Left Quadrant
FACIAL

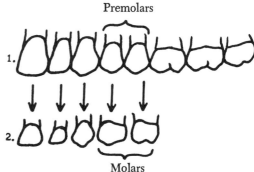

Premolars

Molars

The permanent, molars are not preceded by deciduous teeth; therefore, they are called _____ teeth.

1. Permanent
2. Primary
Maxillary
Left Quadrant
FACIAL

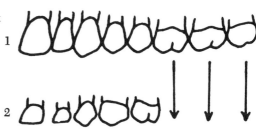

Anterior teeth have incisal edges, but the posterior teeth have occlusal surfaces. On premolar teeth, the view corresponding to the incisal view of the anteriors is called the _____ view.

SECTION 1.1 MAXILLARY FIRST PREMOLAR

The permanent maxillary premolars show evidence of four lobes. The lobes are positioned and named in a manner similar to the lobes described on the maxillary anterior teeth. How many lobes are there on the facial surface of a maxillary premolar? _____

Permanent
Maxillary
Right
1st Premolar
1. FACIAL
2. LINGUAL

1   2

The three lobes that form the facial portion of a maxillary premolar are called the _____, _____, and _____ lobes. The fourth lobe is the _____ lobe.

Permanent
Maxillary
Right
1st Premolar
FACIAL

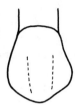

---

mesiofacial, central-facial, distofacial, lingual

In each quadrant, the two teeth immediately anterior to the first molar generally contain two cusps. However, in the mandibular quadrants one of these teeth frequently contains three cusps. Thus, the preferred term for each of the eight teeth is _____ (a. bicuspid *or* b. premolar).

---

b. premolar

Since "bi" denotes "two," the term "bicuspid" means two-cusped. "Premolar" means in front of or anterior to the molars. Since the mandibular second premolar often has three cusps, the term premolar is preferred and will be used in the remainder of this text.

The mesial and distal borders (occlusal view) converge toward the lingual, which is _____ (narrower/wider) than the facial.

Permanent
Maxillary
Right
1st Premolar
OCCLUSAL

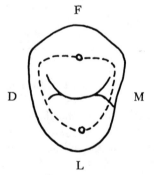

On the two-cusped premolars, one of the cusps is located toward the facial, called the <u>facial cusp.</u> The other cusp is located toward the lingual and is called the _____ cusp.

Permanent
Maxillary
Right
1st Premolar
1. OCCLUSAL
2. DISTAL

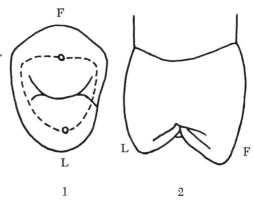

When two or more cusps are compared, the cusp with the <u>greatest **mesiodistal measurement** is the widest</u>. As seen from the occlusal view, which of the two cusps on a maxillary first premolar is the widest? _____

Permanent
Maxillary
Right
1st Premolar
OCCLUSAL

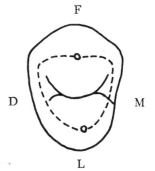

The length of a cusp is determined <u>by its length in the occlusocervical direction</u>. Which view of a maxillary first premolar best shows the comparative length of its two cusps?

_____

Permanent
Maxillary
Right
1st Premolar
1. OCCLUSAL
2. DISTAL

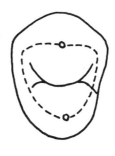
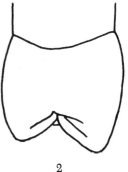

The **occlusocervical measurement** of a cusp is the perpendicular distance from the cusp tip to the plane that contains the point of deepest cut by an occlusal groove. If **a** passes through the deepest cut of an occlusal groove, what is the length of the facial cusp?

_____

Permanent
Maxillary
Right
1st Premolar
MESIAL

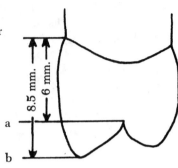

2.5 mm

The facial cusp of a maxillary first premolar is wider than the lingual cusp because it has a greater measurement in the _____ direction.

  a. mesiodistal
  b. occlusocervical
  c. mesiolingual

---

mesiodistal

The facial cusp of the maxillary first premolar has a greater measurement in the occlusocervical direction, but it is the measurement in the mesiodistal direction that determines which cusp is wider. The term "wider" means the "greater mesiodistal measurement" when it is used to compare cusp size. The cusp with the greater measurement in the occlusocervical direction is the "longer" cusp.

When one considers the size of the two cusps of the maxillary first premolar, the facial cusp is both _____ and _____ than the lingual cusp.

Permanent
Maxillary
Right
1st Premolar
1. OCCLUSAL
2. DISTAL

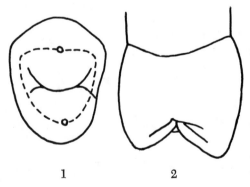

1   2

The ridges of the facial cusp descend from the cusp tip in a pattern that is common to most cusps. How many ridges are in this pattern? _____

Permanent
Maxillary
Right
1st Premolar
OCCLUSAL

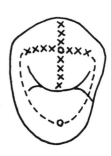

Name the ridges of the facial cusp.

1. _____ ridge of the facial cusp.
2. _____ ridge of the facial cusp.
3. _____ ridge of the facial cusp.
4. _____ ridge of the facial cusp.

Permanent
Maxillary
Right
1st Premolar
OCCLUSAL

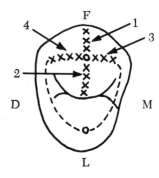

1. Facial; 2. Lingual; 3. Mesial; 4. Distal

Four ridges are located on the larger of the two cusps of the maxillary first premolar, the _____ cusp.

Permanent
Maxillary
Right
1st Premolar
OCCLUSAL

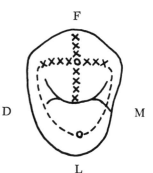

The facial ridge of the facial cusp is broad and prominent. It descends in a cervical direction onto the _____ surface.

Permanent
Maxillary
Right
1st Premolar
OCCLUSAL

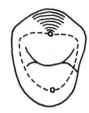

Does the lingual ridge of the facial cusp descend onto the lingual surace? _____

Permanent
Maxillary
Right
1st Premolar
OCCLUSAL

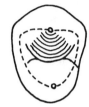

The lingual ridge of the facial cusp runs from the tip of the cusp to the central area of the _____ surface.

Permanent
Maxillary
Right
1st Premolar
OCCLUSAL

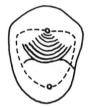

Any ridge on a posterior tooth that descends from the cusp tip and runs to the central area of the occlusal surface is called a **triangular ridge.** Does the facial edge of the facial cusp on a permanent maxillary first premolar qualify as a triangular ridge? _____ (yes/no)

Permanent
Maxillary
Right
1st Premolar
OCCLUSAL

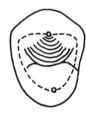

The facial ridge of the facial cusp on a maxillary first premolar is not a triangular ridge, for it does not run toward the central area of the _____ surface.

Permanent
Maxillary
Right
1st Premolar
OCCLUSAL

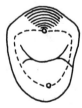

On the maxillary first premolar, the mesial ridge of the facial (buccal) cusp descends from the cusp tip and is continuous with the mesial marginal ridge near the _____ point angle.

Permanent
Maxillary
Right
1st Premolar
OCCLUSAL

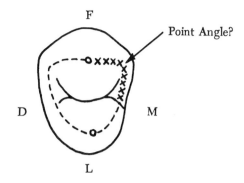

The mesial ridge of the facial cusp joins at an acute angle with the _____ ridge.

Permanent
Maxillary
Right
1st Premolar
OCCLUSAL

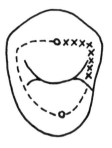

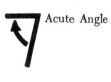

The distal ridge descends from the facial cusp tip and joins at an acute angle with the _____ ridge.

Permanent
Maxillary
Right
1st Premolar
OCCLUSAL

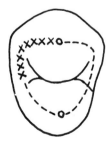

255

Like the facial cusp, the smaller lingual cusp also has _____ (number) ridges emerging from its tip.

Permanent
Maxillary
Right
1st Premolar
OCCLUSAL

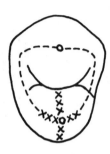

The mesial ridge of the lingual cusp joins the _____ ridge to form a rounded, sweeping curve at the mesiolinguocclusal point angle.

Permanent
Maxillary
Right
1st Premolar
OCCLUSAL

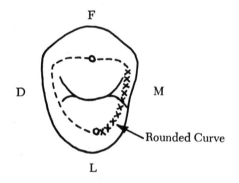

Rounded Curve

The distal ridge of the lingual cusp joins the distal marginal ridge near the _____ point angle.

Permanent
Maxillary
Right
1st Premolar
OCCLUSAL

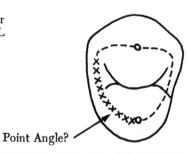

Point Angle?

One of the four ridges of the lingual cusp descends to the lingual surface, becoming the prominence of that surface. Extending to the lingual surface from the lingual cusp tip is the _____.

Permanent
Maxillary
Right
1st Premolar
OCCLUSAL

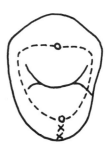

lingual ridge

The facial ridge of the lingual cusp runs from the tip of the lingual cusp to the central area of the _____ surface.

Permanent
Maxillary
Right
1st Premolar
OCCLUSAL

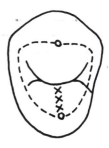

occlusal

Which ridge of the lingual cusp is a triangular ridge? _____

Permanent
Maxillary
Right
1st Premolar
OCCLUSAL

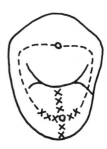

facial

How many triangular ridges are present on a maxillary first premolar? _____

two

Some texts use a slightly different nomenclature for the triangular ridges of the premolars. The lingual ridge of the facial cusp may be called the facial triangular ridge because it is located on the facial cusp. The facial ridge of the lingual cusp may be called the lingual triangular ridge. The nomenclature used in this program is preferred.

Name the following ridges:

a. _____ ridge of the _____ cusp.

b. _____ ridge of the _____ cusp.

Permanent
Maxillary
Right
1st Premolar
OCCLUSAL

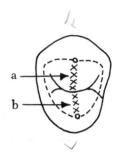

a
b

a. lingual (triangular) ridge of the facial cusp
b. facial (triangular) ridge of the lingual cusp

The large depression (or valley) on the occlusal surface is called the **occlusal sulcus.** The sulcus is included within the limits of the occlusal table. The inclines that meet at an angle form the sulcus. Thus, the occlusal sulcus is surrounded by the cusps and the inclines of the two _____ ridges.

Permanent
Maxillary
Right
1st Premolar
OCCLUSAL

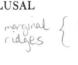

marginal ridges {

m.r.

Occlusal Table

Sulcus is Stippled

---

marginal

The bottom of the occlusal sulcus is marked by developmental grooves. At the central area of the sulcus, the **central groove** divides the two _____ ridges.

Permanent
Maxillary
Right
1st Premolar
OCCLUSAL

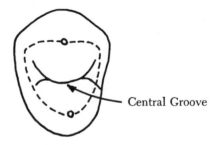

Central Groove

Two grooves meet the central groove at its mesial end, the mesial **marginal groove** and the mesiofacial **triangular groove**. Which groove is located more toward the facial?

Permanent
Maxillary
Right
1st Premolar
OCCLUSAL

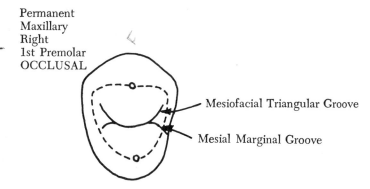

Mesiofacial Triangular Groove

Mesial Marginal Groove

a. mesial marginal groove.
b. mesiofacial triangular groove.

b. mesiofacial triangular groove

The mesial marginal groove extends onto the mesial surface, but first it crosses the ––––––– ridge.

Permanent
Maxillary
Right
1st Premolar
OCCLUSAL

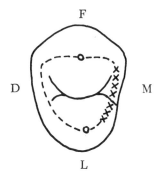

mesial marginal

The central groove extends distally to the distal marginal ridge, where it branches to form the distofacial triangular groove and the distal marginal groove. Which is the distofacial triangular groove: a or b?

Permanent
Maxillary
Right
1st Premolar
OCCLUSAL

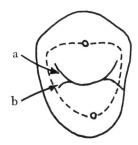

The distal marginal groove extends onto the distal marginal ridge but not onto the _____ surface.

Permanent
Maxillary
Right
1st Premolar
OCCLUSAL

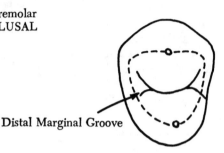

Distal Marginal Groove

Label the five grooves (a through e) on the occlusal surface of a maxillary first premolar.

a. _____
b. _____
c. _____
d. _____
e. _____

Permanent
Maxillary
Right
1st Premolar
OCCLUSAL

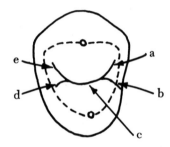

a. mesiofacial triangular groove; b. mesial marginal groove; c. central groove; d. distal marginal groove; e. distofacial triangular groove

At the confluence of these grooves, a small **pit is often found**. On the maxillary first premolar, there are two pits, one at each end of the _____ groove.

Permanent
Maxillary
Right
1st Premolar
OCCLUSAL

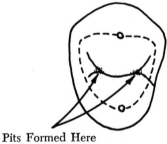

Pits Formed Here

Whenever two or more developmental grooves meet, a _____ is likely to be formed.

The pits at either end of the central groove are named the distal and the _____ pit.

Permanent
Maxillary
Right
1st Premolar
OCCLUSAL

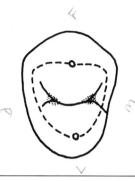

MATRIX TEST 1

Directions . . .

Place an X in the square that matches the left hand column with the top row. Mark your answers and *turn to Page 287.*

Maxillary First Premolar	Facial	Lingual	Mesial	Distal
From the occlusal view, the mesial and distal sides converge toward the:				
Which is the widest cusp?				
Which is the longest cusp?				
Which cusp has a facial ridge that is a triangular ridge?				
A developmental groove extends onto which proximal surface?				

ANSWERS ON PAGE 287

REVIEW TEST 1

Choose the correct answer, make a note of it for each question, *and then turn to Page 283 to check your answers.*

1. Name the ridge indicated by the arrow.

   a. Distal ridge of the lingual cusp.
   b. Distal ridge of the facial cusp.
   c. Mesial ridge of the facial cusp.

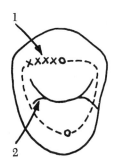

2. Name the groove indicated by the arrow.

   a. Distofacial triangular groove.
   b. Distal marginal groove.
   c. Mesial marginal groove.

3. The wider of two cusps is the cusp with the greater measurement in which direction?

   a. Occlusocervical
   b. Mesiodistal

4. The triangular ridge of a lingual cusp extends from the cusp tip to the _____

   a. Central groove.
   b. Mesial marginal ridge.
   c. Distal marginal groove.

ANSWERS ON PAGE 283

The <u>facial aspect</u> of the permanent maxillary first premolar is outlined by four borders, one being the occlusal. The other three borders are the _____, _____, and _____.

Permanent
Maxillary
Right
1st Premolar
FACIAL

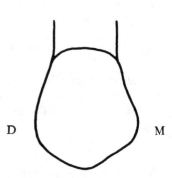

D   M

mesial, distal, cervical

The facial aspect of the maxillary first premolar is similar to that of the maxillary canine. Occlusocervically, the maxillary first premolar is slightly _____ (longer/shorter) than the canine.

Permanent
Maxillary
Right
1. 1st Premolar
2. Canine
FACIAL

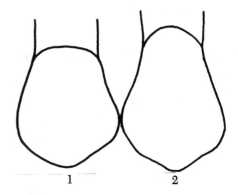

1   2

shorter

The tip of the facial cusp separates the occlusal border into two parts. These are the _____ and _____ ridges of the facial cusp.

Permanent
Maxillary
Right
1st Premolar
FACIAL

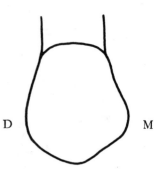

D   M

The mesial and distal ridges of the facial cusp can be distinguished by their shape. Which of the two is straighter? _____ Which is convex? _____

Permanent
Maxillary
Right
1st Premolar
FACIAL

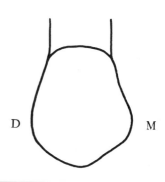

D   M

The tip of the facial cusp is not centered with the long axis of the tooth; instead, it is located _____ (mesially/distally) from the long axis.

Permanent
Maxillary
Right
1st Premolar
FACIAL

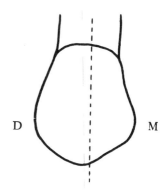

D   M

On the maxillary first premolar, the proximal contacts are located in the middle third of the crown, slightly _____ (<u>cervical</u>/occlusal) <u>to the junction of the middle and occlusal thirds</u>.

Permanent
Maxillary
Right
1st Premolar
FACIAL

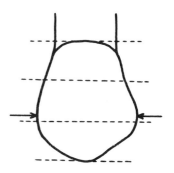

In the incisocervical or occlusocervical direction, the
location of the proximal
contacts varies with the
tooth. On some teeth, the
contacts are in the incisal
third of the crown, on others in the middle third.
However, on all teeth, the
widest part of the crown,
mesiodistally, is at the
level of the _____ .

Permanent
Maxillary
Right
1. 1st Premolar
2. Lateral Incisor
FACIAL

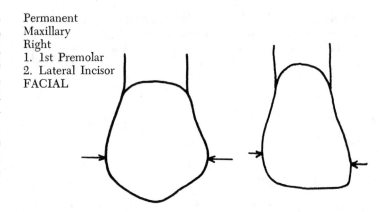

proximal contacts (contact areas)

From the facial aspect of a maxillary first premolar, which
distance is greater?

The distance between the tip of the facial cusp and the mesiocclusal angle . . . . GO TO TOP OF PAGE 267

The distance between the tip of the facial cusp and the distocclusal angle . . . . GO TO NEXT FRAME

▶ From preceding frame   *distocclusal is incorrect*

Since the tip of the facial
cusp is located toward the
distal from the midline of the
crown, <u>the distance between
the cusp tip and the mesiocclusal angle is greater.</u> In
other words, the mesial
ridge of the facial cusp is
longer than the distal ridge.

Permanent
Maxillary
Right
1st Premolar
FACIAL

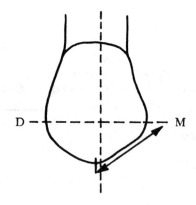

RETURN TO PRECEDING FRAME AND ANSWER AGAIN.

From the facial aspect, which of the two contact areas is formed by a sharper angle?

_____

Permanent
Maxillary
Right
1st Premolar
FACIAL

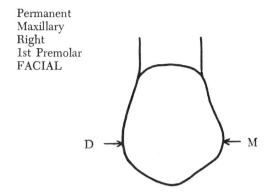

D →   ← M

mesial

On the maxillary first premolar, the mesial surface joins the facial surface to form the rounded but distinct _____ line angle.

Permanent
Maxillary
Right
1st Premolar
1. FACIAL
2. OCCLUSAL

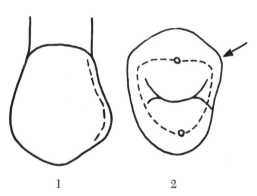

1   2

mesiofacial

The <u>distofacial line angle is less distinct than the mesiofacial line angle.</u> The distal and facial surfaces blend together to create a rounded form that contributes to the broad, rounded distal contact area.

Permanent
Maxillary
Right
1st Premolar
1. FACIAL
2. OCCLUSAL

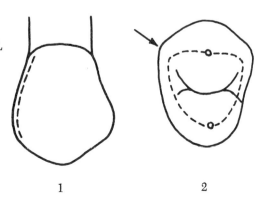

1   2

Remember, the drawings in the program are two-dimensional representations of three-dimensional objects. The conversion from three to two dimensions causes some distinctions to be lost and may distort slightly the appearance of some features.

Also, the discussion of the anatomical features of the teeth describes the average as determined by observing a large sample of individual teeth. A specimen tooth can deviate from the average and remain within the classification of a typical specimen.

Compare the two heavily shaded areas. From the contact area cervically, which border is more nearly straight? _____

Permanent
Maxillary
Right
1st Premolar
FACIAL

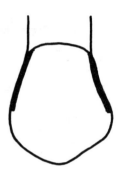

distal

Of the mesial and distal borders of the facial surface, which is <u>concave</u>? _____

Permanent
Maxillary
Right
1st Premolar
FACIAL

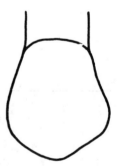

Use the guidelines to sketch a drawing of the maxillary first premolar, but follow this description: Distal straight; rounded distal angle; slightly curved distal cusp ridge; straight mesial cusp ridge; rounded but distinct mesial angle; concave mesial border.

Now compare your sketch with the one in the next frame.

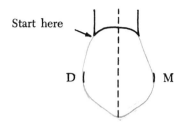

Start here

D | M

Permanent
Maxillary
Right
1st Premolar
FACIAL

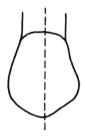

The prominent facial ridge of the facial cusp gives the facial surface its great bulk. The facial ridge runs continuously to the cervical line. Cervically, the facial ridge blends with the _____ ridge.

Permanent
Maxillary
Right
1st Premolar
FACIAL

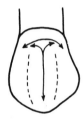

On either side of the facial ridge, **facial grooves** mark the boundaries of the three facial lobes. On the facial surface of a maxillary first premolar, which lobe is the most prominent? _____

Permanent
Maxillary
Right
1st Premolar
FACIAL

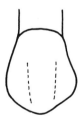

On the facial surface, the two faint _____ separate the facial lobes.

Permanent
Maxillary
Right
1st Premolar
FACIAL

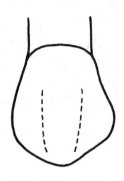

At the cervical border, the facial surface is convex. The cervical line has its crest of convexity toward the _____ (occlusal/apical).

SECTION 2.1   MAXILLARY FIRST PREMOLAR: LINGUAL VIEW

The facial view of the maxillary first premolar completely hides the mesial, distal, and lingual portions of the crown. From the lingual view, the lingual surface, parts of the mesial and distal surfaces, and a portion of the facial cusp are visible. This is because the crown _____ toward the lingual, and, in length, the lingual cusp is _____ than the facial cusp.

Permanent
Maxillary
Right
1st Premolar
LINGUAL

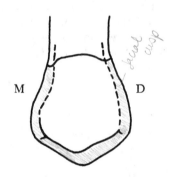

M   D

Mesial and distal ridges are found on both the _____ and _____ cusps.

Permanent
Maxillary
Right
1st Premolar
LINGUAL

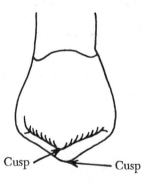

Cusp   Cusp

Unlike the ridges of the facial cusp, the mesial and distal ridges of the lingual cusp form a rounded curve in joining the mesial and distal marginal ridges. Following this pattern, the lingual surface is rounded mesiodistally, making the mesiolingual and distolingual line angles _____ (sharp/indistinct).

Permanent
Maxillary
Right
1st Premolar
1. OCCLUSAL
2. LINGUAL

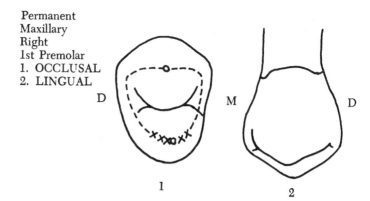

The lingual cusp tip is not in the same faciolingual plane as the facial cusp tip. Compared with the facial cusp tip, is the lingual cusp tip more toward the mesial or distal? _____

Permanent
Maxillary
Right
1st Premolar
OCCLUSAL

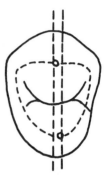

On the maxillary first premolar, which two line angles are more distinct? (mesiofacial and distofacial/mesiolingual and distolingual) _____

Permanent
Maxillary
Right
1st Premolar
OCCLUSAL

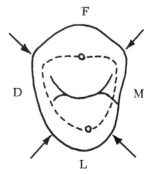

Compare the cervical lines of the facial and lingual views. The convexity of the cervical line on the facial surface is directed in the (occlusal/apical) _____ direction; also the curvature is greater on the _____ surface.

Permanent
Maxillary
Right
1st Premolar
1. FACIAL
2. LINGUAL

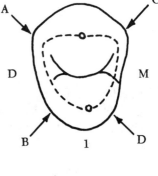

SECTION 2.2 MAXILLARY FIRST PREMOLAR: PROXIMAL VIEW

A portion of the facial and lingual surfaces of the crown can be seen from a mesial or distal view of a maxillary first premolar. The point angles (A, B, C, D) and line angles (a, b, c, d) mark the limits of the proximal surfaces. The facial and lingual borders of the two proximal surfaces are the four _____ angles.

Permanent
Maxillary
Right
1. OCCLUSAL
2. MESIAL
3. DISTAL

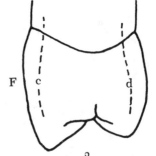

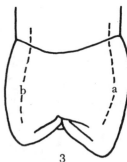

One major difference between the mesial and distal surfaces of the maxillary first premolar is the presence of a **mesial marginal groove** that extends from the occlusal surface onto the _____ surface.

Permanent
Maxillary
Right
1st Premolar
1. MESIAL
2. DISTAL

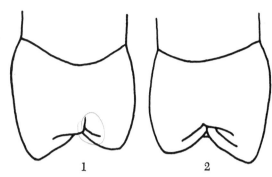

1   2

As is generally true of all teeth, the cervical line has a crest of curvature that is more occlusally (or incisally) located on the _____ (mesial/distal) surface.

Permanent
Maxillary
Right
1st Premolar
1. MESIAL
2. DISTAL

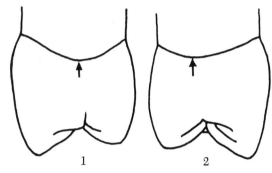

1   2

The mesial marginal groove extends onto the mesial surface of the maxillary first premolar. To do so, this groove passes through the _____ ridge.

Permanent
Maxillary
Right
1st Premolar
MESIAL

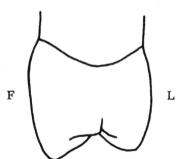

F   L

The end of the mesial marginal groove is lingual to the contact area and terminates in the _____ third of the crown.

Permanent
Maxillary
Right
a. 1st Premolar
MESIAL
b. Canine
c. 1st Premolar
d. 2nd Premolar
OCCLUSAL

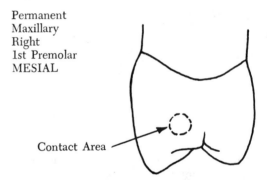

Is the extension of the mesial marginal groove located to the facial or lingual of the contact area? _____

Permanent
Maxillary
Right
1st Premolar
MESIAL

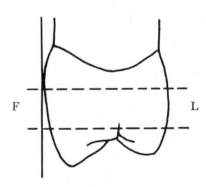

Contact Area

From a mesial view, the facial outline is convex. The height of contour is located in the _____ third of the crown.

Permanent
Maxillary
Right
1st Premolar
MESIAL

F   L

The lingual outline is also convex, the height of contour occurring in the _____ third.

Permanent
Maxillary
Right
1st Premolar
MESIAL

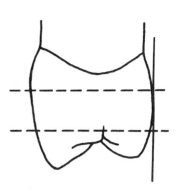

The mesial surface of the maxillary first premolar is both convex and concave. The convexity occurs in the area of the marginal ridge and includes the contact area. The concavity occurs between the contact area and cervical line. In the drawing (right) is the mesial surface toward A or B?

Permanent
Maxillary
Right
1st Premolar
LINGUAL

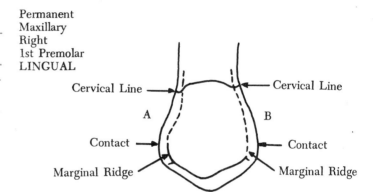

A

Three characteristic features of the maxillary first premolar are (a) the extension of the mesial marginal groove onto the mesial surface, (b) the lingual cusp is shorter than the facial cusp and (c) there is a **mesial concavity** or depression cervical to the contact area. Which of the two diagrams represents a maxillary first premolar? _____ (Fig. 1/Fig. 2)

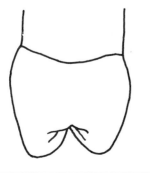

1

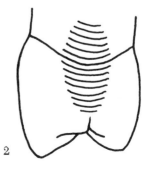

2

Figure 2

If the facial and lingual cusps of a specimen tooth appeared approximately equal in height, perhaps due to wear, the tooth could be identified as a maxillary first premolar by the _____ located cervical to the mesial contact area.

Permanent
Maxillary
Right
1st Premolar
MESIAL

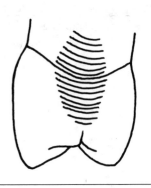

mesial concavity

In contrast to the mesial surface, the distal surface of the crown of a maxillary first premolar does not characteristically have a concavity cervical to the proximal contact area. In the drawing, the distal is toward _____ (A/B).

Permanent
Maxillary
Right
1st Premolar
LINGUAL

Cervical Line ———→   ←——— Cervical Line

A   B

Contact ——→   ←—— Contact

Marginal Ridge ——→   ←—— Marginal Ridge

B

The distal marginal groove does not cut across the distal marginal ridge and onto the distal surface. On a few teeth, an extension of the distal marginal groove may be visible, but it is slight. The drawing shows a maxillary first premolar seen from the _____ view.

Permanent
Maxillary
Right
1st Premolar

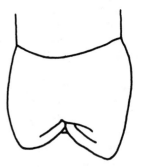

The curvature of the cervical line on the mesial and distal is consistent with the pattern established by anterior teeth. From both the mesial and distal views, the cementoenamel junction curves toward the _____ with the greater amount of curvature on the _____.

Permanent
Maxillary
Right
1st Premolar
1. MESIAL
2. DISTAL

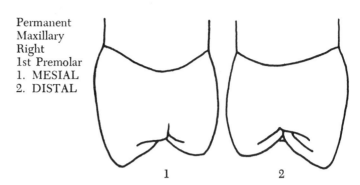

occlusal, mesial

Of the four diagrams, which two show the maxillary left first premolar from the distal aspect?

_____

Permanent
Maxillary
Left
1st Premolars

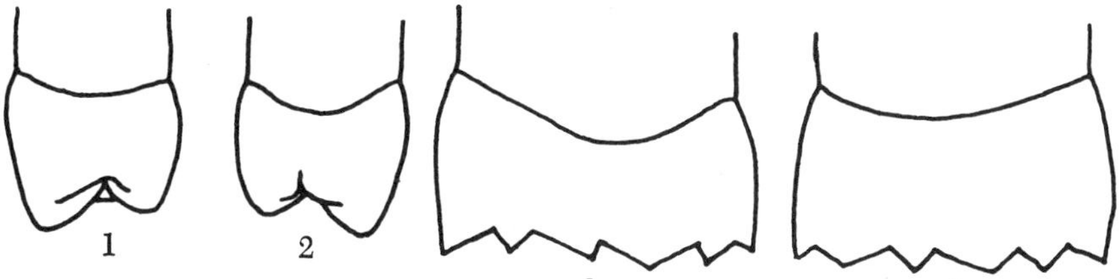

1   2   3   4

Figure (1) and Figure (4)

What are the universal (military) code numbers for the teeth shown in Figures 1-4?

Figure 1 _____
Figure 2 _____
Figure 3 _____
Figure 4 _____

Permanent
Maxillary
1st Premolars

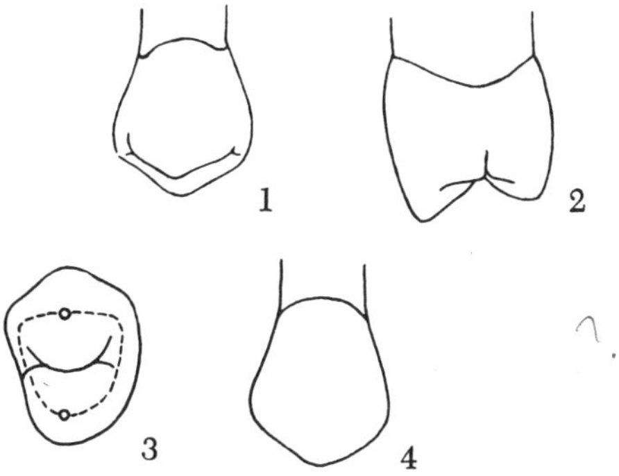

1   2

3   4

Figure 1: 5; Figure 2: 5; Figure 3: 12;
Figure 4: 12

MATRIX TEXT 2

Directions . . .

Write the correct response (one or more words) in the space that matches the left hand column with the top row.

Write your response and *turn to Page 289.*

FILL IN ALL BLANK CELLS

Maxillary First Premolar	Mesial	Distal
Which ridge of the facial cusp is shorter and which is longer?		
Which surface has a cervical line with more curvature?		
Occlusocervical location of this contact area . . .		
Does the developmental groove extend onto this surface?		

REVIEW TEST 2

Maxillary First Premolar

Choose the correct answers, *make a note of them, then turn to Page 290.*

1. The lingual cusp tip is displaced from the facial cusp slightly to the:

   a. Distal
   b. Mesial

2. The cervical line is more convex on which surface?

   a. Facial
   b. Lingual

3. The more distinct line angle:

   a. Mesiofacial
   b. Distofacial

4. The shape of the mesial surface (from contact area to cervical line):

   a. Concave
   b. Convex
   c. Straight

5. List the three distinguishing characteristics of the maxillary first premolar.

   a. _____
   b. _____
   c. _____

6. In which third (cervical, middle, or occlusal) is the height of contour located on each of these surfaces?

   a. Lingual _____
   b. Facial _____

ANSWERS ON PAGE 290.

SECTION 3.0   MAXILLARY SECOND PREMOLAR

The size and shape of the maxillary second premolar is generally similar to the maxillary first premolar.

    Variation in the relative sizes of the two maxillary premolars will occur because the second premolar deviates from the average form more often than the first premolar. Although the crown size of a maxillary second premolar is variable, it generally has approximately the same dimensions as the maxillary _____.

---

first premolar

On the maxillary first premolar, the lingual cusp is shorter than the facial cusp. However, in relative length, the two cusps of the second premolar are approximately _____.

Permanent
Maxillary
Right
1. 1st Premolar
2. 2nd Premolar
MESIAL

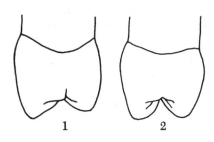

1   2

---

equal (or synonym)

On the maxillary second premolar, if one cusp is slightly shorter, the shorter of the two is the _____ cusp.

Permanent
Maxillary
Right
2nd Premolar
MESIAL

F 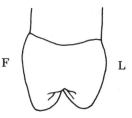 L

---

lingual

The facial cusp of the second premolar lacks the pointed cusp tip seen on the first premolar. Thus, in length (depth of occlusal groove to cusp tip), the facial cusp of the second premolar is _____ than that of the first premolar.

Permanent
Maxillary
Right
1. 1st Premolar
2. 2nd Premolar
MESIAL

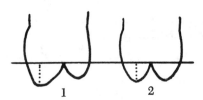

1   2

On the occlusal, <u>the groove pattern of the second premolar is less distinct than that of the first premolar</u>. On the maxillary second premolar, the central groove is short and _____ (straight/irregular).

Permanent
Maxillary
Right
1. 2nd Premolar
2. 1st Premolar
OCCLUSAL

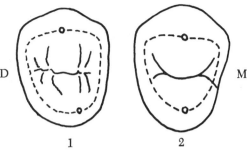

D   M

1   2

On the occlusal surface of the second premolar, shallow linear **supplemental grooves** radiate from the central groove. With the presence of these supplemental grooves, the mesiofacial and distofacial triangular grooves are less positive and may be more difficult to identify. Which of the two diagrams represents the occlusal view of the maxillary second premolar? (Fig. 1 or Fig. 2)

Permanent
Maxillary
Right
Premolars

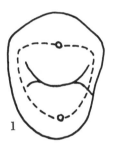 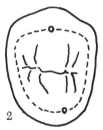

1   2

Figure 2 is correct

On the second premolar, a <u>developmental groove</u> does not cross the mesial marginal ridge and descend onto the mesial surface. The <u>extension of a developmental groove onto the mesial surface is a characteristic only of the maxillary _____ _____.</u>

Permanent
Maxillary
Right
1. 1st Premolar
2. 2nd Premolar
OCCLUSAL

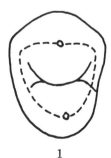 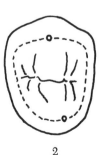

1   2

What is the difference between the relative length of the facial and lingual cusps on the maxillary first premolar when compared to the relative length of the facial and lingual cusps on the maxillary second premolar? _____

Permanent
Maxillary
Right
1., 2. 1st Premolar
3., 4. 2nd Premolar
1., 3. DISTAL
2., 4. MESIAL

1

2

3

4

The facial and lingual cusps on the maxillary second premolar are nearly equal in length.

Of the two maxillary premolars, which has the longer facial cusp? _____

Permanent
Maxillary
Right
1. 1st Premolar
2. 2nd Premolar
MESIAL

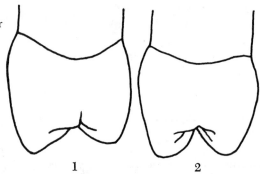

1

2

The mesial surface of the maxillary second premolar differs from the mesial surface of the first premolar. As mentioned, the mesial marginal groove does not extend onto the mesial surface on the maxillary _____ premolar.

Permanent
Maxillary
Right
1. 1st Premolar
2. 2nd Premolar
MESIAL

1

2

The <u>mesial surface on the crown of the maxillary second premolar shows less</u> overall curvature when <u>viewed from the facial or lingual</u> as shown by the mesiolingual line angle. In this respect, the mesial surfaces of the two maxillary premolars are _____ (similar/dissimilar).

Permanent
Maxillary
Right
1. 1st Premolar
2. 2nd Premolar
LINGUAL

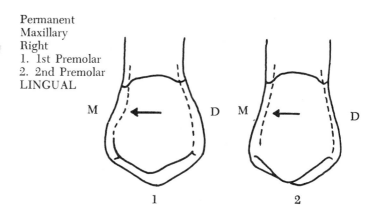

On the facial and lingual surfaces, the cervical line is curved toward the _____; on the mesial and distal surfaces, it is slightly curved toward the _____.

Which maxillary premolar has cervical lines that are slightly less curved? _____ _____

Permanent
Maxillary
1. 1st Premolar
2. 2nd Premolar
a. FACIAL
b. LINGUAL
c. MESIAL
d. DISTAL

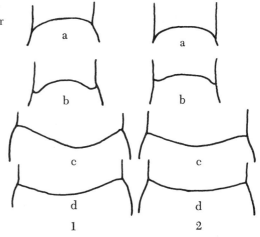

As is true for all posterior teeth, <u>the proximal contact areas on the maxillary premolars are not centered in the faciolingual direction.</u> In the faciolingual direction, the proximal contacts of posterior teeth are located slightly toward the _____.

Permanent
Maxillary
Right
3. 1st Molar
4. 2nd Premolar
5. 1st Premolar
6. canine
OCCLUSAL

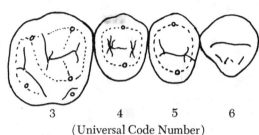

| 3 | 4 | 5 | 6 |

(Universal Code Number)

Similar to the maxillary first premolars, the occlusocervical location of the mesial and distal contact areas on the second premolar is slightly _____ to the junction of the _____ and _____ thirds.

Permanent
Maxillary
Left
11. Canine
12. 1st Premolar
13. 2nd Premolar
14. 1st Molar
FACIAL

(Universal Code Number)

| 11 | 12 | 13 | 14 |

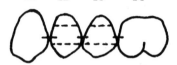

cervical, occlusal, middle

MATRIX TEXT 3

Directions . . .

Place an X in the square that matches the left hand column with the top row. Mark your answer and *then turn to Page 291.*

	First Premolar	Second Premolar	Neither/ Both
Longer buccal cusp . . .			
Mesial marginal groove extends onto mesial surface . . .			
More supplemental grooves . . .			
Cervical line less contoured . . .			
Mesial surface has less curvature . . .			

REVIEW TEST 3

Choose the correct answers and make a note of them. *On Page 292 check your answers.*

1. The tooth shown is which maxillary premolar (mesial view):

    a. First
    b. Second

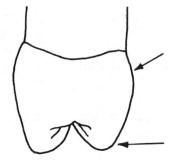

2. This cusp is the:

    a. Buccal
    b. Lingual

3. This maxillary premolar is the:

    a. First
    b. Second

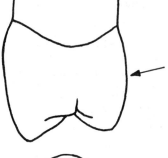

4. The tooth shown is the maxillary:

    a. Second premolar
    b. First premolar

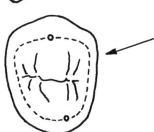

ANSWERS ON PAGE 292

TEST ANSWER SECTION

MATRIX TEST 1
(From Page 262)

If any items were missed, *turn to Frame indicated for review.*
If all are correct, *turn to Page 263 for the first Review Test.*

Maxillary First Premolar	Facial	Lingual	Mesial	Distal
From the occlusal view, the mesial and distal sides converge toward the:		X (P. 250)		
Which is the widest cusp?	X (P. 251)			
Which is the longest cusp?	X (PP. 251–253)			
Which cusp has a facial ridge that is a triangular ridge?		X (PP. 254, 257)		
A developmental groove extends onto which proximal surface?			X (P. 259)	

REVIEW TEST 1
(From Page 263)

Correct Answers:

1. *b* 2. *b* 3. *b* 4. *a*

IF YOU GOT ALL QUESTIONS CORRECT, give yourself a pat on the back because you have just completed Section 1. Research has shown that your concentration and readiness to study will improve if you take a short break now and do something that is interesting to you, not related to dental anatomy, and available to you right now. This might mean going for a walk, reading the paper or magazine, or doing sit-ups! You choose what is most interesting to you right now, you've earned it. *When you return, continue on Page 264, the beginning of Section 2.*

IF YOU MISSED ONE OF THE QUESTIONS, read the directions for reviewing that question below. Review and then retake the test on Page 263.

1. IF YOU MISSED QUESTION 1, review the naming of the cusp ridges on Pages 252–253.

2. IF YOU MISSED QUESTION 2, review the grooves on Pages 259–260.

3. IF YOU MISSED QUESTION 3, review the measurement of cusp width on Page 251.

4. IF YOU MISSED QUESTION 4, review the concept of triangular ridges on Pages 254 and 258 and then the ridges of the lingual cusp on Page 257.

IF YOU MISSED TWO OR MORE QUESTIONS, *please return to Page 245 and review this section again.* The methods of naming ridges, cusps and grooves are basics that you will need. Also, you can impress your friends by naming off all their triangular ridges. Review and then retake the test on Page 263.

MATRIX TEST 2

(From Page 278)

If any items were missed, *turn to the page indicated for review.*
If all are correct, *turn to Page 279 for the second Review Test.*

Maxillary First Premolar	Mesial	Distal
Which ridge of the facial cusp is shorter and which is longer?	Longer (P. 266)	Shorter (P. 266)
Which surface has a cervical line with more curvature?	X (P. 277)	(P. 277)
Occlusocervical location of this contact area . . .	middle third (cervical to junction of occlusal and middle thirds) (PP. 265–266)	middle third (cervical to junction of occlusal and middle thirds) (PP. 265–266)
Does the developmental groove extend onto this surface?	Yes (P. 273)	No (P. 276)

REVIEW TEST 2
(From Page 279)

Correct Answers:

1. *b* 2. *a* 3. *a* 4. *a* 5. *a: Mesial marginal groove extends onto mesial surface b: Lingual cusp is shorter than the facial cusp c: Mesial surface below contact area has a concavity 6. a. Lingual: middle, b. Facial: cervical*

IF YOU GOT ALL QUESTIONS CORRECT, congratulations, you have completed one of the more challenging Review Tests! Take a break and do something you have been wanting to do all day. This will provide a reward and a boost to your study progress. *Continue on Page 280.*

IF YOU MISSED ANY PART OF ONE OF THE QUESTIONS, read the directions for reviewing that question below. Review and then retake the test on Page 279. As you review, be certain to answer the questions in the text again as you read.

1. IF YOU MISSED QUESTION 1, review Page 271 on the alignment of cusps.

2. IF YOU MISSED QUESTION 2, review Pages 271–272 on the curvature of the cervical line on the facial surface.

3. IF YOU MISSED QUESTION 3, review Pages 267–268.

4. IF YOU MISSED QUESTION 4, review Page 268.

5. IF YOU MISSED QUESTION 5, review Pages 275–276 where there is a summary of the distinctive features of the maxillary first premolar and skim this section if additional information is needed.

6. IF YOU MISSED QUESTION 6, examine the drawings in Pages 274–275 and answer the questions concerning them on those pages.

IF YOU MISSED PARTS OF TWO OR MORE QUESTIONS, go back to Page 264 and review this section. Be sure to answer the questions again using a mask because this will help you to prepare for retaking the review test on Page 279. Research on study habits has indicated that you will learn more by answering questions on the subject matter you are learning, than if you merely read and reread it. If you learn the characteristics of the maxillary first premolar it will be a lot easier to learn the features of the other premolars because this section will compare and contrast them. So place your premolar cusps firmly in occlusion and *do some reviewing, then retake the test on Page 279.*

MATRIX TEST 3
(From Page 285)

If any items were missed, *turn to the page indicated for review.*
If all were correct, *turn to Page 286 for the Review Test.*

	First Premolar	Second Premolar	Neither/ Both
Longer buccal (facial) cusp...	X (P. 280)		
Mesial marginal groove extends onto mesial surface . . .	X (P. 281)		
More supplemental grooves . . .		X (P. 281)	
Cervical line less contoured . . .		X (P. 283)	
Mesial surface has less curvature...		X (PP. 282–283)	

REVIEW TEST 3
(From Page 286)

Correct Answers:

1. *b* 2. *b* 3. *a* 4. *a*

IF YOU GOT ALL QUESTIONS CORRECT, very good, give yourself a break and then continue on Page 301, Section 4.

IF YOU MISSED ANY ONE OF THE QUESTIONS, read the directions for reviewing that question below. Review and then retake the test on Page 286.

1. IF YOU MISSED QUESTION 1, note the difference in cusp length and the placement of the mesial marginal groove (onto mesial surface on the first premolar) on Pages 282–283 where first and second premolars are compared.

2. IF YOU MISSED QUESTION 2, review the cusp lengths on Page 280.

3. IF YOU MISSED QUESTION 3, review the differences between first and second premolars on Pages 280 and 282 (cusp lengths) and Pages 282–283 (mesial marginal groove of first premolar extends to mesial surface).

4. IF YOU MISSED QUESTION 4, review the occlusal surface of the second premolar and its supplemental groove pattern on Page 281.

IF YOU MISSED TWO OR MORE QUESTIONS, *please turn to Page 280,* the beginning of Section 3, and review this section again. When you review, answer all of the embedded questions, using any piece of paper, an envelope, or your favorite box top to shield the answers). Review and then retake the test on Page 286 before continuing.

If any items were missed, *turn to the page indicated for review.*
If all are correct, *turn to Page 317 for Review Test 4.*

Mandibular First Premolar	Mesial	Distal
Longer facial cusp ridge . . .		X (P. 309)
Broader contact area . . .		X (P. 305)
Occlusal fossa that contains a developmental groove with a lingual extension . . .	X (P. 308)	
Marginal ridge with a slope most nearly parallel to the slope of the lingual ridge of the facial cusp . . .	X (P. 314)	
Proximal aspect showing least curvature of the cervical line . . .		X (P. 314)

REVIEW TEST 4
(From Page 317)

Correct Answers:

1. *a*   2. *b*   3. *a*   4. *a*

IF YOU GOT ALL ANSWERS CORRECT, you should be heaped with praise for the insightful way in which you can, first, understand the test questions, and, second, get them right! May you be blessed with many years of success. You deserve a break. Why don't you take some time now to reward yourself for a job well done. When you return, continue on Page 318, Section 5.

IF YOU MISSED ONE OF THE QUESTIONS, read the directions for reviewing below. Review and then retake the review test on Page 317.

1. IF YOU MISSED QUESTION 1, study the drawings of the occlusal surface on Pages 306–307 and note the absence of a central groove. Read Pages 307–308 also.

2. IF YOU MISSED QUESTION 2, review the fact that the facial cusp tip is either centered or displaced to the mesial on Pages 309–310. Review the lingual cusp size on Pages 301–303.

3. IF YOU MISSED QUESTION 3, review the transverse ridge on Page 306.

4. IF YOU MISSED QUESTION 4, review the centering of the facial cusp tip on Pages 312–313 or the lingual cusp alignment on Page 314.

IF YOU MISSED TWO OR MORE QUESTIONS, why don't you give the section another try by returning to Page 301 and reviewing the section again. Retake Review Test 4 on Page 317 also.

MATRIX TEST 5

(From Page 333)

If any items were missed, *turn to the page indicated for review.*
If all are correct, *turn to Page 334 for Review Test 5.*

Mandibular Second Premolar	Mesial	Distal
Occlusal fossae located at the . . .	X (P. 322)	X (PP. 322–323)
Larger of the two lingual cusps . . .	X (PP. 321–322)	
Marginal ridge at lower level . . .		X (P. 331)
Central pit displaced toward the . . .		X (P. 330)

REVIEW TEST 5
(From Page 334)

Correct Answers:

1. *a* 2. *b* 3. *b* 4. *a* 5. *a,b,d,f,g*

IF YOU GOT ALL QUESTIONS COMPLETELY CORRECT, you have completed this section, and should take a study break. Go right now and free your mind from the thoughts of dental anatomy. When you return you will be better prepared to concentrate again. You will start Section 6, Page 335, when you return.

IF YOU MISSED ONE QUESTION (OR ONE PART OF A QUESTION), read the directions for review below. When you review try to seriously answer the questions in the text again as you reread a section or page. Retake Review Test 5 on Page 334.

1. IF YOU MISSED QUESTION 1, go back to Pages 252–253 and examine the drawing of the maxillary first premolar. The cusp ridges are named in the same way on all premolars. Also, examine the drawings on Pages 321–322. The buccal cusp is, of course, the facial cusp.

2. IF YOU MISSED QUESTION 2, review the developmental grooves on Page 323.

3. IF YOU MISSED QUESTION 3, review the grooves on Pages 322–323.

4. IF YOU MISSED QUESTION 4, review the cusp names on Pages 321–322 and 328–329.

5. IF YOU MISSED A PART OF QUESTION 5, review that part below:
   a. Five lobes—Page 318
   b. Two lingual cusps—Pages 319–320
   c. Less developed lingual cusp—Page 329
   d. Shorter facial cusp—Pages 326–327
   e. Transverse ridge—(First premolar) Pages 307 and 322
   f. Cusp tip displacement—Page 327
   g. Tooth tilt—Page 330

6. IF YOU MISSED QUESTION 6, we must have missed it too!

IF YOU MISSED TWO OR MORE QUESTIONS OR PARTS OF QUESTIONS, review the section again, starting on Page 318. Think of the fun you'll have finding out which of your friends has "Y," "H," or "U" type.

MATRIX TEST 6
(From Page 349)

If any questions were missed, *turn to the page indicated for review.*
If all answers were correct, *turn to Page 350 and continue with Review Test 6.*

	Maxillary		Mandibular	
	First Premolar	Second Premolar	First Premolar	Second Premolar
Most commonly a single-rooted tooth.	(PP. 341–342)	X (P. 345)	X (PP. 345–346)	X (PP. 346–347)
Tooth whose mesial surface has the most prominent longitudinal groove.	X (P. 343)	(P. 345)	(P. 346)	(P. 346)
Amount of contour equals 1 mm. on lingual surface.	(PP. 339–340)	(PP. 339–340)	X (P. 340)	X (P. 340)
Two teeth which usually have oval to nearly round horizontal root form.			X (PP. 346–347)	X (PP. 346–347)
Premolars whose single root has a rounded or blunt apex (seen from the proximal view).	X (PP. 345–346)	X (PP. 345–346)	(P. 347)	(P. 347)

REVIEW TEST 6
(From Page 350)

Correct Answers:

1. *a*   2. *b*   3. *c*   4. *The second premolar has its crown tilted toward the lingual.*

IF YOU GOT ALL QUESTIONS CORRECT, very good work! You only have one section to go! Take a short break first, such as getting up and stretching (or whatever interests you). Continue on Page 351, Section 7.

IF YOU MISSED ONE OF THE QUESTIONS, review that question as directed below. Then, retake the review test, Page 350.

1. IF YOU MISSED QUESTION 1, restudy the diagrams on Page 337 and answer the questions in Pages 337–338 (embrasures).

2. IF YOU MISSED QUESTION 2, restudy the diagrams on Page 337 and the questions on Pages 337–338 (proximal contacts).

3. IF YOU MISSED QUESTION 3, study the heights of contour on Pages 339–340.

4. IF YOU MISSED QUESTION 4, restudy the illustration and information on Page 341. Perhaps you will also want to look back at Page 330.

IF YOU MISSED TWO OR MORE QUESTIONS, you know what you have to do, Page 335.

MATRIX TEST 7

(From Page 356)

If any items were missed, *turn to the page indicated for review.*
If all were correct, *turn to Page 357 for Review Test 7.*

Pulp of Premolars	Max. First Premolar	Mand. First Premolar	Max. Second Premolar	Mand. Second Premolar
Most common number of root canals.	two (P. 351)	one (P. 354)	one (P. 353)	one (P. 354)
If the tooth has a less common number of root canals, what number of canals would that be?	one (P. 351)	two (P. 354)	two (P. 352)	two (P. 354)
Number of pulp horns in pulp chamber.	two (P. 352)	one (P. 353)	two (P. 352)	two (P. 353)
Names of usual root canals (if more than one).	Facial Lingual (P. 351)	one only (P. 354)	one only (P. 352)	one only (P. 354)

REVIEW TEST 7
(From Page 357)

Correct Answer:

1. *a. Mesiodistal*

If necessary, check your answer and review Pages 351–352 (maxillary premolars) and Page 354 (mandibular premolars). And, then, you also deserve your own self-administered reward for finishing this chapter.

SECTION 4.0   MANDIBULAR FIRST PREMOLAR

The mandibular premolars are located immediately posterior to the permanent mandibular canines. Since the permanent mandibular central incisors are teeth number 24 and 25 (universal code), what numbers are assigned to the permanent mandibular first premolars? _____

Permanent
Mandibular Arch
OCCLUSAL

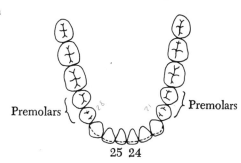

Premolars {   } Premolars

25 24

21, 28

Similar to the maxillary premolars, the mandibular first premolar has a four-lobe pattern. Three of the lobes are seen on the _____ portion of the crown; the fourth lobe represents the _____ portion.

Permanent
Mandibular
Right
1st Premolar
a. FACIAL
b. LINGUAL

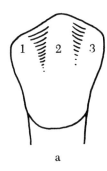
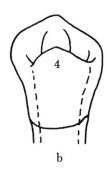

a

b

facial, lingual

Like the maxillary premolars, the mandibular first premolar has two cusps, called the _____ and _____ cusps.

Permanent
Mandibular
Right
1st Premolar
MESIAL

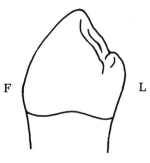

F   L

301

Only one of the two cusps of the mandibular first premolar is functional. The shorter, non-functional cusp does not usually occlude with maxillary teeth. Which is the functional cusp? _____

Permanent
Mandibular
Right
1st Premolar
MESIAL

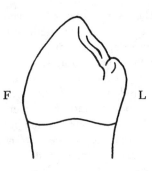

F   L

In some respects, the mandibular first premolar resembles a canine. The lingual feature of a mandibular first premolar that resembles a large cingulum on a canine is the _____.

Permanent
Mandibular
Right
1st Premolar
MESIAL

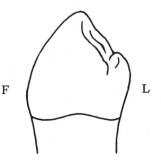

F   L

The facial cusp of the mandibular first premolar is large and considered a **centric cusp**; however, the lingual cusp is small and considered a _____ cusp.

Permanent
Mandibular
Right
1st Premolar
MESIAL

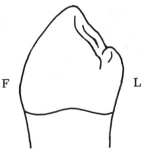

F   L

Centric cusps of mandibular premolars are those that contact their antagonists and determine the position of the mandible in maximum opposing tooth contact (*centric occlusion*).

Choose the letter (a or b) corresponding to the centric cusp shown on the right _____.

Permanent
Mandibular
Right
1st Premolar
MESIAL

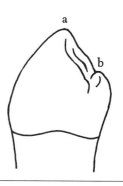

a

Viewed from the distal, the premolars normally occlude so that the mandibular facial cusps strike the _____.

a. central portion of the occlusal surface of their antagonists.

b. facial portion of the facial cusps of their antagonists.

Permanent
1st Premolars
DISTAL
OCCLUDED

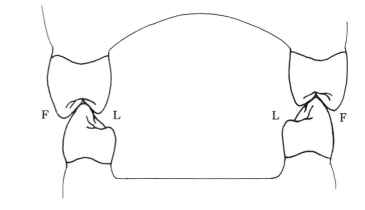

a. central portion

From the occlusal view, the geometric outline of the crown is nearly a rounded diamond shape with a mesiodistal width that is narrower in the _____ (facial/lingual) portion.

Permanent
Mandibular
Right
1st Premolar
OCCLUSAL

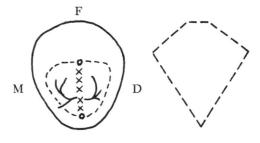

Which crown surface (occlusal view) combines with the occlusal surface to form the major part of the tooth? _____

Permanent
Mandibular
Right
1st Premolar
OCCLUSAL

M   D

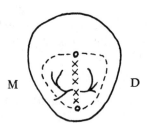

Compared to the maxillary premolars, the more lingual location of the facial cusp tip on the mandibular first premolar results in an occlusal surface that is relatively _____ (small/large).

Permanent
Mandibular
Right
1st Premolar
OCCLUSAL

M   D

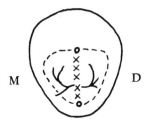

The <u>facial ridge of the facial cusp descends in the cervical direction as part of the facial surface.</u> It adds to the prominence of the _____ lobe.

Permanent
Mandibular
Right
1st Premolar
1. OCCLUSAL
2. FACIAL

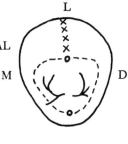

L

M   D   D   M

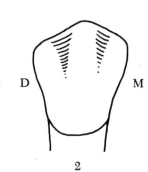

1   2

The <u>mesial and distal ridges of the facial cusp descend toward the proximal contact areas where they become continuous with the mesial and distal</u> _____.

Permanent
Mandibular
Right
1st Premolar
OCCLUSAL

F

M   D

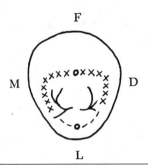

L

From the occlusal view, the large arc of the distal outline creates a broad contact area. The <u>mesial outline turns more acutely than the distal and forms</u> a _____ (relative size) contact area.

Permanent
Mandibular
Right
1st Premolar
OCCLUSAL

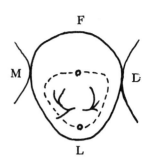

smaller (or less rounded)

The maxillary premolars have <u>central grooves that separate the triangular ridges.</u> Notice, however, that the mandibular first premolar *does not* usually <u>have a division of the two triangular ridges.</u> Instead, the triangular ridges characteristically cross the occlusal surface uninterrupted. Any union of two triangular ridges produces <u>a single ridge called the</u> **transverse ridge.**

Permanent
Maxillary
Right
1. 1st Premolar
2. 2nd Premolar
Mandibular
3. 1st Premolar
OCCLUSAL

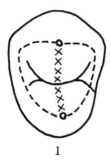

1

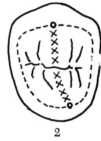

2

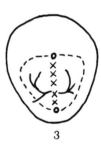

3

In the most common form of the mandibular first premolar <u>the occlusal table (bounded by the cusp ridges and marginal ridges) is triangular shaped and bisected by a prominent</u> _____ ridge.

Permanent
Mandibular
Right
1st Premolar
OCCLUSAL

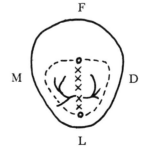

Occlusal Table

305

Because of the reduced form of the lingual cusp, the major portion of the lingual half of the occlusal table is bounded by the mesial and distal _____.

Permanent
Mandibular
Right
1st Premolar
OCCLUSAL

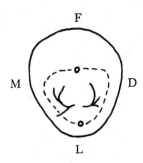

The prominent triangular ridge of the facial cusp and the small facial ridge of the lingual cusp unite to form a _____ ridge.

Permanent
Mandibular
Right
1st Premolar
OCCLUSAL

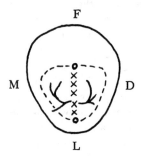

You may occasionally find specimens of mandibular first premolars that do not have an uninterrupted transverse ridge, because they have a more prominent central _____.

Permanent
Mandibular
Right
1st Premolar
OCCLUSAL

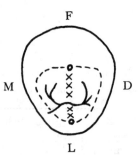

Of the maxillary premolars and the mandibular first premolar, which usually has an uninterrupted transverse ridge? _____

Permanent
Maxillary
Right
1. 1st Premolar
2. 2nd Premolar
Mandibular
3. 1st Premolar
OCCLUSAL

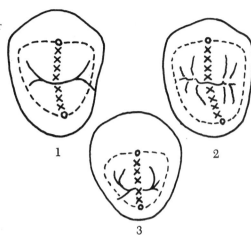

What cusp ridge contributes the largest part to the transverse ridge of the mandibular first premolar? _____ ridge of the _____ cusp.

Permanent
Mandibular
Right
1st Premolar
OCCLUSAL

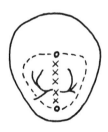

The occlusal surface of the mandibular first premolar has two fossae (the mesial and distal fossae). The mesial and distal ridges of the cusps and the marginal ridges surround the two **occlusal fossae** which are separated by the _____.

Permanent
Mandibular
Right
1st Premolar
OCCLUSAL

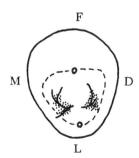

307

Since the two occlusal fossae of the mandibular first premolar are separated by the transverse ridge, <u>the groove patterns of the maxillary premolars and mandibular first premolar are</u> ————— (similar/different).

Permanent
Mandibular
Right
1st Premolar
OCCLUSAL

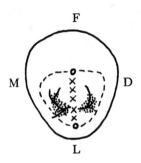

different

Although the groove pattern is variable, most mandibular first premolars have a mesial groove contained within the mesial fossae. The <u>mesial groove runs in a faciolingual direction and is continuous with its lingual extension, the mesiolingual groove.</u>

Which groove separates the mesial marginal ridge from the mesial ridge of the lingual cusp? —————

Permanent
Mandibular
Right
1st Premolar
OCCLUSAL

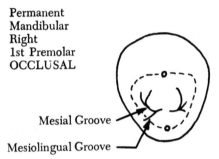

Mesial Groove

Mesiolingual Groove

mesiolingual

Which of the following grooves is not usually present on a mandibular first premolar?

a. mesial groove
b. central groove
c. mesiolingual groove

Permanent
Mandibular
Right
1st Premolar
OCCLUSAL

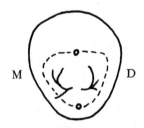

SECTION 4.1 MANDIBULAR FIRST PREMOLAR: FACIAL VIEW

The facial aspect of the mandibular first premolar has a general resemblance to the facial aspect of the mandibular canine. On which of the two teeth is the cusp tip slightly more rounded? _____

Permanent
Mandibular
Right
1. 1st Premolar
2. Canine
FACIAL

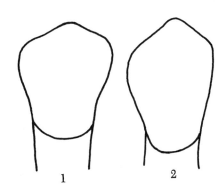

1   2

first premolar

Of the mesial and distal ridges on the facial cusp of the mandibular first premolar, which is longer? _____

Permanent
Mandibular
Right
1st Premolar
FACIAL

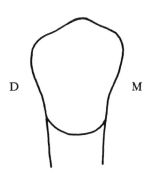

D   M

distal

In which arch is the tip of the facial cusp on the first premolar located toward the distal (from the longitudinal axis of the crown)? _____.

Permanent
Maxillary
Right
4. 2nd Premolar
5. 1st Premolar
6. Canine
Mandibular
Right
29. 2nd Premolar
28. 1st Premolar
27. Canine
FACIAL

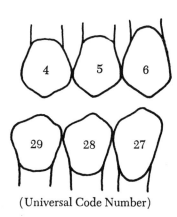

(Universal Code Number)

Examine teeth 5, 6, 27, 28 from the facial (see preceeding drawing). How many have cusps with a distal ridge longer than the mesial ridge? _____

two . . . . .GO TO NEXT FRAME
three . . . . .GO TO BOTTOM OF THIS PAGE

▶ From preceding page

two is incorrect

From the facial, both the mandibular canine and the mandibular first premolar have cusps with a distal ridge longer than the mesial ridge. In the maxillary arch, a similar relationship exists between the mesial and distal ridges of the canine. Of the four teeth, 5, 6, 27, and 28, only tooth number 5, the maxillary first premolar, has a facial cusp with the mesial ridge longer than the distal ridge.

Permanent
Maxillary
Right
4. 2nd Premolar
5. 1st Premolar
6. Canine
Mandibular
Right
29. 2nd Premolar
28. 1st Premolar
27. Canine
FACIAL

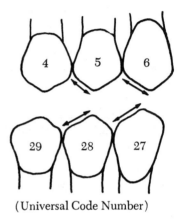

(Universal Code Number)

▶ From top of this page

three is correct

The facial surface of the mandibular first premolar exhibits two concave areas, called facial grooves. The two facial grooves are evidence of the three anatomical divisions called _____ .

Permanent
Mandibular
Right
1st Premolar
FACIAL

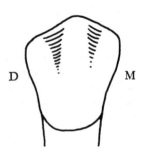

On the mandibular first premolar, the facial grooves are particularly evident because of the prominence of the ———— lobe.

Permanent
Mandibular
Right
1st Premolar
FACIAL

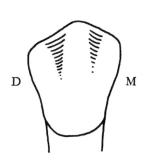

D   M

central-facial

The mesial and distal contact areas are broad, rounded areas located approximately at the same level in the occlusocervical direction. Occlusocervically, the proximal contacts of the mandibular first premolar are located in the middle third of the crown, usually slightly ———— to the junction of the middle and ———— thirds.

Permanent
Mandibular
Right
1st Premolar
FACIAL

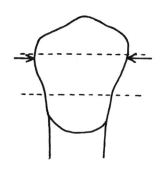

cervical, occlusal

SECTION 4.2 MANDIBULAR FIRST PREMOLAR: LINGUAL VIEW

Because of the distinct lingual convergence of the crown and the reduced development of the lingual cusp, more than the lingual surface is visible from the lingual aspect of the mandibular first premolar. The surfaces visible are the lingual surface, most of the mesial and distal surfaces, and a large portion of the ———— surface.

Permanent
Mandibular
Right
1st Premolar
LINGUAL

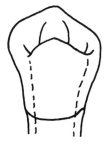

311

From the lingual view, the most visible occlusal feature of the mandibular first premolar is the well developed _____ of the facial cusp.

Permanent
Mandibular
Right
1st Premolar
LINGUAL

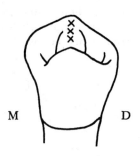

lingual ridge (triangular ridge)

From the lingual aspect, the lingual surface of the crown includes only that part of the crown lying between the _____ and _____ _____ _____.

Permanent
Mandibular
Right
1st Premolar
LINGUAL

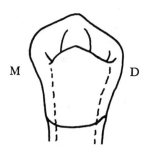

mesiolingual and distolingual line angles

In the mesiodistal direction, the lingual surface of the mandibular first premolar is best described by which two of the following adjectives: wide, narrow, convex, flat, long?

Permanent
Mandibular
Right
1st Premolar
1. LINGUAL
2. OCCLUSAL

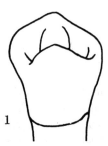
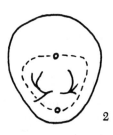

narrow, convex

Originating in the mesial fossa of the occlusal surface, a developmental groove extends lingually to separate the mesial marginal ridge from the lingual cusp. This groove, a unique feature of the mandibular first premolar, is called the _____ groove.

Permanent
Mandibular
Right
1st Premolar
LINGUAL

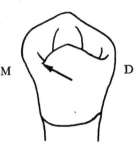

From the proximal views, the tip of the facial cusp is nearly in line with the long axis of the root in the _____ direction.

Permanent
Mandibular
Right
1st Premolar
1. MESIAL
2. DISTAL

F   L   F

1   2

In position in the arch (Fig. 1), the first premolar has a <u>slight facial tilt</u>. The <u>shape of the facial surface as seen from a proximal view appears to allow the contour of the crown to be continuous with the surrounding gingival tissue</u>. When viewed out of the mouth, in an upright position (Fig. 2), however, the facial height of contour appears accentuated by the sharp inclination of the _____ cusp.

Permanent
Mandibular
Right
1. & 2. 1st Premolar
MESIAL

1

F   L

2

F   L

9°

From a proximal view in relation to the long axis of the tooth, the tip of the lingual cusp is located in a very _____ (central/lingual) position.

Permanent
Mandibular
Right
1st Premolar
MESIAL

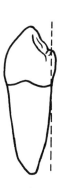

In the faciolingual direction, perpendicular to the long axis of the tooth, the <u>lingual height of contour</u> _____ (extends beyond/is in line with) the root of the mandibular first premolar.

Permanent
Mandibular
Right
1st Premolar
MESIAL

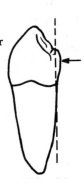

extends beyond

<u>A key distinction between the mesial and distal surfaces of the mandibular first premolar is the degree of linguocervical inclination</u> of the marginal ridges. Which marginal ridge more <u>nearly parallels the slope of the lingual ridge of the facial cusp?</u> _____

Permanent
Mandibular
Right
1. MESIAL
2. DISTAL

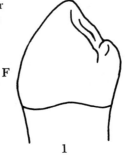
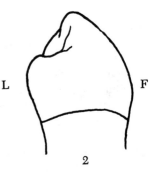

mesial

The <u>cervical line is slightly curved toward the occlusal on both the mesial and distal surfaces</u>. From which proximal aspect does the <u>cervical line exhibit less curvature?</u> _____

Permanent
Mandibular
Right
1st Premolar
1. MESIAL
2. DISTAL

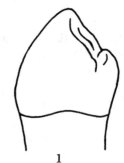
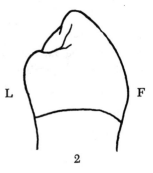

The features of the mandibular first premolar show a great deal of variation between different people. The prominence of the transverse ridge and the size of the lingual cusp are features which vary. Which drawing to the right shows a more prominent transverse ridge from a mesial view, A or B? _____

Permanent
Mandibular
Right
A & B 1st Premolar
MESIAL

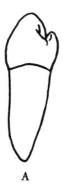

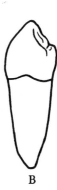

A   B

B

MATRIX TEST 4

Directions . . .

Place an X in the space that matches the left hand column with the top row. Mark your answers and *then turn to* Page 293.

Mandibular First Premolar	Mesial	Distal
Longer facial cusp ridge . . .		
Broader contact area . . .		
Occlusal fossa that contains a developmental groove with a lingual extension . . .		
Marginal ridge with a slope most nearly parallel to the slope of the lingual ridge of the facial cusp . . .		
Proximal aspect showing least curvature of the cervical line . . .		

ANSWERS ON PAGE 293

REVIEW TEST 4

Choose the correct answers and make a note of them. Then, *turn to page 294 to check them.*

Choose the Correct Statement From Each Pair

1. **a.** Mandibular first premolars usually have no central groove.
   b. All permanent first premolars usually have no central groove.

2. **a.** In the facial view of the mandibular first premolar, the tip of the facial cusp is displaced slightly toward the distal from the midline of the crown.
   b. Of all the premolars you have studied so far, the mandibular first premolar has the smallest lingual cusp.

3. **a.** On the mandibular first premolar, the transverse ridge is made up of the lingual ridge of the facial cusp and the facial ridge of the lingual cusp.
   b. The transverse ridge of the mandibular first premolar is made up of the mesial and distal ridges of the facial cusp.

4. **a.** On the mandibular first premolar, the tip of the facial cusp is nearly centered over the root in a faciolingual direction.
   b. On the mandibular first premolar, the tip of the lingual cusp is in line with the height of contour on the lingual surface.

ANSWERS ON PAGE 294

The mandibular second premolar often shows one more lobe than the other premolars. Therefore, how many lobes would you expect to find on the mandibular second premolar?

_____

Permanent
Mandibular
Right
2nd Premolar
1. FACIAL
2. LINGUAL

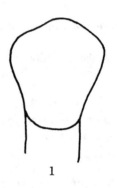 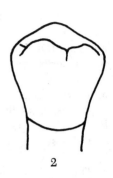

1   2

five

The facial portion of the mandibular second premolar has three lobes, and the lingual portion often has _____ lobes.

5 loBES

Permanent
Mandibular
Right
2nd Premolar
1. FACIAL
2. LINGUAL

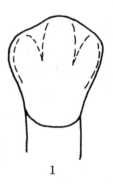 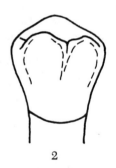

1   2

two

In the occlusal view, the mandibular second premolar is nearly square in shape with little of the lingual convergence seen on the mandibular first premolar. Which of the drawings at the right is of a second premolar, A or B?

_____

Permanent
Mandibular
Premolars
OCCLUSAL

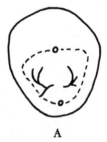 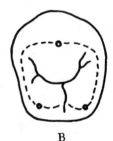

A   B

318

When you examine all of the permanent premolars, you see that two of the four show little, if any, lingual convergence in an occlusal view, the maxillary second premolar and the _____ premolar. (The latter premolar also has three rather than two cusps, typically).

Permanent
Maxillary
Right
1. 1st Premolar
2. 2nd Premolar
Mandibular
3. 1st Premolar
4. 2nd Premolar
OCCLUSAL

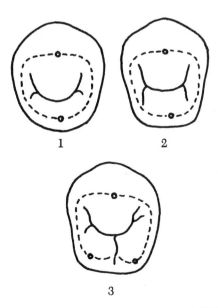

mandibular second premolar

Actually, the occlusal surface of the mandibular second premolar occurs as one of three types. Each "Y," "H," and "U type," is named for its **occlusal groove pattern.** Figure 1 shows the _____ type, Figure 2 the _____ type, and Figure 3 the _____ type.

Permanent
Mandibular
Right
2nd Premolar
OCCLUSAL

Figure 1, "U"; Figure 2, "H"; Figure 3, "Y"

Of the three types of mandibular second premolars, the most common is the three-cusp or ________ type.

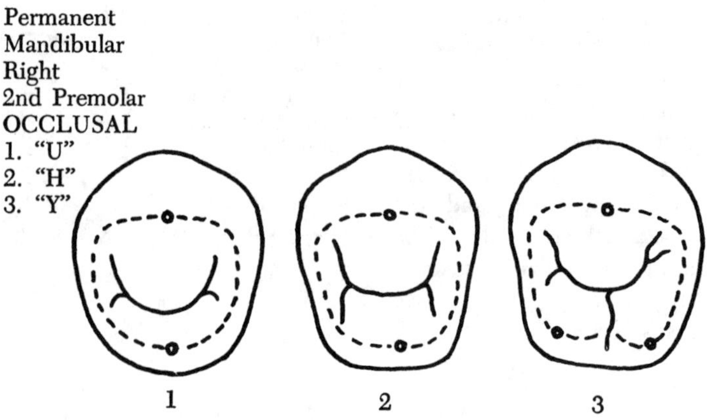

Permanent
Mandibular
Right
2nd Premolar
OCCLUSAL
1. "U"
2. "H"
3. "Y"
1
2
3

"Y"

In contrast to the "Y" type, the "H" and "U" types have ________ (number) cusps.

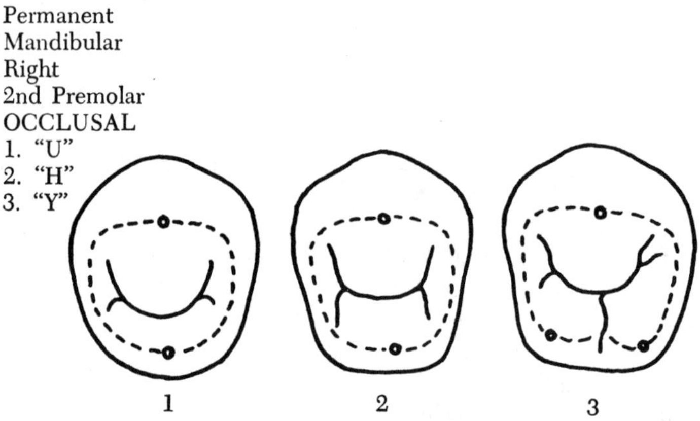

Permanent
Mandibular
Right
2nd Premolar
OCCLUSAL
1. "U"
2. "H"
3. "Y"
1
2
3

---

two

On two-cusped mandibular premolars, the "H" type groove pattern is the more common. Therefore, the most common type on mandibular second premolars is the ________ type; the least common is the ________ type.

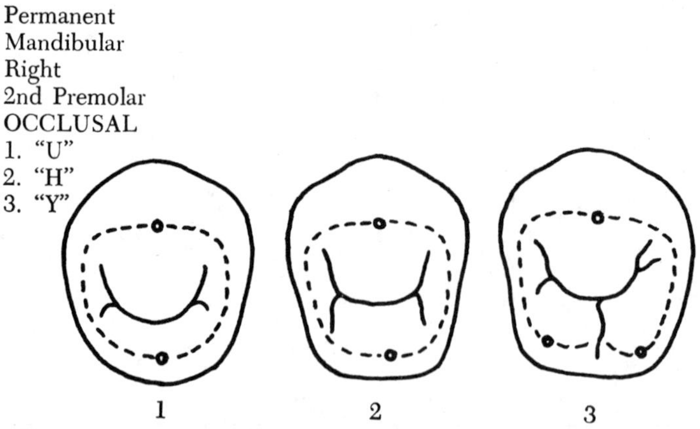

Permanent
Mandibular
Right
2nd Premolar
OCCLUSAL
1. "U"
2. "H"
3. "Y"
1
2
3

When three cusps are present, which portion of the crown has two cusps? _____ (facial/lingual)

Permanent
Mandibular
Right
2nd Premolar
OCCLUSAL

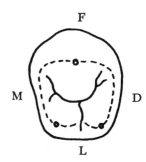

lingual

The two lingual cusps on the "Y" type result in a greater lingual development. Which one of the following terms best describes the outline of the occlusal table on the "Y" type: circular—square—ovoid?

Permanent
Mandibular
Right
2nd Premolar
OCCLUSAL

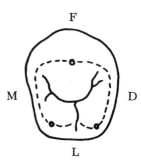

square

Because the "Y" type of groove pattern is the most common of the three types, it will be described in detail. Although the "H" and "U" types are less common, they are considered as typical specimens of the mandibular second premolar.

Of the two lingual cusps (the mesiolingual and distolingual), which is the largest?_____

Permanent
Mandibular
Right
2nd Premolar
OCCLUSAL

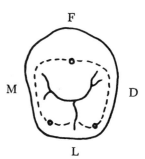

Arrange the three cusps of the mandibular second premolar in order according to size, largest to smallest.

Largest _____

Next largest _____

Smallest _____

On the "Y" type mandibular second premolar, how many triangular ridges run toward the center of the occlusal surface? _____

Permanent
Mandibular
Right
2nd Premolar
OCCLUSAL

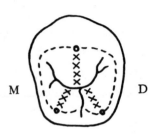

M   D

The three triangular ridges partition the occlusal table. Toward the mesial, a mesial fossa is bound mesially by the mesial marginal ridge and distally by the triangular ridges of the _____ and _____ cusps.

Permanent
Mandibular
Right
2nd Premolar
OCCLUSAL

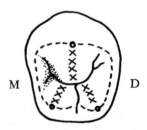

M   D

The mesial border of the distal fossa is formed by the triangular ridges of the _____ and _____ cusps.

Permanent
Mandibular
Right
2nd Premolar
OCCLUSAL

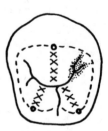

One of three developmental grooves, the lingual groove passes between the two lingual cusps, ending on the _____ surface.

Permanent
Mandibular
Right
2nd Premolar
OCCLUSAL

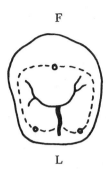

The mesial groove originates at the central pit and runs in a mesiofacial direction through the mesial _____.

Permanent
Mandibular
Right
2nd Premolar
OCCLUSAL

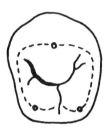

The distal groove originates at the central pit and runs in a distofacial direction through the _____.

Permanent
Mandibular
Right
2nd Premolar
OCCLUSAL

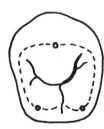

Similar to that of the mandibular first premolar, the facial surface of the mandibular second premolar is inclined toward the lingual. Because of the increased faciolingual diameter of the second premolar, the tip of the facial cusp is located slightly toward the _____ from the faciolingual midline of the crown.

Permanent
Mandibular
Right
1. 2nd Premolar
2. 1st Premolar
MESIAL

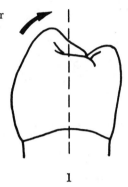
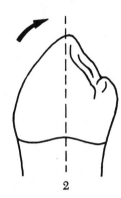

1   2

From which proximal view of the mandibular second premolar is a greater portion of the occlusal surface visible? _____

Permanent
Mandibular
Right
2nd Premolar
1. MESIAL
2. DISTAL

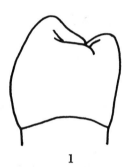
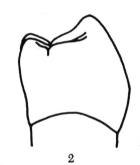

1   2

Which is the smallest cusp? _____

Permanent
Mandibular
Right
2nd Premolar
OCCLUSAL

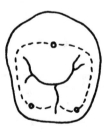

The three developmental grooves on the three-cusped mandibular second premolar originate at the point of common intersection called the _____.

central pit

Name the three developmental grooves of the three-cusped mandibular second premolar.

1. ______________________
2. ______________________
3. ______________________

mesial, distal, and lingual

Complete the following matrix by supplying the appropriate letter or numeral for each space.

PERMANENT MANDIBULAR SECOND PREMOLAR GROOVE PATTERN TYPES

	name of type	number of cusps
most common		
less common		
least common		

Answers:

PERMANENT MANDIBULAR SECOND PREMOLAR GROOVE PATTERN TYPES

	name of type	number of cusps
most common	Y	3
less common	H	2
least common	U	2

The occlusal table of the two-cusped mandibular second premolars is partioned by two _____ ridges.

Permanent
Mandibular
Right
2nd Premolar
OCCLUSAL
1. "H"
2. "U"

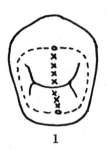 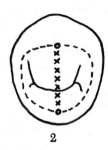

1   2

triangular

On the "H" and "U" occlusal types, a groove separates the triangular ridges and <u>terminates in the mesial and distal fossae.</u> As on the maxillary premolars, this groove is called the _____ groove.

Permanent
Mandibular
Right
2nd Premolar
OCCLUSAL
1. "H"
2. "U"

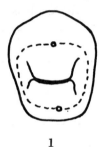

1   2

central

SECTION 5.1 MANDIBULAR SECOND PREMOLAR: FACIAL VIEW

From the facial aspect most features of the mandibular second premolar are similar to the first premolar. However, there is a small difference in the length of their facial cusps. Recall <u>that cusp length is defined as the measurement from the cusp tip to the depth of the occlusal grooves.</u> On which of these teeth is the facial cusp slightly shorter?

Permanent
Mandibular
Right
1. 1st Premolar
2. 2nd Premolar
FACIAL

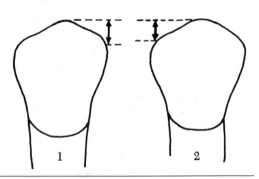

On the mandibular second premolar, the angle formed by the mesial and distal ridges of the facial cusp is less pointed. This blunter angulation is a result of the cusp tip of the second molar being _____ (shorter/longer).

Permanent
Mandibular
Right
1. 1st Premolar
2. 2nd Premolar
FACIAL

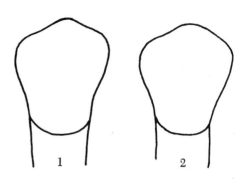

Compared to the mandibular first premolar, the position of the facial cusp of the mandibular second premolar is more toward the _____ (lingual/facial).

Permanent
Mandibular
Right
1., 3. 2nd Premolar
2., 4. 1st Premolar
1., 2. MESIAL
3., 4. OCCLUSAL

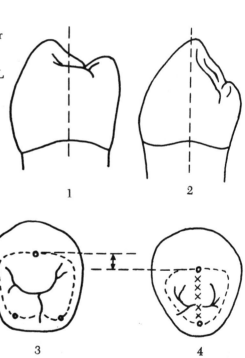

SECTION 5.2 MANDIBULAR SECOND PREMOLAR: LINGUAL VIEW

The lingual aspects of the mandibular first and second premolars are distinctly different. On the drawing of the lingual aspect, indicate which portion of the second premolar is the lingual· surface by sketching in the mesiolingual and distolingual line angles.

Permanent
Mandibular
Right
2nd Premolar
1. LINGUAL
2. OCCLUSAL

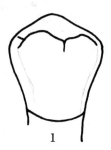
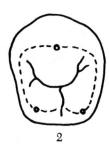

1   2

Compare your drawing with the illustration below.

In your own words describe the size of the lingual surface of the mandibular second premolar as compared to the lingual surface of the mandibular first premolar.

Permanent
Mandibular
Right
1. 2nd Premolar
2. 1st Premolar
LINGUAL

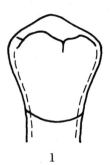
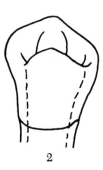

1   2

Your description should indicate that the lingual surface of the second premolar is wider in the mesiodistal direction and longer in the occlusocervical direction.

The lingual surface of the mandibular second premolar is marked by a groove running between the cusps. This groove is called the _____ groove.

Permanent
Mandibular
Right
2nd Premolar
LINGUAL

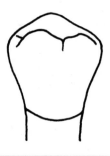

The lingual groove separates the two lingual cusps, the larger _____ cusp and the smaller _____ cusp.

SECTION 5.3 MANDIBULAR SECOND PREMOLAR: PROXIMAL VIEW

Of the three cusps on the mandibular second premolar, is the widest also the longest? _____ (yes/no)

Permanent
Mandibular
Right
2nd Premolar
LINGUAL

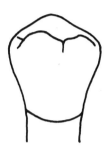

yes

The greater lingual development on the mandibular second premolar causes the mesial and distal marginal ridges to be nearly

Permanent
Mandibular
Right
2nd Premolar
1. MESIAL
2. DISTAL

   a. perpendicular to the long axis of the tooth.

   b. parallel to the lingual ridge of the facial cusp.

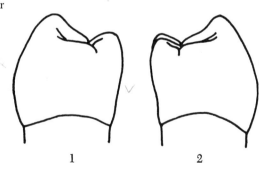

1   2

In place in the mouth, the mandibular first premolar is tipped slightly to the facial, (as is the mandibular canine). However, the second premolar, and the mandibular teeth posterior to it, are tipped toward the lingual.

The contours of the premolar crowns become continuous with the surrounding gingival tissue in this way. Also, this makes the occlusal planes of the premolars more _____ (in line/out of line).

Permanent
Mandibular
Right
1. 2nd Premolar
2. 1st Premolar
MESIAL

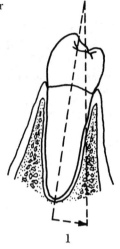
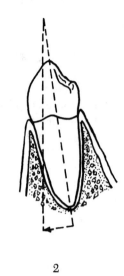

1   2

From an occlusal view, the location of the central pit, in a faciolingual direction, is _____ (central/toward the lingual).

Permanent
Mandibular
Right
2nd Premolar
OCCLUSAL

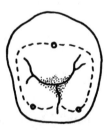

In the mesiodistal direction, the central pit is displaced slightly toward the _____ (mesial/distal).

Permanent
Mandibular
Right
2nd Premolar
OCCLUSAL

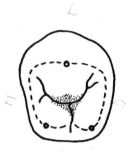

On the mandibular second premolar, which marginal ridge is at a lower level in the occlusocervical direction? _____

Permanent
Mandibular
Right
2nd Premolar
1. MESIAL
2. DISTAL

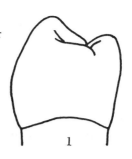
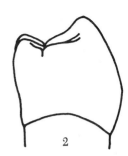

1   2

In the mandibular arch, the premolars somewhat resemble either a canine, or a molar. Of these two classes of teeth, the mandibular second premolar more closely resembles a _____ .

Permanent
Mandibular
Right
1. Canine
2. 1st Premolar
3. 2nd Premolar
4. 1st Molar
MESIAL

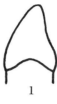

1   2

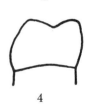

3   4

Indicate whether each of the diagrams represents a <u>maxillary or mandibular, first or second premolar.</u> (All are drawn with crowns toward the top of the page even if they are maxillary.)

Permanent
Premolars
MESIAL

Figure 1 _____ _____ *premolar*
Figure 2 _____ _____ *premolar*
Figure 3 _____ _____ *premolar*
Figure 4 _____ _____ *premolar*

F   1   2   L

3   4

In position in the mandibular arch, the mandibular second premolar has its crown tipped slightly toward the _____ (facial/lingual).

---

lingual

The second premolar is tipped to the lingual, whereas the crown of the mandibular first premolar is tipped toward the facial.

MATRIX TEXT 5

Directions . . .

Place an X in the square that matches the left hand column with the top row. Mark your answers and *turn to Page 295.*

Mandibular Second Premolar	Mesial	Distal
Occlusal fossae located at the . . .		
Larger of the two lingual cusps . . .		
Marginal ridge at lower level . . .		
Central pit displaced toward the . . .		

ANSWERS ON PAGE 295

REVIEW TEST 5

Choose the correct answers and make a note of them. *Turn to Page 296 to check your answers.*

Use this diagram for questions 1-4

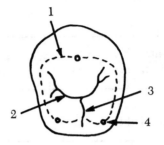

Identify each of the four features:

1. **a.** Mesial ridge of the buccal cusp.
   b. Distal ridge of the buccal cusp.

2. **a.** Central groove.
   b. Mesial groove.

3. **a.** Distolingual groove.
   b. Lingual groove.

4. **a.** Distolingual cusp.
   b. Distal cusp.

5. Which of the following describe the mandibular second premolar as compared to the mandibular first premolar:

   a. composed of five lobes most frequently.
   b. most frequently has two lingual cusps.
   c. has a less well developed lingual cusp.
   d. has a slightly shorter facial cusp.
   e. most frequently has a single highly developed transverse ridge.
   f. tip of facial cusp displaced toward the facial from the faciolingual midline of the tooth.
   g. the root of the tooth is tilted with its apex more toward the facial than its crown.

ANSWERS ON PAGE 296

SECTION 6.0 PROXIMAL CONTACTS, EMBRASURES AND CROWN CONTOURS OF THE PREMOLARS

Recall that the proximal contacts provide stability to the dental arch by helping to support the individual tooth.

Permanent
Maxillary
Anterior
FACIAL

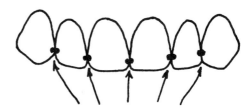

Contact Areas

The spaces or potential spaces that surround the contact areas are called the interdental areas and the _____.

Permanent
Maxillary
Right
a. 1st Molar
b. 2nd Premolar
c. 1st Premolar
1. FACIAL
2. OCCLUSAL

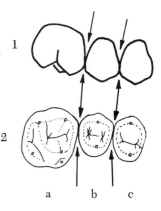

embrasures

The embrasures are named according to their location in relation to the contact. The embrasures located incisally or occlusally of the contact are called the incisal or occlusal embrasures. The embrasures located facially are called _____ embrasures, and those located lingually are called _____.

Permanent
Maxillary
Right
1. 2nd Molar
2. 1st Molar
3. 2nd Premolar
OCCLUSAL

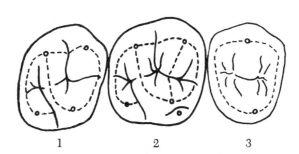

The proximal contact area is located in (1) the **incisocervical** or **occlusocervical dimension** and (2) the **faciolingual dimension**. In the diagram to the right, dimension A is the _____ dimension, and B is the _____ dimension.

Permanent
Maxillary
Right
2nd Premolar
PROXIMAL

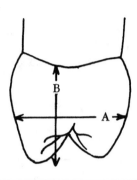

The faciolingual location of the proximal contact and the configuration of two embrasures are seen from an occlusal or incisal view. The two embrasures outlined in an occlusal view are the _____ and _____ embrasures.

Permanent
Maxillary
Right
1. 1st Molar
2. 2nd Premolar
OCCLUSAL

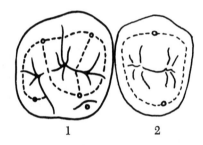

1   2

The relative depth of the facial and lingual embrasures is determined by the location of the contact faciolingually. If the contact is located more facially, the embrasure with the greater depth is the _____ embrasure.

Permanent
Maxillary
Right
1. 1st Molar
2. 2nd Premolar
OCCLUSAL

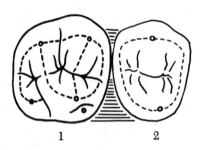

1   2

The drawings on the right show the proximal contacts of all teeth in both the incisocervical (occlusocervical) and faciolingual dimensions.

Study the drawings and then answer the questions in the next five frames. Refer back to these drawings as necessary to answer the questions.

In the region of the anterior teeth, the facial and lingual embrasures have approximately equal depth. The proximal contacts between anterior teeth are _____ (centered/more to the facial) in the faciolingual dimension.

Permanent
1. Maxillary
2. Mandibular
Left Quadrants
FACIAL

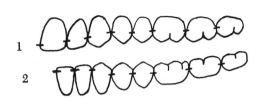

1

2

Inciso- or Occlusocervical Location of Contacts

Permanent
Maxillary
Right Quadrant and
Left Central Incisor
OCCLUSAL

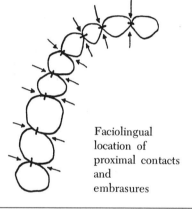

Faciolingual location of proximal contacts and embrasures

In the region of the posterior teeth, the lingual embrasures are deeper than facial embrasures. This is because the proximal contacts between posterior teeth are toward the _____ (facial/lingual) surface in the faciolingual dimension.

Faciolingually, all proximal contacts are either displaced slightly toward the _____ or are _____ on the faciolingual axis of the crown.

The relative depth of facial and lingual embrasures is determined by the location of the contact in the _____ dimension.

The incisocervical or occlusocervical location of the proximal contacts may be seen by examining a _____ view of the teeth.

In the incisocervical or occlusocervical dimension, if you examine the location of the proximal contacts from the anterior teeth back to the posterior teeth, you will see that the contacts tend to be located in or near the incisal third between anteriors and in or near the _____ third on the posteriors.

Both the mesial and distal contacts on each of the eight premolars are located occlusocervically, just cervical to the junction of the occlusal and middle thirds. Therefore, the contact areas on each of the premolars are in the _____ third of the crown.

Permanent
Maxillary
Left
1. Canine
2. 1st Premolar
3. 2nd Premolar
4. 1st Molar
Mandibular
5. Canine
6. 1st Premolar
7. 2nd Premolar
8. 1st Molar
FACIAL

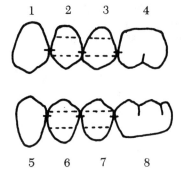

It is important to study the curved contours of crowns because there are many occasions for the dentist to operate on these contours in restoring or replacing crown surfaces. There is clinical evidence that smooth and properly contoured (not too convex) crown surfaces promote tooth cleaning and gingival health.

The curved contours of the crown are normally continuous with the gingiva, as shown in the drawing. This form seems to help make the _____ (cervical/occlusal) areas of the teeth cleanable.

Permanent
Mandibular
Right
1st Premolar
FACIOLINGUAL
    SECTION

F   L

One of the best ways to study the contour of crowns is to focus on the **height of contour.** The height of contour is an imaginary line encircling the entire crown of the tooth. The proximal contacts of a tooth lie _____ (along/above) the height of contour.

Permanent
Mandibular
Right
1st Premolar
MESIAL

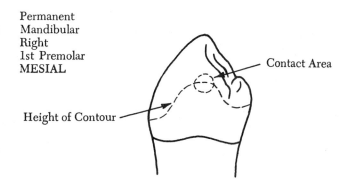

Contact Area

Height of Contour

cervical

along

Maxillary posterior teeth have the height of contour in the middle third on the _____ surface.

Permanent
Maxillary
Right
2nd Molar
MESIAL

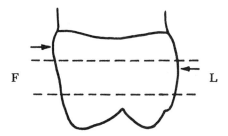

F   L

lingual

In proximal view, maxillary teeth give the impression that the amount of contour is greater on the facial than on the lingual surface (especially true for anterior teeth). However, careful examination will show that the contour, both facially and lingually, for all maxillary teeth measures approximately _____ mm.

Permanent
Maxillary
Right
1. Central Incisor
2. 1st Premolar
MESIAL

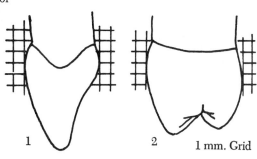

1   2   1 mm. Grid

Both the maxillary posterior teeth and the mandibular posterior teeth have the height of contour on the facial surface in the _____ third and the lingual height of contour the _____ third.

Permanent
1. Mandibular Left
1st Premolar
DISTAL
2. Maxillary Right
1st Premolar
MESIAL

1   2

cervical, middle

The amount of contour on the facial surfaces of mandibular posteriors is similar to that on the facial surfaces of the maxillary posterior teeth. This contour measures approximately _____ mm.

Permanent
Mandibular
Left
1. 1st Premolar
2. 1st Molar
DISTAL

1   2
1 mm. Grid

The mandibular posterior teeth have lingual contours that measure nearly double those of the maxillaries. The amount of contour on the lingual surface of mandibular posterior teeth approaches _____ mm in measurement.

Permanent
Mandibular
Right
1st Molar
MESIAL

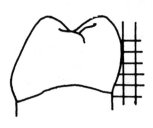

When examining the mandibular second pre-molar in position in the oral cavity, the observed lingual height of contour may appear closer to the occlusal surface than the anatomical contour would suggest. This is because the mandibular second premolar (and the mandibular molars) are inclined, so that their crowns are tilted toward the _____ (facial/lingual/distal).

Permanent
Mandibular
Right
2nd Premolar
MESIAL

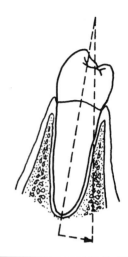

lingual

The height of contour is located in the middle third on the lingual surface of all maxillary and mandibular _____ (anterior/posterior) teeth.

posterior

SECTION 6.1 ROOT ANATOMY OF THE PREMOLARS

The maxillary first premolar is the only pre-molar that commonly occurs in two different root types—single-rooted and bifurcated—but the most common root type is the _____ type.

Permanent
Maxillary
Right
1st Premolars
1. Bifurcated
2. Single rooted
MESIAL

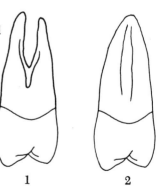

341

The bifurcation commonly occurs in either the apical or middle third of the root. Generally, the root is bifurcated for approximately half its length. Therefore, the bifurcation most commonly occurs in the _____ third and less commonly the _____ third of the root.

Permanent
Maxillary
Right
1st Premolars
MESIAL

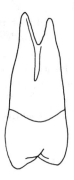
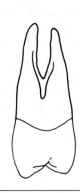

When present, the bifurcation is in the mesiodistal direction. The two terminal roots are therefore the _____ and _____ roots.

Permanent
Maxillary
Right
1st Premolar
1. MESIAL
2. FACIAL

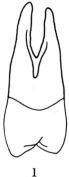
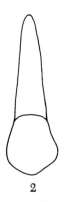

1   2

A horizontal section shows that both terminal roots of the maxillary first premolar are oval to nearly round.

Permanent
Maxillary
Right
1st Premolar
MESIAL

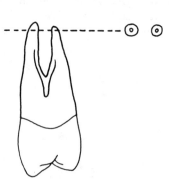

In the longitudinal direction, both terminal roots are nearly straight, but it is not uncommon to find a slight deflection of each root to either the facial or lingual. Which drawing shows a straight lingual root and a facial root with a facial deflection? _____

Permanent
Maxillary
Left
1st Premolars
DISTAL

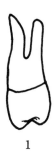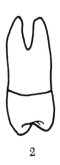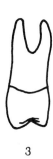

1 2 3

Figure 1

The mesial surface of the root trunk on a maxillary first premolar has a deep developmental groove that runs from the bifurcation to the cervical line and continues onto the cervical portion of the mesial crown surface as a concavity.

On the distal surface, the longitudinal groove is greatly reduced. In the cervical region of the distal surface of the root trunk, the faciolingual curvature is flat or slightly convex. In the horizontal section (Fig. 2), the mesial surface is toward _____ (A/B).

Permanent
Maxillary
Right
1st Premolar
1. MESIAL
2. HORIZONTAL SECTION

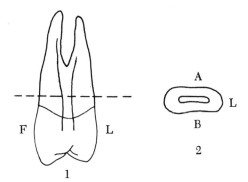

B

A horizontal section of the root trunk (Fig. 2), shows that the facial and lingual surfaces are convex. Which surface is more narrow—the facial or lingual? _____.

Permanent
Maxillary
Right
1st Premolar
1. MESIAL
2. HORIZONTAL
   SECTION

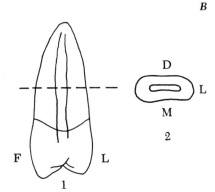

The mesial and distal surfaces on the single-rooted form of the maxillary first premolar are marked by longitudinal grooves similar to those on the root trunk of the bifurcated form. The longitudinal groove is more highly developed on the _____ surface.

Permanent
Maxillary
Right
1st Premolar
1. MESIAL
2. HORIZONTAL SECTION

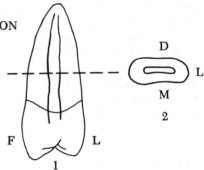

The cervical portion of the root structure on the two forms of the maxillary first premolar is generally similar. In the longitudinal direction, the cervical portions of the facial and lingual surfaces are _____ (straight/convex).

Permanent
Maxillary
Right
1st Premolar
1. Bifurcated
2. Single Rooted
MESIAL

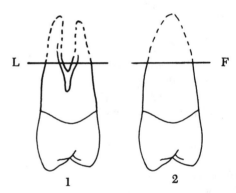

The mesial and distal surfaces have longitudinal curvatures in the cervical portion that are nearly straight or very slightly convex. Of the two pairs of opposite root surfaces (mesial, distal/facial, lingual), on which pair is the longitudinal curvature more pronounced?

_____

Permanent
Maxillary
Right
1st Premolar
1. FACIAL
2. MESIAL

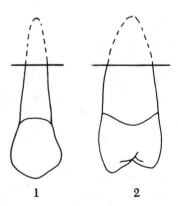

344

The maxillary *second* premolar has a root which is generally _____ (single/multi-rooted).

The root of the maxillary second premolar closely resembles the single-rooted form of the maxillary first premolar. The key distinction is the extent of the longitudinal groove on the mesial surface.

The maxillary second premolar does not have a longitudinal groove as highly developed as the first premolar. Also, the distal surfaces on the two teeth are more nearly alike. Both proximal root surfaces on the maxillary second premolar have a longitudinal groove and, therefore, a curvature in the faciolingual direction that is nearly flat to _____.

Permanent
Maxillary
Right
2nd Premolar
1. MESIAL
2. HORIZONTAL SECTION
1st Premolar
3. MESIAL
4. HORIZONTAL
   SECTION

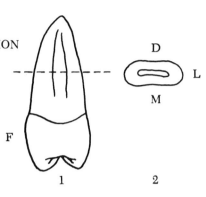

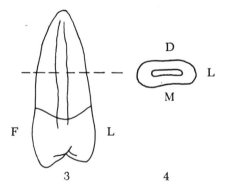

In terms of pointed or rounded, the apex of the maxillary second premolar (mesial or distal view) is _____.

Permanent
Maxillary
Right
2nd Premolar
MESIAL

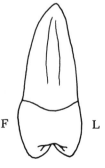

345

The mandibular first premolar is normally _____ -rooted.

Permanent
Mandibular
Right
1st Premolar
1. FACIAL
2. MESIAL

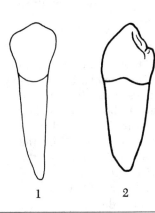

1   2

single

Most frequently the mesial and distal surfaces on a mandibular premolar tend to be convex in the faciolingual direction. A shallow longitudinal groove may be present on the proximal root surfaces. When present, the grooves cause the central part of these surfaces to be slightly concave or nearly flat in the faciolingual direction. Which drawing illustrates the more common form on the mesial and distal root surfaces of a mandibular premolar? _____

Permanent
Mandibular
Right
1st Premolar
1. MESIAL
2. MESIAL

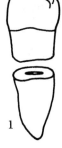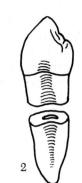

1   2

Figure 1

The root of the mandibular second premolar is similar in form to the mandibular first premolar, but is _____ (larger/smaller) in all directions.

Permanent
Mandibular
Right
1. 1st Premolar
2. 2nd Premolar
MESIAL

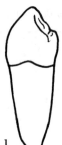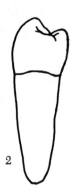

1   2

The mandibular premolar root tends to have a more oval shape as seen from a horizontal section (Fig. 3), when longitudinal grooves are not present. The longitudinal curvature of the facial surface is irregular, having both convexities and concavities. The lingual, mesial, and distal surfaces are more evenly contoured in the longitudinal direction and tend to be flat or very slightly convex. The longitudinal curvatures result in a root with a distinct taper on all four surfaces and an apex more pointed than the apexes on the single-rooted premolars in the maxillary arch. Considering the root forms on the premolars, in which arch could a premolar be more easily rotated in its alveolus? _____

Mandibular arch ..GO TO TOP OF PAGE 348
Maxillary arch.........GO TO NEXT FRAME

Permanent
Mandibular
Right
2nd Premolar
1. LINGUAL
2. DISTAL
3. HORIZONTAL
   SECTION

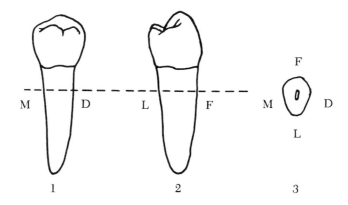

♦ From preceding frame

maxillary arch is incorrect

Recall that the maxillary arch includes the bifurcated first premolar which would be tricky to rotate.

RETURN TO PRECEDING FRAME AND ANSWER AGAIN.

Here is a comparison of the root structures of the premolars in each arch.

Maxillary arch
    Frequently bifurcated (especially first premolars).
    Broad in the faciolingual direction.
    Distinct longitudinal grooves.

Mandibular arch
    Single-rooted.
    Tends to be oval in horizontal section.

More slender than those of the maxillary arch.
Tapered in longitudinal direction.
Shallow or no longitudinal grooves.

The root forms of the premolars in the maxillary arch would be generally resistant to rotation in their alveoli. In the mandibular arch, the root forms of the premolars would tend to allow rotation.

The apex on each of the single-rooted permanent premolars, particularly the maxillary second premolar, may have a slight deviation toward the molars. The deviation of the apex of the premolars is, therefore, in the _____ direction.

Permanent
Mandibular
Right
2nd Premolar
FACIAL

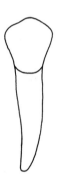

distal

On the mandibular premolars, the facial and lingual surfaces are smoothly convex. The mesial and distal surfaces may show a horizontal curvature with a slight central concavity created by the _____.

Permanent
Mandibular
Right
2nd Premolar
1. FACIAL
2. HORIZONTAL SECTION

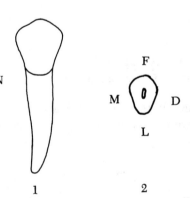

1   2

longitudinal groove

NOW GO TO THE NEXT PAGE FOR MATRIX TEST 6.

MATRIX TEST 6

Directions . .

Place an X in the square that matches the left hand column with the top row.

Turn to Page 297 and check your answers.

	Maxillary		Mandibular	
	First Premolar	Second Premolar	First Premolar	Second Premolar
Most commonly a single-rooted tooth.				
Tooth whose mesial surface has the most prominent longitudinal groove.				
Amount of contour equals 1 mm. on lingual surface.				
Two teeth which usually have an oval to nearly round horizontal root form.				
Premolars whose single root has a rounded or blunt apex (seen from the proximal view).				

ANSWERS ON PAGE 297

349

REVIEW TEST 6

Make a note of your answers and check them on Page 298.

1. Choose the CORRECT statement.
   a. The lingual embrasures are deeper than the facial embrasures on the premolars.
   b. The facial embrasures are deeper than the lingual embrasures on the premolars.

2. Choose the CORRECT statement.
   a. The proximal contacts of the premolars are located, in the occlusocervical dimension, just occlusal to the junction of the occlusal and middle thirds.
   b. The proximal contacts of the premolars are located in the occlusocervical dimension, just cervical to the junction of the occlusal and middle thirds.

3. On the facial and lingual surfaces of the premolars, where are the heights of contour located:
   a. In the cervical third on the facial and in the cervical third on the lingual.
   b. In the middle third on the facial and in the cervical third on the lingual.
   c. In the cervical third on the facial and in the middle third on the lingual.

4. Describe the alignment of the mandibular second premolar in position in the alveolar bone.

ANSWERS ON PAGE 298.

SECTION 7.0 PULP ANATOMY OF THE PREMOLARS

A maxillary first premolar may have one or two terminal roots, but in either case two root canals are generally present. Similar to the relative positions of the terminal roots on a bifurcated root structure, the root canals are located toward the _____ and _____.

Permanent
Maxillary
1st Premolar
FACIOLINGUAL
SECTION

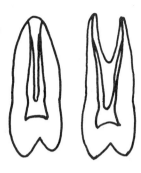

facial, lingual

If the drawings constitute a representative sample of all maxillary first premolars, you may deduce that about _____% have only one canal.

Permanent
Maxillary
1st Premolars
FACIOLINGUAL
SECTIONS

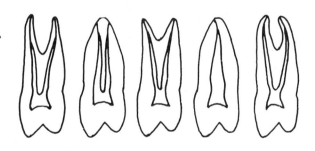

20

In the case of the single canal, it is wider in the _____ direction.

Permanent
Maxillary
1st Premolar
1. FACIOLINGUAL SECTION
2. MESIODISTAL SECTION

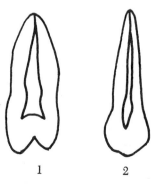

1   2

351

Whether a maxillary premolar has one or two terminal roots, the number of pulp horns corresponds to the number of cusps. How many pulp horns will be present in the pulp chamber of a maxillary premolar? _____

two

As seen in mesiodistal section, the pulp cavity form of the maxillary first premolar is similar to that of a maxillary _____ (canine/incisor).

Permanent
Maxillary
1st Premolar
MESIODISTAL
SECTION

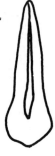

canine

A horizontal section taken at the level of the cervical line on a maxillary premolar cuts through the pulp chamber. On maxillary premolars, the floor of the pulp chamber is located _____ (apical/oclusal) to the cervical line.

Permanent
Maxillary
1st Premolar
1. FACIOLINGUAL
    SECTION
2. HORIZONTAL
    SECTION

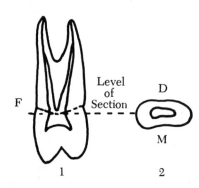

apical

With the exception of the relative frequency of teeth with a single root canal, the form of the pulp chamber on the maxillary second premolar is similar to that of the maxillary first premolar. As suggested by the relative frequency of the bifurcated roots, which maxillary premolar is most likely to have a single root canal? _____

As shown by the drawings, approximately 60% of the maxillary second premolars have _____ (number) root canals.

Permanent
Maxillary
2nd Premolars
FACIOLINGUAL
   SECTIONS

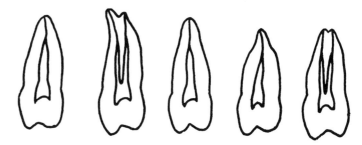

one

The pulp cavities of the mandibular first and second premolars are similar in form, the chief distinction being the pulp chamber. As suggested by the cusp development on the two teeth, one pulp chamber has two well-developed pulp horns; the other has one. Which mandibular premolar would have a facial and lingual pulp horn?

_____

Permanent
Mandibular
1. 1st Premolar
2. 2nd Premolar
FACIOLINGUAL
   SECTIONS

F 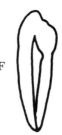 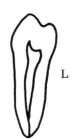 L

Because of the cusp development on the mandibular first premolar, which pulp horn is usually absent or very small? _____

Permanent
Mandibular
1st Premolar
FACIOLINGUAL SECTION

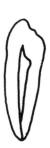

A faciolingual longitudinal section of the mandibular first premolar shows a spindle-shaped pulp canal with one horn, the _____ pulp horn.

Permanent
Mandibular
1st Premolar
FACIOLINGUAL SECTION

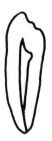

Because the mandibular premolar has a single root canal, the division between the pulp chamber and root canal is indistinct. Premolars with a single root canal have a pulp chamber with no _____ (roof/floor/walls).

Permanent
Mandibular
1st Premolar
FACIOLINGUAL SECTION

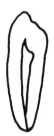

Similar to the root canals of the mandibular canine, the root canal of a mandibular premolar is widest in which horizontal direction?

Permanent
Mandibular
1st Premolar
1. FACIOLINGUAL SECTION
2. MESIODISTAL SECTION

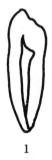

1   2

A bifurcated root canal is rare in the mandibular premolars. When found, the bifurcation generally occurs in the _____ portion of the root.

Permanent
Mandibular
1st Premolar
FACIOLINGUAL
    SECTION

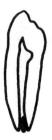

Occasionally, lateral branches of the root canal will be present in the apical portion of the root. These branches are called _____.

Permanent
Mandibular
1st Premolar
FACIOLINGUAL
   SECTION

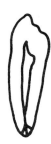

---

accessory canals

Which represents the form of the pulp cavity of a mandibular *first* premolar as seen in faciolingual section? _____

Figure 1 . . . . .GO TO NEXT FRAME
Figure 2 . . . .GO TO BOTTOM OF THIS PAGE

Permanent
Mandibular
Premolars
FACIOLINGUAL
   SECTIONS OF
   PULP CAVITIES

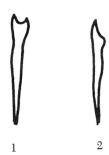

          1   2

◗ From preceding frame

Figure 1 is incorrect

The mandibular first premolar usually has one pulp horn. You chose the illustration with two pulp horns, which is typical of the mandibular second premolar.

Permanent
Mandibular
1. 2nd Premolar
2. 1st Premolar
FACIOLINGUAL
   SECTIONS

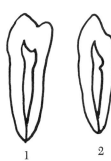

          1   2

TURN TO PAGE 356 AND TAKE MATRIX TEST 7.

◗ From middle of this page

Figure 2 is correct

MATRIX TEST 7

Directions . .

Write in the correct word(s) in the square that matches the left hand column with the top row *and turn to Page 299.*

Pulp of Premolars	Max. First Premolar	Mand. First Premolar	Max. Second Premolar	Mand. Second Premolar
Most common number of root canals.				
If the tooth has a less common number of root canals, what number of canals would that be?				
Number of pulp horns in pulp chamber.				
Names of usual root canals (if more than one).				

ANSWERS ON PAGE 299

REVIEW TEST 7

SURPRISE!

As a gesture of good will for the effort you have put into studying this volume, this last review test has been made as brief as possible.

1. When the premolars have a single root canal, that root canal is narrower in which direction?
   a. Mesiodistal
   b. Faciolingual
   c. Occlusocervical
   d. Sideways

ANSWER ON PAGE 300.

4
THE PERMANENT MOLARS

SECTION 1.0 ERUPTION OF THE MOLARS

The eruption of the permanent molars is related to the growth and development of the maxilla and mandible. Since the permanent incisors, canines, and premolars succeed the primary dentition, the permanent molars erupt in positions _____ (anterior/posterior) to the original positions of the primary dentition.

1. Permanent
2. Primary
Maxillary
Left Quadrant
FACIAL

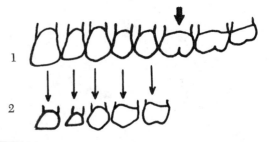

posterior

The permanent teeth replacing the primary dentition are called succedaneous teeth. Permanent molars are called _____ teeth.

non-succedaneous

The permanent first molars are the first permanent teeth to erupt. At the time of eruption, the permanent maxillary first molar is in contact mesially with the

_____ _____
(dentition)   (arch)

_____.
(tooth)

1. Permanent
2. Primary
Maxillary
Left Quadrants
FACIAL

After the eruption of the permanent dentition, the permanent maxillary first molar is in contact mesially with the _____

(dentition)

_____ _____.

(arch)   (tooth)

Permanent
Maxillary
Left
FACIAL

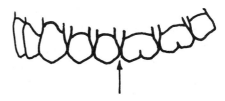

permanent maxillary second premolar

The eruption sequence of the permanent dentition was discussed in Chapter 1. Check your recall by answering these questions.

    a. At what age, approximately, do the permanent first molars erupt? _____.

    b. In which arch does the permanent first molar usually erupt first? _____.

a. six, b. mandibular

On molar teeth, each lobe is represented by a cusp. Both the permanent maxillary first molar and the permanent mandibular first molar have _____ (number) lobes.

Permanent
1. Maxillary
2. Mandibular
Right
1st Molar
OCCLUSAL

1   2

F   F

D   M   D

L   L

five

SECTION 1.1 MAXILLARY FIRST MOLAR: OCCLUSAL VIEW

There is a great deal of variation in the development of the cusp of Carabelli on the mesiolingual surface of the mesiolingual cusp of the maxillary first molar. It may be completely absent, appear as a groove or as a cusp. For this reason, the maxillary first molar may be thought of as having only how many major cusps? _____.

Permanent
Maxillary
Right
1st Molar
1. Five cusps
2. Four cusps
OCCLUSAL

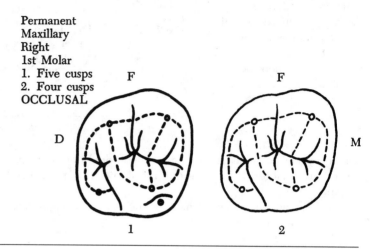

1   2

four

The two facial cusps of the maxillary first molar are named the _____ cusp and the _____ cusp.

Permanent
Maxillary
Right
1st Molar
OCCLUSAL

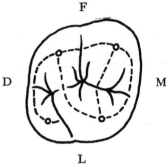

mesiofacial (mesiobuccal), distofacial (distobuccal)

The two lingual cusps are called the _____ cusp and the _____ cusp.

Permanent
Maxillary
Right
1st Molar
OCCLUSAL

When highly developed, the fifth cusp of the permanent maxillary first molar (the cusp of Carabelli) is seen lingual to the _____ cusp.

Permanent
Maxillary
Right
1st Molar
OCCLUSAL

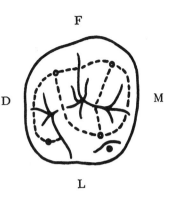

The occlusal surface of the maxillary first molar varies a good deal from person to person. The occlusal outline may appear square (Fig. 1) or rhomboidal (Fig. 2) or quadrilateral (Fig. 3). This means that, unlike any other tooth in the permanent dentition, the mesiodistal width at the lingual is equal to (and at times slightly greater than) the width at the _____.

Permanent
Maxillary
Right
1st Molar
OCCLUSAL
1. Square
2. Rhomboidal
3. Quadrilateral

1   2   3

When the occlusal outline is rhomboidal, the junctions of which sides (facial, lingual, mesial, distal) of the rhomboid form acute angles? _____ and _____, _____ and _____.

Permanent
Maxillary
Right
1st Molar
OCCLUSAL

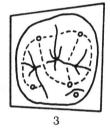

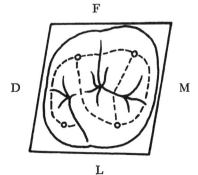

361

There are several major features that characterize the occlusal view of the maxillary first molar:

1. Lines connecting the cusp tips of the three largest cusps form a triangle.
2. The faciolingual diameter is equal to or greater than the mesiodistal width.
3. There is usually a pronounced oblique ridge from the distofacial cusp to the mesiolingual cusp.
4. The distolingual cusp is less developed than the three larger cusps.
5. A small fifth cusp, the cusp of Carabelli, is frequently present.

Each of these will be discussed in turn.

Permanent
Maxillary
Right
1st Molar
OCCLUSAL

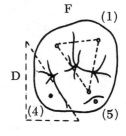
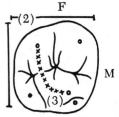
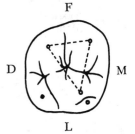
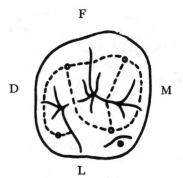

What are the names of the three major cusps that form a triangle if lines are drawn to connect their cusp tips? ————, ———, —————.

Permanent
Maxillary
Right
1st Molar
OCCLUSAL

Of the three major cusps on the maxillary first molar, which is the widest mesiodistally? —————.

   a.   mesiofacial
   b.   mesiolingual

Permanent
Maxillary
Right
1st Molar
OCCLUSAL

Maxillary molars have crowns with a faciolingual size that is equal to or greater than the _____ width of the crown.

Permanent
Maxillary
Right
1st Molar
OCCLUSAL

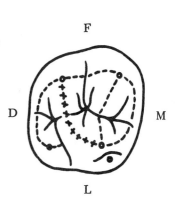

Maxillary molars have a characteristic **oblique ridge**. An oblique ridge is the union of two ridges running obliquely across the occlusal surface. On the maxillary first molar, the oblique ridge is made up of the distal ridge of the mesiolingual cusp and the _____ ridge of the distofacial cusp.

Permanent
Maxillary
Right
1st Molar
OCCLUSAL

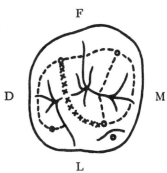

Oblique ridges are found only on the molar teeth in one arch and running in the same direction. Therefore, oblique ridges are found only on the molars of the _____ arch and always run between the _____ facial cusp and the _____ lingual cusp.

Permanent
Maxillary
Right
1st Molar
OCCLUSAL

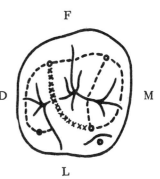

Complete the following list of the five cusps of the maxillary first molar in the order of their size, largest to smallest (mesiodistal measurement).

    a. mesiolingual
    b. _____
    c. _____
    d. _____
    e. cusp of Carabelli

Permanent
Maxillary
Right
1st Molar
OCCLUSAL

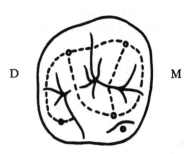

D   M

b. mesiofacial; c. distofacial; d. distolingual

On the drawing, sketch the path of the **oblique** ridge.

    Compare your work with the drawing on the previous page.

Permanent
Maxillary
Right
1st Molar
OCCLUSAL

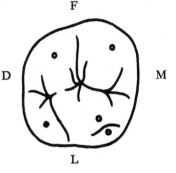

F   D   M   L

GO TO THE NEXT FRAME AFTER COMPARING YOUR DRAWING.

The smaller distolingual cusp of the maxillary first molar forms somewhat of a shelf that is lower in elevation than the rest of the occlusal surface. This triangular shelf has one side that is distolingual to and parallel with the _____ (oblique/marginal) ridge.

Permanent
Maxillary
Right
1st Molar
OCCLUSAL

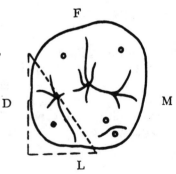

F   D   M   L

To review, complete the following list of the three major characteristics of the occlusal view of the maxillary first molar:

1. _____.
2. _____.
3. _____.
4. The distolingual cusp is less developed than the three larger cusps and forms a triangular area distolingual to the oblique ridge.
5. The small fifth cusp is frequently present.

Permanent
Maxillary
Right
1st Molar
OCCLUSAL

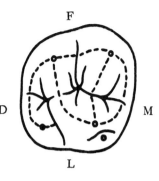

1. The three largest cusps form a triangle. 2. Faciolingual diameter equal to or greater than the mesiodistal. 3. There is a prominent oblique ridge.

Name the small fifth cusp which is often present on the permanent maxillary first molar: _____.

Permanent
Maxillary
Right
1st Molar
OCCLUSAL

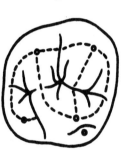

The facial ridges of the two facial cusps descend in the cervical direction to become part of the _____.

Permanent
Maxillary
Right
1st Molar
OCCLUSAL

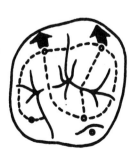

The lingual ridges of the two facial cusps are triangular ridges; therefore, they descend to the central area of the _____ _____.

Permanent
Maxillary
Right
1st Molar
OCCLUSAL

F

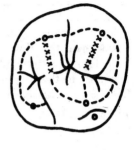

D

M

L

Keeping in mind the rules for naming ridges and the cusps involved, name the four ridges that form the faciocclusal line angle of the maxillary first molar _____ _____ _____ _____.

Permanent
Maxillary
Right
1st Molar
OCCLUSAL

F

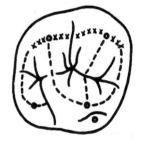

D

M

L

mesial and distal ridges of the mesiofacial cusp;
mesial and distal ridges of the distofacial cusp

Name the ridges labeled in the drawing:

a. _____.
b. _____.
c. _____.
d. _____.
e. _____.

Permanent
Maxillary
Right
1st Molar
OCCLUSAL

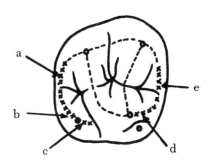

a. distal marginal ridge; b. distal ridge of the
distolingual cusp; c. mesial ridge of the
distolingual cusp; d. mesial ridge of the
mesiolingual cusp; e. mesial marginal ridge

On the maxillary first molar, mesial and distal ridges of the
cusps, the mesial marginal ridge and the distal marginal ridge
form the boundary of the _____ _____.

Permanent
Maxillary
Right
1st Molar
OCCLUSAL

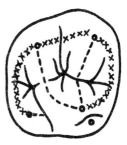

The ridges crossing the occlusal surface of the maxillary first molar divide that surface into _____ (number) fossae.

Permanent
Maxillary
Right
1st Molar
OCCLUSAL

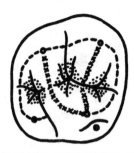

three

The fossae on either side of the central fossa are called the mesial and distal fossa. Therefore, the oblique ridge separates the _____ fossa from the _____ fossa.

Permanent
Maxillary
Right
1st Molar
OCCLUSAL

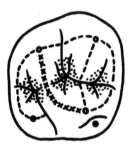

distal, central

The lingual ridge of the mesiofacial cusp and the facial ridge of the mesiolingual cusp separate the central fossa from the _____ fossa.

Permanent
Maxillary
Right
1st Molar
OCCLUSAL

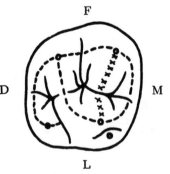

Within each of the three fossae, a pointed depression (called a pit) is found at the intersection of two or more developmental ——.

Permanent
Maxillary
Right
1st Molar
OCCLUSAL

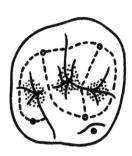

The occlusal pits of the maxillary first molar are named for the fossa in which they are found. The pits labeled A, B, and C are the ———— pit, ———— pit, and ———— pit.

Permanent
Maxillary
Right
1st Molar
OCCLUSAL

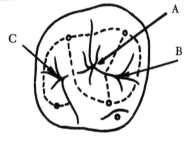

A. central; B. mesial; C. distal

The coalescence of the mesiofacial and distofacial lobes is marked by the facial groove which originates at the central pit and runs in the ———— direction.

Permanent
Maxillary
Right
1st Molar
OCCLUSAL

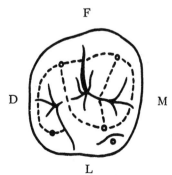

369

The oblique ridge, if highly developed, is not crossed by a groove (Fig. 1). However, if the oblique ridge is not as prominent (Fig. 2), both the mesial and distal grooves originate at the central pit and terminate at the mesial and distal pits. The mesial and distal grooves together form the central groove. Which part of the central groove may cross the oblique ridge? _____.

Permanent
Maxillary
Right
1st Molar
OCCLUSAL

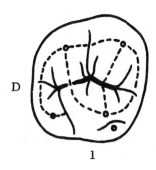

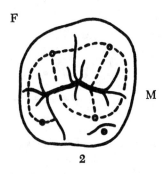

1   2

The union of the two ridges forming the oblique ridge is relatively complete. Because the distal groove may or may not cross the oblique ridge, the distal groove is often separated into two parts.

Of the mesial and distal developmental grooves which is more distinct? _____.

Permanent
Maxillary
Right
1st Molar
OCCLUSAL

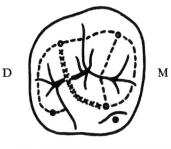

The mesial and distal grooves form the two parts of the central groove. For the maxillary first molar, the term "central groove" refers to the one running in the mesiodistal direction between the _____ _____ and the _____ _____.

Permanent
Maxillary
Right
1st Molar
OCCLUSAL

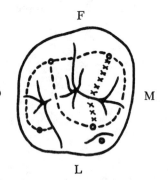

In addition to the mesial groove, the mesial fossa contains three grooves that are confluent at the mesial pit: the mesiofacial triangular groove, the mesiolingual triangular groove, and the mesial marginal groove.

The grooves marked A, B, and C are . . .

A. _____.
B. _____.
C. _____.

Permanent
Maxillary
Right
1st Molar
OCCLUSAL

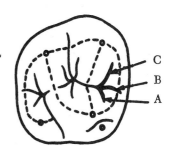

A. mesiolingual triangular; B. mesial marginal;
C. mesiofacial triangular

Five grooves run through the distal fossa. One of these is the distal groove. The longest, most distinct is the distolingual groove. It extends onto the lingual surface and separates the mesiolingual cusp from the _____ cusp.

Permanent
Maxillary
Right
1st Molar
OCCLUSAL

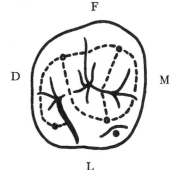

distolingual

The grooves (labeled A, B, and C) originate at the distal pit and are named similar to the corresponding grooves in the mesial fossa; these are the . . .

A. _____ groove,
B. _____ groove, and the
C. _____ groove.

Permanent
Maxillary
Right
1st Molar
OCCLUSAL

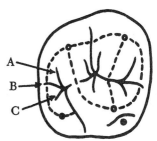

The accessory fifth cusp of the maxillary first molar is separated from the mesiolingual cusp by the mesiolingual developmental groove. The mesiolingual developmental groove _____ (is/is not) within the occlusal surface.

Permanent
Maxillary
Right
1st Molar
OCCLUSAL

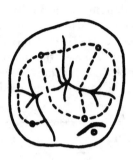

is

The mesiolingual cusp of the maxillary first molar is separated from the distolingual cusp by the _____ groove and from the fifth cusp by the _____ groove.

Permanent
Maxillary
Right
1st Molar
OCCLUSAL

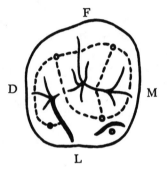

distolingual, mesiolingual (in that order)

GO TO THE NEXT PAGE FOR MATRIX TEST 1

MATRIX TEST 1

Directions . . .

Place an X in the square that matches the left hand column with the top row. Turn to Page 417 to check your answers.

	Mesio-facial	Mesio-lingual	Disto-lingual	Disto-facial
Cusp with widest mesiodistal measurement				
Two cusps joined by oblique ridge				
The cusp which is least developed of the four major cusps				
Cusp nearest the cusp of Carabelli				
Cusps with ridges that surround the central fossa				

ANSWERS ON PAGE 417

373

REVIEW TEST 1

Make a note of your answers. Turn to Page 418 to check them.

1. Select the true statement.
    a. At the time of eruption, the permanent maxillary first molar is in contact mesially with the permanent maxillary second premolar.
    b. From the occlusal aspect of a rhomboid-shaped maxillary first molar, the mesiofacial angle of the rhomboid shape is often acute.

2. Which of the following statements is more correct?
    a. The permanent maxillary first molar has three lobes.
    b. An oblique ridge is found only on maxillary molars and always runs between the mesiolingual and distofacial cusps.

3. Select the true statement.
    a. On the permanent maxillary first molar, the mesial groove is usually more distinct than the distal groove.
    b. The occlusal fossae of the permanent maxillary first molar are called the mesial, distal, central, and lingual fossae.

4. The faciocclusal line angle of the maxillary first molar is formed by the . . .
    a. Mesial and distal ridges of the mesiofacial and distofacial cusps.
    b. Mesial and distal ridges of the mesiofacial cusp and the mesial ridge of the distofacial cusp.

5. Here is an exercise to help you name the grooves on the occlusal portion of the maxillary first molar.
    Write in the names of the lettered grooves as shown in the illutration.
    a. _____
    b. _____
    c. _____
    d. _____
    e. _____
    f. _____

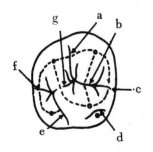

ANSWERS ON PAGE 418.

SECTION 2.0 MAXILLARY FIRST MOLAR: FACIAL VIEW

In general, the outline of the facial view of the maxillary first molar is closest to which of these shapes? _____ (circle/trapezoid/square)

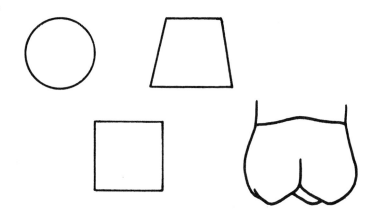

trapezoid

Originating at the central pit and emerging from between the two facial cusps is the _____ groove.

Permanent
Maxillary
Right
1st Molar
1. OCCLUSAL
2. FACIAL

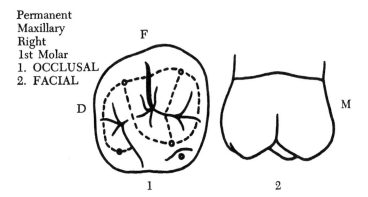

facial

The intersection of the mesial and facial surfaces tends to form an _____ angle, while the intersection of the facial and distal surfaces forms an _____ angle.

Permanent
Maxillary
Right
1st Molar
1. OCCLUSAL
2. FACIAL

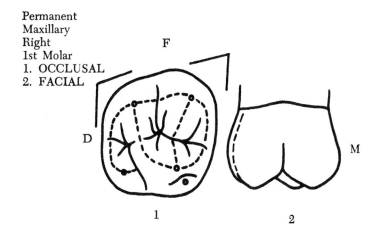

From a facial view, a portion of the distal surface can be seen particularly on those maxillary first molars with a rhomboidal occlusal surface.

Permanent
Maxillary
Right
1st Molar
FACIAL

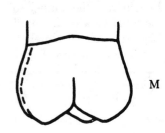

D   M

The facial groove terminates in a dip in the facial contour occlusocervically in the _____ third of the crown.

Permanent
Maxillary
Right
1st Molar
FACIAL

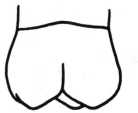

D   M

middle

As the facial groove progresses in the cervical direction from the occlusal, it gradually becomes _____ (more/less) distinct.

Permanent
Maxillary
Right
1st Molar
FACIAL

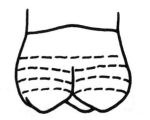

D   M

less

The terminal end of the facial groove is sometimes marked by a small pointed pit. What is the logical name for that pit? _____.

Permanent
Maxillary
Right
1st Molar
FACIAL

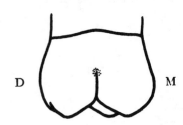

D   M

Compare the mesiodistal contour of the facial surface at (a) the height of contour with that at (b) the junction of the occlusal and middle thirds. The difference in shape is the concavity caused by the ⎯⎯⎯⎯⎯.

Permanent
Maxillary
Right
1st Molar
FACIAL

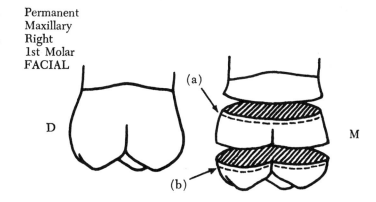

The convexity on either side of the facial groove is formed by the ⎯⎯⎯⎯⎯ ⎯⎯⎯⎯⎯ of each facial cusp.

Permanent
Maxillary
Right
1st Molar
FACIAL

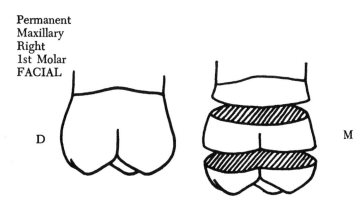

At the height of contour (mesiodistal direction), the form of the facial surface is ⎯⎯⎯⎯⎯.

Permanent
Maxillary
Right
1st Molar
FACIAL

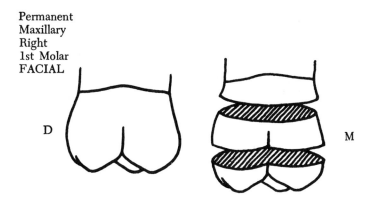

377

Of the two facial cusps on the maxillary first molar, which cusp is wider mesiodistally? _____.

Permanent
Maxillary
Right
1st Molar
FACIAL

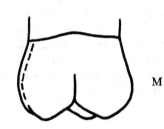

D   M

In the "V" shaped concavity between the distal ridge of the mesiofacial cusp and the mesial ridge of the distofacial cusp, one sees a portion of one of the lingual cusps. Which cusp is it? _____.

Permanent
Maxillary
Right
1st Molar
1. FACIAL
2. OCCLUSAL

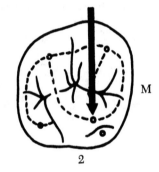

D

M

1   2

SECTION 2.1   MAXILLARY FIRST MOLAR: LINGUAL VIEW

The lingual outline of the maxillary first molar is the same as the facial outline. A portion of the _____ surface can be seen from the lingual.

Permanent
Maxillary
Right
1st Molar
LINGUAL

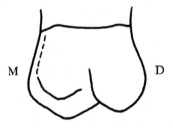

M   D

From the lingual view, the crown is trapezoid in outline. The trapezoid is narrower at the _____ (occlusal/cervical).

Permanent
Maxillary
Right
1st Molar
LINGUAL

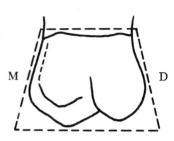

Earlier, you learned the names of the two developmental grooves that appear on the lingual surface of the maxillary first molar: the (A) _____ _____ and the (B) _____ _____.

Permanent
Maxillary
Right
1st Molar
LINGUAL

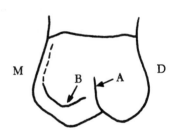

A. distolingual groove; B. mesiolingual groove

The distolingual groove originates at an occlusal pit and terminates in a pit on the lingual surface. Therefore, the distolingual groove of the maxillary first molar runs from the _____ pit to the _____ pit.

Permanent
Maxillary
Right
1st Molar
LINGUAL

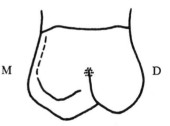

Of the two lingual cusps, one is the longest and the other the shortest of the four major cusps on the maxillary first molar. Complete the list of the four major cusps in order, longest to shortest.

Permanent
Maxillary
Right
1st Molar
LINGUAL

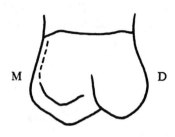

M   D

    a.   _____ (longest)
    b.   distofacial
    c.   mesiofacial
    d.   _____ (shortest)

a. mesiolingual; d. distolingual

SECTION 2.2   MAXILLARY FIRST MOLAR: PROXIMAL VIEW

From the proximal views, the mesiofacial, mesiolingual, distofacial, and distolingual line angles bound the proximal surfaces of the maxillary first molar. To the right and left of these line angles, portions of the _____ and _____ surfaces are visible.

Permanent
Maxillary
Right
1st Molar
1. MESIAL
2. DISTAL

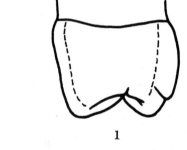

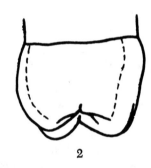

1   2

facial, lingual

From the proximal views, which surface is more uniformly convex in the occlusocervical direction? _____ (facial/lingual)

Permanent
Maxillary
Right
1st Molar
1. MESIAL
2. DISTAL

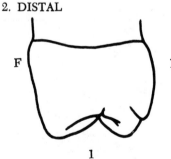

F   L

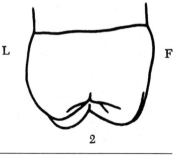

L   F

1   2

On the maxillary first molar, the lingual height of contour is in the _____ third of the crown.

Permanent
Maxillary
Right
1st Molar
1. MESIAL
2. LINGUAL

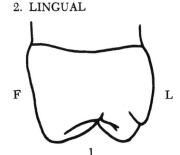

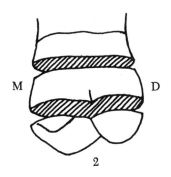

The rounded fold of enamel that forms the occlusal border of the mesial surface is the _____ _____.

Permanent
Maxillary
Right
1st Molar
1. MESIAL
2. OCCLUSAL

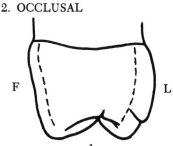

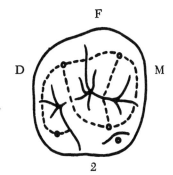

Which of the following describes the form of the mesial marginal ridge as seen from the mesial view? _____.

    a. The mesial marginal ridge nearly parallels the curvature of the cervical line.

    b. The mesial marginal ridge has a slight central concavity between the mesiofacial and mesiolingual cusps.

Permanent
Maxillary
Right
1st Molar
MESIAL

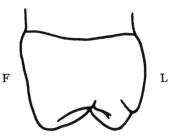

Compared to the cervical line on anterior teeth and premolars, the cervical line on the maxillary first molar has _____ (more/less) curvature.

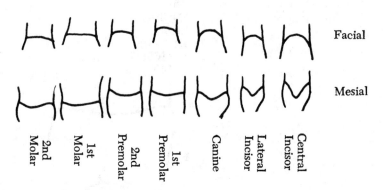

Facial

Mesial

2nd Molar · 1st Molar · 2nd Premolar · 1st Premolar · Canine · Lateral Incisor · Central Incisor

---

less

The mesial contact area is located, occlusocervically, in the _____ third of the crown and, faciolingually, slightly _____ to the faciolingual midline of the crown.

Permanent Maxillary Right 1st Molar MESIAL

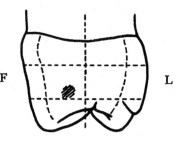

F L

---

middle, facial

Cervical to the mesial contact area is a shallow, irregular shaped concave region extending nearly to the cervical line and often crossing the mesiofacial line angle onto the _____ surface.

Permanent Maxillary Right 1st Molar MESIAL

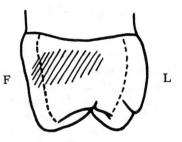

F L

Compare the mesial and distal views of the maxillary first molar. Which exposes more of the occlusal surface? _____.

Permanent
Maxillary
Right
1st Molar
1. MESIAL
2. DISTAL

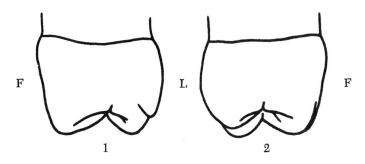

1   2

The increased exposure of the occlusal surface from the distal view is due to the short distolingual cusp and the lower level of the

_____   _____

_____.

Permanent
Maxillary
Right
1st Molar
1. MESIAL
2. DISTAL

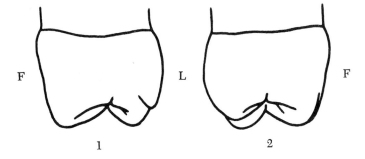

1   2

Because of the distal taper of the facial surface, the faciolingual measurement of the distal surface is slightly _____ (more/less) than that of the mesial surface.

Permanent
Maxillary
Right
1st Molar
OCCLUSAL

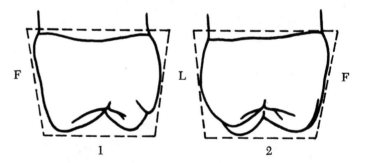

less

From a proximal view, the crown of the maxillary first molar is wider, faciolingually at the _____ (occlusal/cervical).

Permanent
Maxillary
Right
1st Molar
1. MESIAL
2. DISTAL

cervical

The distal surface of the maxillary first molar has a small concave area located in the _____ (facial/lingual) portion of its _____ (middle/cervical) third.

Permanent
Maxillary
Right
1st Molar
DISTAL

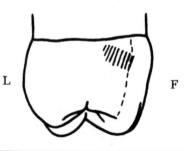

The location of the distal contact area is similar to that of the mesial contact area; that is,

    a. occlusocervial direction _____

    b. faciolingual direction _____

Permanent
Maxillary
Right
1st Molar
DISTAL

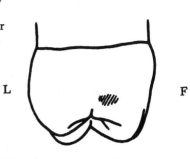

L   F

a. middle third; b. slightly facial to the midline

MATRIX TEXT 2

Directions . . .

Place an X in the square that matches the left hand column with the top row.

Mark your answers in the book, and turn to Page 420.

Maxillary First Molar	Facial	Lingual	Mesial	Distal
What surfaces are visible from the facial aspect? (complete or part)				
What surfaces are visible from the lingual aspect? (complete or part)				
Which proximal view exposes more of the occlusal?				
What surfaces have their widest measurement at the occlusal?				
Which surfaces are marked by a developmental groove that terminates in a pit?				

ANSWERS ON PAGE 420

REVIEW TEST 2

Make a note of your answers so you can check them on Page 421.

1. The order of the four major cusps of the maxillary first molar, longest to shortest is:
   a. mesiofacial, mesiolingual, distofacial, distolingual.
   b. mesiolingual, distofacial, distolingual, mesiofacial.
   c. mesiolingual, distofacial, mesiofacial, distolingual.

2. What cusps are visible from the facial view of the maxillary first molar?
   a. mesiofacial, distofacial, distolingual.
   b. mesiofacial, distofacial, mesiolingual.
   c. mesiofacial, distofacial.

3. Which facial cusp of the maxillary first molar is narrower?
   a. mesiofacial.
   b. distofacial.

4. Which of the following proximal surfaces have contact areas which are displaced some-what to the lingual from the midline of the crown?
   a. mesial
   b. distal
   c. both
   d. neither

ANSWERS ON PAGE 421

Because the maxillary second molar resembles the maxillary first molar, only the essential differences will be covered.

In the occlusocervical direction, the crown of the second molar is _____ (longer/shorter) than the first molar.

Permanent
Maxillary
Right
1. 1st Molar
2. 2nd Molar
FACIAL

D   M

1   2

shorter

What is the relationship between the faciolingual measurement of the maxillary first and second molars?

    a.   The first molar has a greater faciolingual measurement.

    b.   The two molars have nearly equal faciolingual measurement.

Permanent
Maxillary
Right
1. 1st Molar
2. 2nd Molar
MESIAL

F   L

1   2

b is correct

In the mesiodistal direction, the maxillary second molar is _____ (wider/narrower) than the first molar.

Permanent
Maxillary
Right
1. 1st Molar
2. 2nd Molar
FACIAL

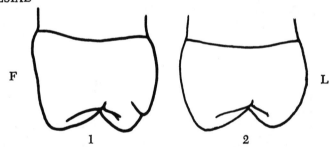

D   M

1   2

In occlusal view, which tooth outline is more narrow mesiodistally? _____ _____.

Permanent
Maxillary
Right
1. 1st Molar
2. 2nd Molar
OCCLUSAL

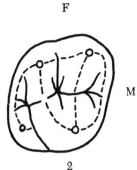

1 2

How many cusps are visible in occlusal view of the second molar? _____.

Permanent
Maxillary
Right
2nd Molar
OCCLUSAL

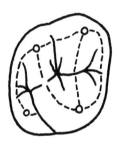

Each lobe is represented by a cusp on molar teeth; thus, the maxillary first molar has _____ (number) lobes, and the maxillary second molar has _____ (number) lobes.

Permanent
Maxillary
Right
2nd Molar
OCCLUSAL

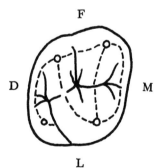

389

On the maxillary second molar, the small accessory cusp of Carabelli _____ (is/is not) present.

Permanent
Maxillary
Right
2nd Molar
1. OCCLUSAL
2. LINGUAL

F

D

M

D

1

2

The cusps of the maxillary second molar are as follows:

A. _____

B. _____

C. _____

D. _____

Permanent
Maxillary
Right
2nd Molar
OCCLUSAL

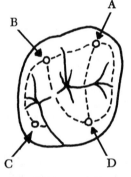

B

A

C

D

A. mesiofacial; B. distofacial; C. distolingual; D. mesiolingual

The maxillary second molar has two types of occlusal patterns: (1) the more common rhomboidal type and (2) the "heart shaped" type. Which occlusal type has more nearly parallel sides which run in the faciolingual direction? _____

Permanent
Maxillary
Right
2nd Molar
OCCLUSAL
1. Rhomboidal
2. Heart Shaped

F

F

D

M

L

1

2

On the rhomboidal type, the outline formed by joining the four cusp tips is a rhomboid. The longer and more nearly parallel sides run in the _____ direction.

Permanent
Maxillary
Right
2nd Molar
OCCLUSAL

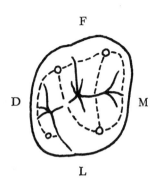

The two largest cusps on the maxillary second molar are the _____ and _____ cusps.

Permanent
Maxillary
Right
2nd Molar
OCCLUSAL

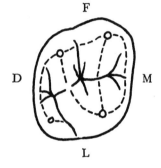

In the study of the premolars, the difference was drawn between developmental and supplemental grooves. Which of these two types of grooves does not mark the major anatomical division of tooth crowns? _____.

The maxillary second molar may have more shallow linear grooves than the first molar. These grooves neither mark the junction of the primary parts of the tooth nor are shown in the standard drawings of the occlusal aspect of the crown. As on the maxillary second premolar, these shallow grooves are called _____ grooves.

Permanent
Maxillary
Right
2nd Molar
OCCLUSAL

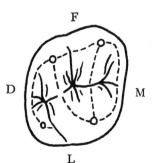

The less common "heart shaped" occlusal type results from the poor development of the _____ cusp.

Permanent
Maxillary
Right
2nd Molar
OCCLUSAL

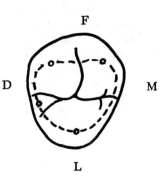

The rhomboidal occlusal pattern of the maxillary second molar resembles the maxillary first molar, but the "heart shaped" occlusal pattern resembles the maxillary _____ (compare Figs. 3 and 4).

Permanent
Maxillary
Right
1. 1st Molar
2. 2nd Molar (Rhomboid)
3. 2nd Molar (Heart-shaped)
4. 3rd Molar
OCCLUSAL

1

2

3

4

How do the measurements of the maxillary second molar compare to those of the maxillary first molar in the following directions?

    a.   faciolingual _____ (larger/smaller/equal)

    b.   mesiodistal _____ (larger/smaller/equal)

    c.   occlusocervical _____ (larger/smaller/equal)

The mesiolingual and distolingual cusps show a progressive shift in position from the maxillary first to third molar. Which cusp has the greater amount of variability in position? _____ .

Permanent
Maxillary
Right
Molars
OCCLUSAL

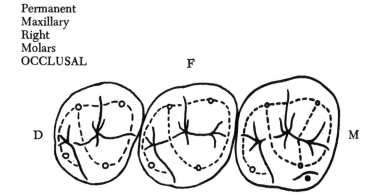

distolingual

The mesiolingual cusp shifts slightly toward the distal. The distolingual cusp shifts toward the mesial and _____ directions.

Permanent
Maxillary
Right
Milars
OCCLUSAL

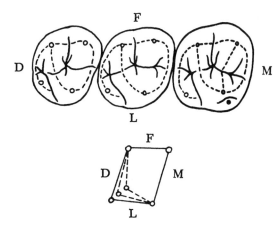

facial

Compared to the first molar, the facial groove of the maxillary second molar is slightly _____ (more distinct/less distinct).

Permanent
Maxillary
Right
1. 1st Molar
2. 2nd Molar
FACIAL

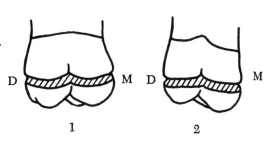

A part of the oblique ridge is seen in the concavity between the two facial cusps, the _____ ridge of the _____ cusp.

Permanent
Maxillary
Right
2nd Molar
FACIAL

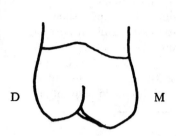

D   M

The two distal cusps of the maxillary second molar are not only smaller than those of the first molar, but in the occlusocervical direction, they are _____.

Permanent
Maxillary
Right
1. 1st Molar
2. 2nd Molar
DISTAL

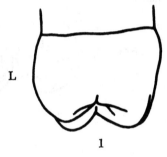

L

1

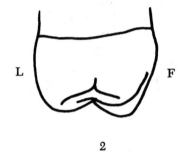

L   F

2

A notable difference between the maxillary first and second molars is that the cusp of Carabelli is not present on the _____ surface of the _____ molar.

Permanent
Maxillary
Right
2nd Molar
LINGUAL

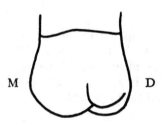

M   D

From the lingual view of the maxillary second molar, which facial cusp is visible below the distolingual cusp? _____ .

**Permanent
Maxillary
Right
2nd Molar
LINGUAL**

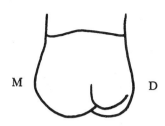

M   D

The maxillary second molar generally resembles the maxillary first molar. Some of the essential differences are . . .

    a.   The maxillary second molar has _____ cusps.

    b.   The second molar is generally smaller than the first molar except in the _____ direction.

    c.   The second molar has two common occlusal patterns, a variation largely due to the smaller size of the _____ cusp.

a. four; b. faciolingual; c. distolingual

TURN TO THE NEXT PAGE FOR THE MATRIX TEST.

MATRIX TEST 3

Directions . . .

Place an X in the square that matches the left hand column with the top row.

Mark your answers in the book and then *turn to Page 422.*

	Maxillary First Molar	Maxillary Second Molar	Neither or Both
Shorter occlusocervically . . .			
Longer faciolingually . . .			
Wider mesiodistally . . .			
Tooth which often has more supplemental grooves . . .			

ANSWERS ON PAGE 422.

SECTION 3.1 MAXILLARY THIRD MOLAR

The form of the third molar varies more than the form of any of the other teeth in the dental arch. The most common form of the maxillary third molar closely resembles the "heart shaped" form of the maxillary second molar and has _____ (number) cusps.

Permanent
Maxillary
Right
3rd Molar
OCCLUSAL
1.-4. Variations
5. Typical Form

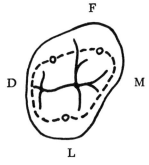

three

Generally, the distolingual cusp is absent on the maxillary third molar. The three remaining cusps maintain the names of the three largest cusps on the maxillary second molar; the _____, _____, and _____ cusps.

Permanent
Maxillary
Right
3rd Molar
OCCLUSAL

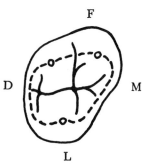

mesiofacial, distofacial, and mesiolingual

Which of the well-developed cusps on the maxillary first and second molars does not develop on the most common form of the maxillary third molar? _____.

Permanent
Maxillary
Right
3rd Molar
OCCLUSAL

Of the maxillary second and third molars, which has the larger facial cusps? _____

Permanent
Maxillary
Right
1. 2nd Molar
2. 3rd Molar
FACIAL

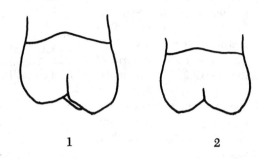

1   2

How many cusps are usually found on the lingual aspect of the third molar? _____

Permanent
Maxillary
Right
3rd Molar
OCCLUSAL

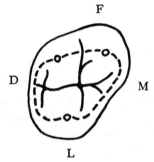

Compared to that of the maxillary second molar, the facial surface of the maxillary third molar is _____ (smaller/larger) in both directions.

Permanent
Maxillary
Right
1. 2nd Molar
2. 3rd Molar
FACIAL

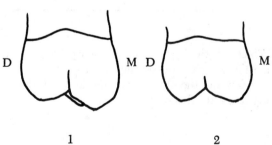

1   2

From the facial view, the facial groove of the maxillary third molar is less distinct than that of the maxillary second molar. Of the three maxillary molars, the molar with the most distinct facial groove is the _____; the molar with the least distinct facial groove is the _____.

Permanent
Maxillary
Right
1. 1st Molar
2. 2nd Molar
3. 3rd Molar
FACIAL

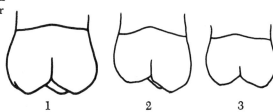

1   2   3

Concerning cusp arrangement, one difference between the maxillary second and third molars is that the third molar frequently has only one _____ cusp.

Permanent
Maxillary
Right
3rd Molar
OCCLUSAL

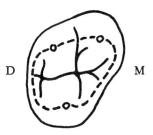

D   M

Similar to the maxillary first and second molars, when a small distolingual cusp is present on the third molar, it is separated from the mesiolingual cusp by the _____ groove.

Permanent
Maxillary
Right
3rd Molar
OCCLUSAL

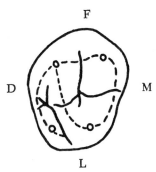

F

D   M

L

Compared to that of the maxillary second molar, the lingual surface of the maxillary third molar has a mesiodistal convexity that is _____ (more pronounced/less pronounced).

Permanent
Maxillary
Right
1. 2nd Molar
2. 3rd Molar
OCCLUSAL

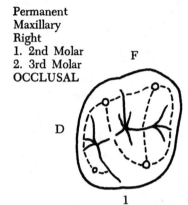

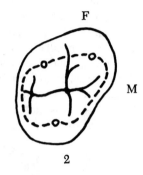

1   2

more pronounced

Compared to those of the maxillary second molar, the measurements of the crown of the typical maxillary third molar are _____ (increased/reduced).

---

reduced

Sometimes, extra ridges descend from the cusp tips of the third molars onto the occlusal surface. Similar to the nomenclature for the shallow linear "extra" grooves on the occlusal surfaces of some teeth, these ridges are called _____ _____.

---

supplemental ridges

Which proximal surface on the maxillary third molar is more uniformly convex? _____

Permanent
Maxillary
Right
3rd Molar
OCCLUSAL

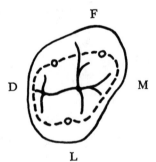

Three significant features of the maxillary third molar are . . .

a. The form of the third molar varies _____ (more/less) than any other tooth.

b. The typical form of the maxillary third molar has _____ cusps.

c. In all dimensions, the maxillary third molar is _____ (larger/smaller) than the second molar.

a. more; b. three; c. smaller

TURN TO THE NEXT PAGE FOR THE REVIEW TEST

REVIEW TEST 3

Make a note of your answers and then turn to Page 423 to check them.

1. In the "heart shaped" variation of the second molar, which cusp is poorly developed?
    a. distolingual
    b. mesiolingual

2. Which is the most common form of the maxillary second molar?
    a. rhomboidal
    b. "heart shaped"

3. In the diagram, the arrow points to the ———————— side of the tooth.
    a. mesial
    b. distal

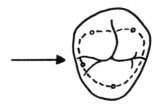

4. Which maxillary molar generally has the facial surface with the least distinct facial groove?
    a. second molar
    b. third molar

5. Which surface of the maxillary third molar is generally more uniformly convex?
    a. mesial
    b. distal

ANSWERS ON PAGE 423.

SECTION 4.0   MANDIBULAR FIRST MOLAR

The mandibular first molar is the largest, strongest tooth in the mandibular arch. It has _____ lobes.

Permanent
Mandibular
Right
1st Molar
OCCLUSAL

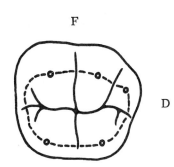

five

How many cusps (lobes) are located to the lingual? _____

Permanent
Mandibular
Right
1st Molar
OCCLUSAL

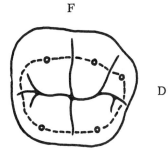

two

Similar to those of the maxillary second molar, the two lingual cusps of the mandibular first molar are called the mesiolingual and _____ cusps.

Permanent
Mandibular
Right
1st Molar
OCCLUSAL

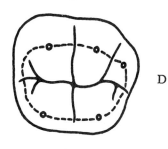

The three remaining cusps are the mesiofacial, distofacial, and distal cusps. Which of the five cusps on the mandibular first molar is the smallest? —————

Permanent
Mandibular
Right
1st Molar
OCCLUSAL

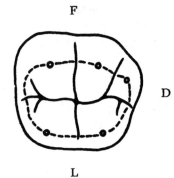

Which of the five cusps of the mandibular first molar is the widest? —————

Permanent
Mandibular
Right
1st Molar
OCCLUSAL

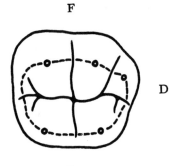

In which direction is the crown of the mandibular first molar wider? ————— (mesiodistal/faciolingual)

Permanent
Mandibular
Right
1st Molar
OCCLUSAL

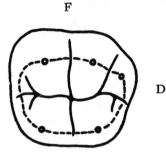

Similar to those of the mandibular first molar, the crowns of the mandibular second and third molars are wider in the mesiodistal direction than in the faciolingual direction.

Which of the following correctly describes the relationship between the mesiodistal and faciolingual measurements of the molars? _____

a. All molars, maxillary and mandibular, are wider mesiodistally than faciolingually.

b. Maxillary molars are wider faciolingually than mesiodistally, but the opposite is true for mandibular molars.

---

b is correct (If you missed this question read the next frame carefully)

The relationship between the mesiodistal and faciolingual measurements of the crowns is one characteristic that differentiates maxillary from mandibular molars.

Remember that maxillary molars are wider faciolingually than mesiodistally, but on mandibular molars the crown is wider in the _____ direction.

Permanent
1. Maxillary
2. Mandibular
Right
1st Molar
OCCLUSAL

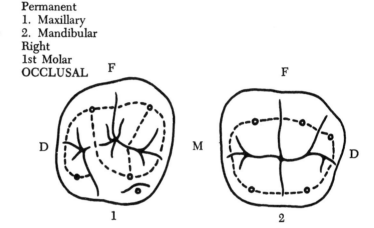

Another important difference between the maxillary and mandibular molars is in the pattern of their occlusal ridges. The maxillary molars have an _____ ridge and the mandibular molars do not.

Permanent
1. Maxillary
2. Mandibular
Right
1st Molar
OCCLUSAL

The occlusal surface of the mandibular first molar is divided into three fossae. Similar to the three fossae of the maxillary first molar, they are called the *mesial, distal,* and *central* fossae.

Permanent Mandibular Right 1st Molar OCCLUSAL

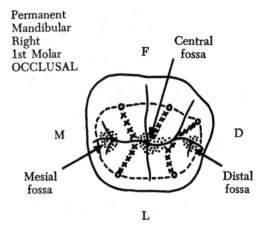

Central fossa

Mesial fossa

Distal fossa

The central fossa is the largest of the three and is separated from the mesial fossa by the triangular ridges of the _____ and _____ cusps.

Permanent Mandibular Right 1st Molar OCCLUSAL

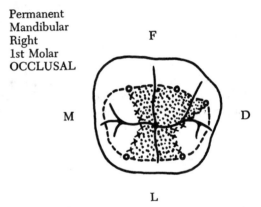

mesiofacial, mesiolingual

The triangular ridges of the distal and distolingual cusps separate the central fossa from the _____ _____.

Permanent Mandibular Right 1st Molar OCCLUSAL

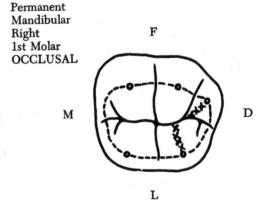

Which cusp of the mandibular first molar has a triangular ridge that does not form a part of the mesial or distal boundary of the central fossa? _____

Permanent
Mandibular
Right
1st Molar
OCCLUSAL

F

M

D

L

The triangular ridge of the distofacial cusp descends into the largest of the three fossae, the _____ fossa.

Permanent
Mandibular
Right
1st Molar
OCCLUSAL

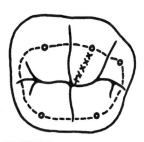

Four developmental grooves originate at the central pit in the central fossa. Of these four (the mesial, distal, facial and lingual developmental grooves), which passes between the mesiolingual and distolingual cusps? _____

Permanent
Mandibular
Right
1st Molar
OCCLUSAL

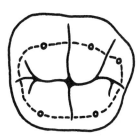

Name each of the developmental grooves of the mandibular first molar described.

a. The _____ groove originates at the central pit and terminates in the mesial fossa.

b. The _____ groove originates at the central pit and separates the mesiofacial and distofacial cusps.

c. The _____ groove originates at the central pit and terminates in the distal fossa.

Permanent Mandibular Right 1st Molar OCCLUSAL

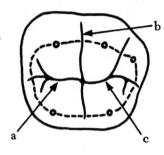

a. mesial; b. facial; c. distal

At a point slightly distal to the central pit, the distofacial developmental groove branches from the distal groove and passes between the distal and _____ cusps.

Permanent Mandibular Right 1st Molar OCCLUSAL

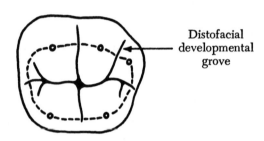

Distofacial developmental grove

distofacial

Similar to the nomenclature for the maxillary molars, the union of the mesial and distal grooves on the mandibular first molar is called the _____ groove.

Permanent Mandibular Right 1st Molar OCCLUSAL

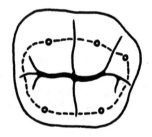

central

Additional shallow supplemental grooves are sometimes seen on the occlusal surface of the mandibular first molar. These supplemental grooves _____ (do/do not) mark the boundaries of the five lobes.

Permanent Mandibular Right 1st Molar OCCLUSAL

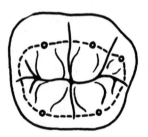

Use your note card mask to cover the next frame. Now, on this outline of the mandibular first molar, sketch the pattern formed by the ten developmental grooves. Use your own recall.

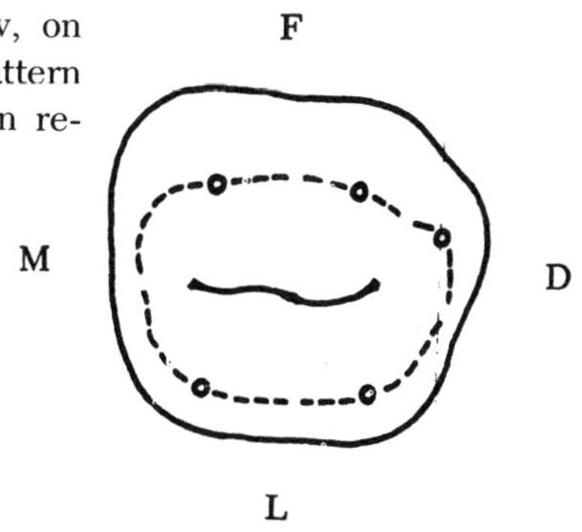

CHECK YOUR DRAWING WITH THIS ILLUSTRATION.

Permanent
Mandibular
Right
1st Molar
OCCLUSAL

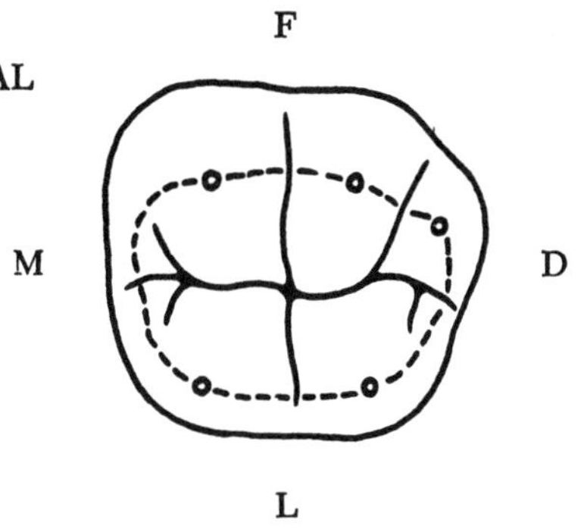

Here is an exercise in cusp and groove identification.

MANDIBULAR FIRST MOLAR

Name the cusps and grooves marked by the labels. *Turn to the next frame to check your answers.*

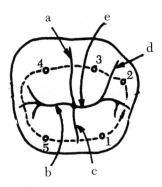

Cusps: 1. _____   4. _____
           2. _____   5. _____
           3. _____

Grooves: a. _____   b & e. _____
           b. _____
           c. _____
           d. _____
           e. _____

MANDIBULAR FIRST MOLAR: ANSWERS

If any items were missed, *turn to the page indicated for review.*

If all items are correct, *turn to the next page and continue.*

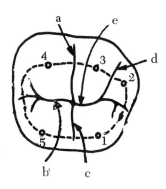

Cusps

1. distolingual	pp. 403–404	4. mesiofacial	pp. 403–404
2. distal	pp. 403–404	5. mesiolingual	pp. 403–404
3. distofacial	pp. 403–404		

Grooves

a. facial	p. 407
b. mesial	p. 407
c. lingual	p. 407
d. distofacial	p. 408
e. distal	p. 407
b&e central	p. 408

The "corners" of the occlusal view are _____ (sharply angled/rounded).

Permanent
Mandibular
Right
1st Molar
OCCLUSAL

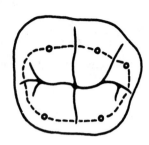

rounded

Unlike the maxillary first molar the mesial and distal surfaces of the mandibular first molar converge slightly toward the lingual. Which half of the mandibular first molar crown is wider in the mesiodistal direction? _____ (facial/lingual)

Permanent
1. Maxillary
2. Mandibular
Right
1st Molar
OCCLUSAL

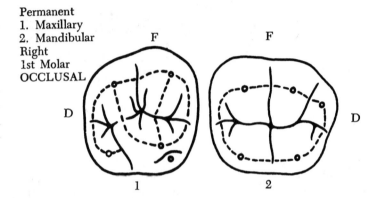

facial

The location of the distal cusp causes a problem in naming the four ridges. Because the mesial and distal ridges of other cusps help to form the borders of the occlusal surface, it is convenient to name the four ridges of the distal cusp as follows:

    lingual ridge — descends onto the occlusal surface;

    facial ridge — descends onto facial surface very slightly facial to the distofacial line angle;

    mesial ridge — forms part of the facioclusal line angle;

    distal ridge — blends with the distal marginal ridge.

Name the ridges indicated by the labels.

1. _____
2. _____
3. _____
4. _____

Permanent
Mandibular
Right
1st Molar
OCCLUSAL

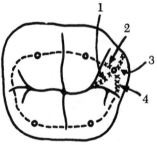

How many cusps on the mandibular first molar have lingual ridges that are triangular ridges? _____

Permanent
Mandibular
Right
1st Molar
OCCLUSAL

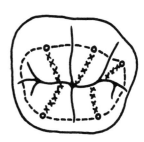

three

Similar to those of the maxillary molars, the mesial marginal ridge and the distal marginal ridge form two of the borders of the _____.

Permanent
Mandibular
Right
1st Molar
OCCLUSAL

M

D

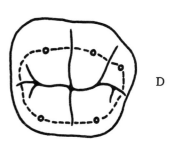

occlusal surface

From the occlusal view, the linguocclusal line angle runs in a nearly straight line in the mesiodistal direction. The faciocclusal line angle is slightly more curved running in the mesiodistal direction; it is slightly convex toward the _____ direction.

Permanent
Mandibular
Right
1st Molar
OCCLUSAL

F

M

D

L

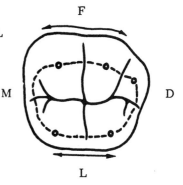

facial

Of the five cusps, which is the longest? _____

Permanent
Mandibular
Right
1st Molar
1. MESIAL
2. LINGUAL

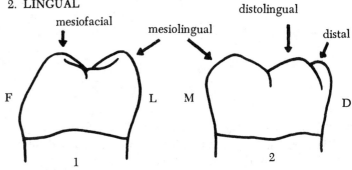

mesiofacial

mesiolingual

distolingual

distal

F

L   M

D

1

2

mesiolingual

The mesiolingual is slightly longer than the distolingual cusp, and the distofacial is slightly longer than the mesiofacial cusp. Which cusp of the mandibular first molar is the shortest? _____

Permanent
Mandibular
Right
1st Molar
FACIAL

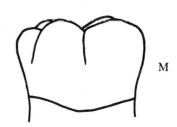

D

M

distal

414

MATRIX TEXT 4

Place an X in the squares that match the left hand column with the top row. Mark your answers and then turn to Page 424.

Cusps of the Mandibular First Molar

	Mesio-facial	Disto-facial	Distal	Disto-lingual	Mesio-lingual
Widest cusp					
Smallest cusp					
Has triangular ridge that descends into the central fossa					
Connected by the oblique ridge					
Longest cusp					

ANSWERS ON PAGE 424.

415

REVIEW TEST 4

Make a note of your answers and turn to Page 425 when you finish, to check them.

1. The distal limit of the mesial fossa is formed by the —
   a. facial ridge of the mesiolingual cusp and the lingual ridge of the distofacial cusp.
   b. lingual ridge of the mesiofacial cusp and the facial ridge of the mesiolingual cusp.

2. The mandigular first molar is widest in the —
   a. mesiodistal direction.
   b. faciolingual direction.

3. List two major differences between the maxillary and mandibular first molars from an occlusal view:
   a. _____
   b. _____

4. Which groove on the mandibular first molar extends on to the facial surface and lies next to the smallest cusp? _____

ANSWERS ON PAGE 425

TEST ANSWER SECTION

MATRIX TEST 1
(From Page 373)

If any items were missed, *turn to the page indicated for review.*
If all are correct, *turn to Page 374 and take Review Test 1.*

	Mesio-facial	Mesio-lingual	Disto-lingual	Disto-facial
Cusp with widest mesiodistal measurement		X (PP. 362-363)		
Two cusps joined by oblique ridge		X (P. 363)		X (P. 363)
The cusp which is least developed of the four major cusps			X (PP. 362, 364, 365)	
Cusp nearest the cusp of Carabelli		X (P. 361)		
Cusps with ridges that surround the central fossa	X (P. 368)	X (P. 368)		X (P. 368)

REVIEW TEST 1
(From Page 374)

CORRECT ANSWERS: 1. b 2. b 3. a 4. a

IF YOU GOT THEM ALL CORRECT, you have just completed a most important section in this chapter. The occlusal features of the maxillary first molar will provide a very useful comparison for the other molars. Before you continue, however, take a few minutes to take a break away from studying and do something that interests you right now. This will help to reward your study progress and to prevent mental fatigue. Stretch, jump around, take a walk, drink some _____, or eat some _____, or look at a _____ magazine (You fill in the blanks—it's your reward). *When you return, continue on Page 375, Section 2.*

IF YOU GOT ONE OF THE QUESTIONS INCORRECT, read the directions for review below. Review and then retake the review test on Page 374.

1. IF YOU MISSED QUESTION 1, recall that the maxillary first molar is the first permanent tooth to erupt (see P. 358), or that the occlusal outline is rhomboidal at times (P. 361).

2. IF YOU MISSED QUESTION 2, review the number of lobes on Pages 359–360, or the oblique ridge on Page 363.

3. IF YOU MISSED QUESTION 3, review the distal groove and its intersection with the oblique ridge on Page 370 or the names of the three fossae on Page 368.

4. IF YOU MISSED QUESTION 4, recall that the faciocclusal line angle is an imaginary line dividing the occlusal and facial surfaces (see Pages 362–366 for the ridges along this line angle).

5. If you missed any of the groove names, turn to the page indicated for review.

NAME	REVIEW PAGE
a. facial groove	P. 369
b. mesial groove (of central groove)	P. 370
c. mesial marginal groove	P. 371
d. mesiolingual groove	P. 372
e. distolingual groove	P. 371
f. distal marginal groove	P. 371
g. distal groove (of central groove)	P. 370
b+g central groove	P. 370

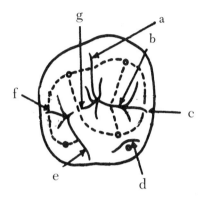

IF YOU MISSED TWO OR MORE QUESTIONS, it will be very helpful to you in later sections of this chapter to have mastered this section on the occlusal aspect of the maxillary first molar. Please return to Page 358 and review this section again, making sure to use a card to shield the answers as you respond to each question in the text. (Read the top paragraph on Page 418 and you'll see what fun you'll have if you get all questions correct when you retake the review test on Page 374 after you have reviewed the entire section).

MATRIX TEST 2
(From Page 386)

If any items were missed, *turn to the page indicated for review.*
If all were correct, turn to Page 387 for the Review Test.

Maxillary First Molar	Facial	Lingual	Mesial	Distal
What surfaces are visible from the facial aspect? (complete or part)	**X** (P. 375)			**X** (P. 375)
What surfaces are visible from the lingual aspect? (complete or part)		**X** (P. 378)	**X** (P. 378)	
Which proximal view exposes more of the occlusal?				**X** (P. 383)
What surfaces have their widest measurement at the occlusal?	**X** (P. 375)	**X** (P. 379)		
Which surfaces are marked by a developmental groove that terminates in a pit?	**X** (P. 376)	**X** (P. 379)		

REVIEW TEST 2
(From Page 387)

CORRECT ANSWERS: 1. c 2. b 3. b 4. d

IF YOU GOT ALL THE QUESTIONS CORRECT, congratulations, you should take a short break and repeat to yourself, "I'm actually learning dental anatomy." *Continue on Page 388, Section 3.*

IF YOU MISSED ONE OF THE QUESTIONS, think of your future clinical work and how important it will be to have mastered this material—perhaps this will help in reviewing the questions, as indicated below. Please retake the review test after you have followed the directions below.

1. IF YOU MISSED QUESTION 1, review the length of cusps on Page 380.

2. IF YOU MISSED QUESTION 2, review the visibility of the mesiolingual cusp and the facial cusps on Page 378.

3. IF YOU MISSED QUESTION 3, look at the illustration in Page 378. Measure the width of each cusp.

4. IF YOU MISSED QUESTION 4, review the facial displacement of the proximal contact areas on Page 382 (mesial) and 385 (distal).

IF YOU MISSED TWO OR MORE QUESTIONS, return to Page 375 and review the important features of the facial, lingual, mesial and distal views of the maxillary first molar. To make it more exciting you might practice identifying those features on someone's real molar—someone you want to get to know better. Review and then retake the review test on Page 387.

MATRIX TEST 3
(From Page 396)

If any items were missed, *turn to the page indicated for review.*
If all are correct, *turn to Page 397 and continue.*

	Maxillary First Molar	Maxillary Second Molar	Neither or Both
Shorter occlusocervically . . .		X (P. 388)	
Longer faciolingually . . .			X (P. 388)
Wider mesiodistally . . .	X (P. 388)		
Tooth which often has more supplemental grooves . . .		X (P. 391)	

REVIEW TEST 3

(From Page 402)

CORRECT ANSWERS: 1. a   2. a   3. b   4. b   5. b

IF YOU GOT THEM ALL CORRECT, you have studied well. Go out and buy yourself a _____, or go to the refrigerator and get a _____, or go for a stroll to _____ and talk with _____. (Fill-in questions can be fun.) A break from study activity will help to reduce fatigue and increase your interest in studying if you do it immediately and consistently when you feel you have accomplished a goal such as passing one of these review tests. *Continue on Page 403, Section 4 when you get back.*

IF YOU MISSED ONE OF THE QUESTIONS, the directions that follow will help you to go back and find out what the problem is. Review and then retake the review test on Page 402.

1. IF YOU MISSED QUESTION 1, answer the questions on Page 392 again.

2. IF YOU MISSED QUESTION 2, read Pages 390–391.

3. IF YOU MISSED QUESTION 3, review the second molar in the "heart shaped" form on Page 392, and the discussion of the distolingual cusp location on Page 393.

4. IF YOU MISSED QUESTION 4, Page 399 will tell it like it is.

5. IF YOU MISSED QUESTION 5, examine the drawing on Page 400 and notice the flatness of part of the mesial surface. The distal is more rounded and convex.

IF YOU MISSED TWO OR MORE QUESTIONS, you will want to review this section again. You will want to fill yourself with wisdom concerning the third molar—the wisdom tooth—a tooth patients will ask about in clinical practice. Start on Page 388, and use a card to help you test yourself to see if you really are mastering the concepts presented. *Retake the review test on Page 402.*

If any items were missed, turn to the page indicated for review.

If all items are correct, turn to Page 416 for the Review Test.

Cusps of the Mandibular First Molar

	Mesio-facial	Disto-facial	Distal	Disto-lingual	Mesio-lingual
Widest cusp	X (P. 404)				
Smallest cusp			X (P. 404)		
Has triangular ridge that descends into the central fossa		X (P. 407)			
Connected by the oblique ridge	(No oblique ridge is present, (P. 405)				
Longest cusp					X (P. 414)

REVIEW TEST 4
(From Page 416)

CORRECT ANSWERS: 1. b 2. a 3. You should have listed two of the following three differences: a. maxillary widest in faciolingual direction b. maxillary has oblique ridge c. maxillary does not have lingual convergence 4. distofacial.

IF YOU GOT ALL QUESTIONS CORRECT, good work! You are approximately half-way through this chapter already. Before you continue, do something unrelated to dental anatomy to clear your mind. *Continue on Page 434 when you return.*

IF YOU MISSED ONE OF THE QUESTIONS, you should review the answer to that question so that you can really master this information on the important mandibular first molar. Read the directions for review below. Review and then retake the review test on Page 416.

1. IF YOU MISSED QUESTION 1, examine the drawing on Page 407. This page doesn't tell you about the distal limit of the mesial fossa specifically, but you should be able to figure that out by identifying the ridges on the distal side of that fossa.

2. IF YOU MISSED QUESTION 2, answer the question again on Page 405.

3. IF YOU MISSED QUESTION 3, study Pages 405 and 412. This is an important list of differences to learn.

4. IF YOU MISSED QUESTION 4, restudy the question and diagram on Page 408.

IF YOU MISSED TWO OR MORE QUESTIONS, you will want to go back and reread (and answer questions) starting at Page 403. This section will help you in any future tooth-identification exams you might have, or, in the clinic. Review and then retake the test on Page 416.

MATRIX TEST 5
(From Page 442)

If any items were missed, *turn to the page indicated for review.*

If all items are correct, *turn to Page 443 for the Review Test.*

Mandibular First Molar	Facial	Lingual	Mesial	Distal
The views from which five cusps are visible . . .	X (P. 434)			X (P. 440)
The proximal surface with the more convex curvature in the faciolingual direction as seen from an occlusal view . . .				X (P. 440)
The portion of the crown with the two most pointed cusps . . .		X (P. 437)		

REVIEW TEST 5
(From Page 443)

CORRECT ANSWERS: 1. a 2. b 3. a

IF YOU GOT ALL ANSWERS CORRECT, you have demonstrated a good understanding of the mandibular first molar. Take a short break and then *continue with Section 6, Page 444.*

IF YOU MISSED ONE OF THE QUESTIONS, read the directions for review below. Review the answer to the appropriate question and then retake the test on Page 443.

1. IF YOU MISSED QUESTION 1, review Pages 435–436.

2. IF YOU MISSED QUESTION 2, review Page 437.

3. IF YOU MISSED QUESTION 3, review Page 439.

IF YOU MISSED TWO OR MORE QUESTIONS, skim back over this very short section again, starting on Page 434. Retake the test on Page 443.

If any items were missed, *turn to the page indicated for review.*

If all items are correct, *turn to Page 455 for the Review Test.*

Mandibular Molars	Mandibular Molars		
	First	Second	Neither
The tooth with three lingual cusps . . .			**X** (P. 404, 445)
The tooth with the more symmetrical form . . .		**X** (P. 445)	
The tooth with the smaller measurements in all dimensions . . .		**X** (P. 444)	
The tooth with the greater amount of lingual convergence on the mesial and distal surfaces . . .	**X** (P. 451)		
The tooth with two developmental grooves of the facial surface . . .	**X** (P. 448)		

REVIEW TEST 6

(From Page 455)

CORRECT ANSWERS: 1. b 2. b 3. b 4. b 5. b

IF YOU GOT ALL QUESTIONS CORRECT, you win big! Go out and enjoy a diversion for a while. You'll like it, and it will serve to refresh your mind and make you feel young again. So take a break first, and then *continue on Page 456*, Section 7 (which is the next to the last section, but also a long one, so you'll want to be ready for it).

IF YOU MISSED ONE OF THE QUESTIONS, (especially if you missed number 6) read the review directions below for the question you missed. Review and then retake the test on Page 455.

1. IF YOU MISSED QUESTION 1, compare the drawings of the second molar on Page 444 (facial) with Page 445 (lingual). You will see only the facial or lingual cusps from their respective views, indicating they are of equal length.

2. IF YOU MISSED QUESTION 2, reread Page 447.

3. IF YOU MISSED QUESTION 3, answer the questions for Page 452.

4. IF YOU MISSED QUESTION 4, note that the question asked for the mandibular tooth with only one antagonist. The maxillary third molar has only one. Examine the drawings on Page 453.

5. IF YOU MISSED QUESTION 5, reread Page 452 on the third molar and its shallow central fossa, and/or Page 450 where the second and first mandibular molars are compared.

IF YOU MISSED TWO OR MORE QUESTIONS, it will be important to you to *review this section again, beginning on Page 444.*

If any items were missed, *turn to the page indicated for review.*

If all were correct, *turn to Page 476 for the Review Test.*

Molars	Facial	Lingual	Mesial or Mesio-facial	Distal or Disto-facial
Largest root of maxillary first molar.		X (P. 461)		
Inclination of lingual root apex, maxillary first molar.	X (P. 464)			
The smallest root of the maxillary first molar.				X (P. 462)
Root with the sharpest apex, maxillary second molar.				X (P. 467)
Largest root, mandibular first molar.			X (P. 471)	
Straighter root (occluso-apical direction) of mandibular first molar.				X (P. 472)
Inclination of roots, mandibular third molar.				X (P. 474)

REVIEW TEST 7
(From Page 476)

CORRECT ANSWERS: 1. a-3, b-2 2. b 3. b 4. b

IF YOU GOT ALL THE QUESTIONS CORRECT, congratulations, you have completed the second to the last section in this chapter. You deserve a break after that relatively long section. Find something immediately available that interests you and enjoy it for a few minutes—read a magazine, take a walk, eat or drink something, etc. *Continue on Page 477 when you return to study.*

IF YOU MISSED ONE OF THE QUESTIONS, read the directions for reviewing that question below. Retake the test on Page 476 after reviewing.

1. IF YOU MISSED QUESTION 1, skim back through Pages 458–459 to review the number of terminal roots.

2. IF YOU MISSED QUESTION 2, read Page 468 on the maxillary third molar.

3. IF YOU MISSED QUESTION 3, examine the drawing and the question on Page 459. Skim the section on the mandibular first molar, Pages 469–473.

4. IF YOU MISSED QUESTION 4, answer the questions and look closely at the drawings on Pages 471–473.

IF YOU MISSED TWO OR MORE QUESTIONS, you should go back and review this section again starting on Page 458.

MATRIX TEXT 8
(From Page 484)

If any items were missed, *turn to the page indicated for review.*

If all were correct, *turn to Page 485 for the Review Test.*

Pulp of Posterior Teeth	Maxillary First Molar	Mandibular First Molar
Most common number of root canals.	four (P. 477)	three (P. 481)
If the tooth has a less common number of root canals, what number of canals would that be?	four (P. 477)	four or two (P. 483)
Number of pulp horns in pulp chamber.	four (P. 477)	five (P. 481)
Names of usual root canals (if more than one).	Mesiofacial Distofacial Lingual (P. 479)	facial canal of Mesial, lingual canal of Mesial, Distal, (P. 481)

REVIEW TEST 8
(From Page 485)

CORRECT ANSWERS: 1. a. $4 + 3 = 7$
                              b. $3 + 4 = 7$
                              c. $2 + 5 = 7$

IF YOU GOT ALL PARTS CORRECT, good job! You have, of course, finished this chapter and have earned a just reward.

IF YOU MISSED ANY PART OF THE QUESTION, review Pages 477–483 and the matrix-test answers on Page 432.

SECTION 5.0   MANDIBULAR FIRST MOLAR: FACIAL VIEW

How many cusps contribute to the facial portion of the mandibular first molar? _____

Permanent
Mandibular
Right
1st Molar
FACIAL

D   M

three

With the tooth in vertical position, the tips of two lingual cusps are seen. They are the _____ and _____ cusps.

Permanent
Mandibular
Right
1st Molar
FACIAL

D   M

mesiolingual, distolingual

Which three cusps contribute to the faciocclusal line angle of the mandibular first molar? _____, _____, and _____.

Permanent
Mandibular
Right
1st Molar
1. FACIAL
2. OCCLUSAL

F

D   M   D

1   2

Although the distal cusp contributes to the facial surface, most of the facial surface is formed by the _____ and _____ cusps.

Permanent
Mandibular
Right
1st Molar
FACIAL

D

M

From the facial view, which facial cusp of the mandibular first molar is more rounded? _____

Permanent
Mandibular
Right
1st Molar
FACIAL

D

M

Two developmental grooves originate in the central fossa and cross the faciocclusal line angle onto the facial surface. Separating the mesiofacial and distofacial cusps is the _____ groove.

Permanent
Mandibular
Right
1st Molar
FACIAL

D

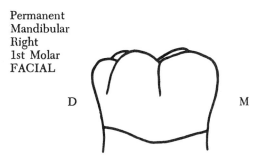

M

The facial groove terminates on the facial surface in the facial pit located in the _____ (occlusal/middle) third of the crown.

Permanent
Mandibular
Right
1st Molar
FACIAL

D

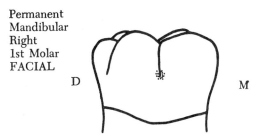

M

Also visible on the facial surface and separating the distal cusp from the distofacial cusp is the _____ _____.

Permanent
Mandibular
Right
1st Molar
FACIAL

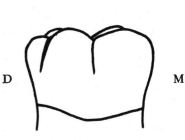

D   M

The distofacial groove gradually becomes less distinct as it descends from the faciocclusal line angle toward the cervical line. Generally, it fades out in the _____ third of the crown.

Permanent
Mandibular
Right
1st Molar
FACIAL

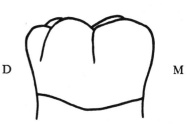

D   M

The facial groove of the mandibular first molar originates at the central pit and terminates at the _____ _____.

Permanent
Mandibular
Right
1st Molar
1. OCCLUSAL
2. FACIAL

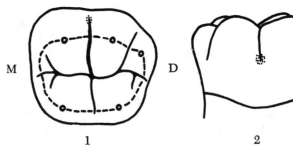

F

M   D   M

1   2

SECTION 5.1 MANDIBULAR FIRST MOLAR: LINGUAL VIEW

From the lingual aspect of the mandibular first molar, three cusps are visible: the _____, _____, and _____ cusps.

Permanent
Mandibular
Right
1st Molar
LINGUAL

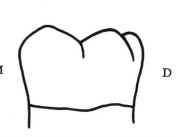

mesiolingual, distolingual, distal

Similar to the facial line angles, the mesiolingual and distolingual line angles of the mandibular first molar are indistinct. At the mesiolingual and distolingual line angles, the contour of the crown in the horizontal dimension is well _____.

Permanent
Mandibular
Right
1st Molar
1. LINGUAL
2. OCCLUSAL

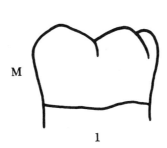

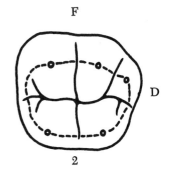

rounded

In contrast to the facial cusps, the mesial and distal ridges of each lingual cusp meet to form a cusp tip that is more _____.

Permanent
Mandibular
Right
1st Molar
LINGUAL

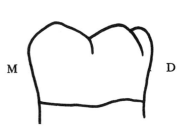

The developmental groove extending onto the lingual surface and separating the two lingual cusps is called the _____ groove.

Permanent
Mandibular
Right
1st Molar
LINGUAL

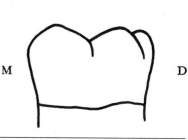

M   D

lingual

The mesial surface is convex from the mesial marginal ridge to the area of the proximal contact. From the contact to the cervical line, the mesial surface is flat or slightly concave. This flatness or concavity on the proximal surface allows room for the tissue called the _____   _____ .

Permanent
Mandibular
Right
1st Molar
LINGUAL

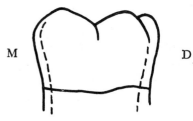

M   D

interdental papilla

To allow space for the interdental papilla, from the contact area to the cervical line, the occlusocervical curvature of the distal surface of the mandibular first molar is _____ or slightly _____ .

Permanent
Mandibular
Right
1st Molar
LINGUAL

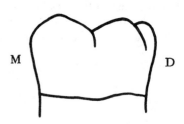

M   D

SECTION 5.2 MANDIBULAR FIRST MOLAR: Proximal View

Of the two marginal ridges on the crown of the mandibular first molar, which is at a higher level above the cervical line? _____

_____   _____

Permanent
Mandibular
Right
1st Molar
1. MESIAL
2. DISTAL

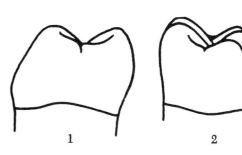

mesial marginal ridge

Which of the marginal ridges on the mandibular first molar is cut more deeply by a developmental groove? _____.

Permanent
Mandibular
Right
1st Molar
1. MESIAL
2. DISTAL

mesial (marginal ridge)

The distal cusp forms a prominent part of the distal surface of the mandibular first molar. Because of the distal cusp, the faciolingual length of the distal marginal ridge is _____ (greater than/less than) that of the mesial marginal ridge.

Permanent
Mandibular
Right
1st Molar
1. MESIAL
2. DISTAL

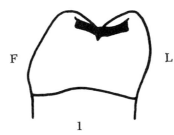
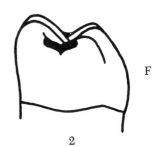

439

In some cases the distal cusp may be reduced so that it appears as a small convexity of the _____ _____ _____.

Permanent
Mandibular
Right
1st Molar
1. DISTAL
2. FACIAL.

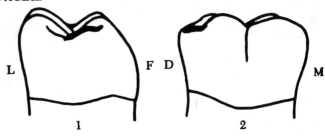

The rounded form of the distal cusp continues from the facial surface onto the distal so that the distal surface is slightly more convex than the mesial surface, in the _____ direction.

Permanent
Mandibular
Right
1st Molar
OCCLUSAL

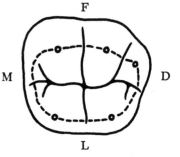

How many cusps (at least in part) are visible from the distal view of the mandibular first molar? _____

Permanent
Mandibular
Right
1st Molar
DISTAL

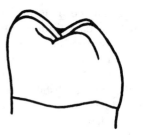

440

The cervical line (facial surface, mandibular first molar) is smoothly curved. On the lingual surface, the cervical line has an irregular curvature. On which of these two surfaces does the cervical line exhibit a smaller degree of curvature? _____.

Permanent
Mandibular
Right
1st Molar
1. LINGUAL
2. FACIAL

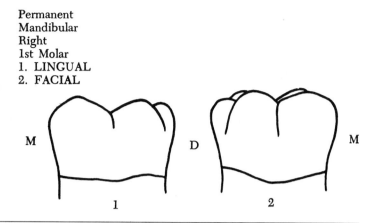

M   D   M

1   2

GO TO NEXT PAGE FOR MATRIX TEST 5.

MATRIX TEST 5

Directions . . .

   Place an X in the squares that match the top row with the left hand column.

   Mark your answers and *turn to Page 426*.

Mandibular First Molar	Facial	Lingual	Mesial	Distal
The views from which five cusps are visible . . .				
The proximal surface with the more convex curvature in the faciolingual direction as seen from an occlusal view . . .				
The portion of the crown with the two most pointed cusps . . .				

ANSWERS ON PAGE 426.

REVIEW TEST 5

Make a note of the correct answers. *Turn to Page 427 to check them.*

1. Of the two developmental grooves that cross the faciocclusal line angle onto the facial surface, which one most often ends in a pit?
   a. facial
   b. distofacial

2. The contour of the crown on the mandibular first molar in the horizontal directions (faciolingual and mesiodistal) at the mesiofacial, distofacial, mesiolingual, and distolingual line angles is . . .
   a. sharply angled
   b. well rounded

3. Of the two marginal ridges on the mandibular first molar, which is at a higher level above the cervical line and more deeply cut by a developmental groove?
   a. mesial
   b. distal

ANSWERS ON PAGE 427.

SECTION 6.0 MANDIBULAR SECOND MOLAR

The mandibular second molar maintains many of the characteristics of the mandibular first molar. This discussion emphasizes the features that distinguish the two teeth. (Features not discussed should be considered common to both teeth.)

Concerning the crown size, the measurements of the mandibular second molar (in all dimensions) are _____ (smaller/greater) than those of the mandibular first molar.

Permanent
Mandibular
Right
1., 2. 1st Molar
3., 4. 2nd Molar
1., 3. OCCLUSAL
2., 4. FACIAL

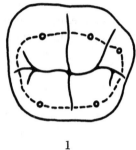

1

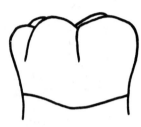

2

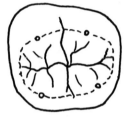

3

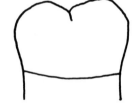

4

smaller

The mandibular second molar has four cusps, suggesting that it has _____ lobes.

Permanent
Mandibular
Right
2nd Molar
OCCLUSAL

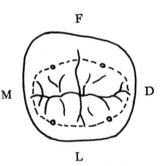

A characteristic of the mandibular second molar is its symmetrical development. More than any other molar, the cusps are nearly _____ in size.

Permanent
Mandibular
Right
2nd Molar
OCCLUSAL

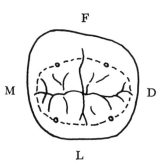

equal (or synonym)

In occlusal view, the faciolingual dimension of the mandibular second molar is broader at the _____ (mesial/distal).

Permanent
Mandibular
Right
2nd Molar
OCCLUSAL

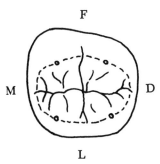

mesial

Similar to the nomenclature for other molars, the two facial cusps are called the _____ and _____ cusps.

    The two lingual cusps of the mandibular second molar are called the _____ and _____ cusps.

Permanent
Mandibular
Right
2nd Molar
LINGUAL

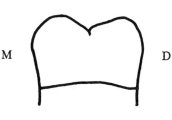

What cusp on the mandibular first molar has no counterpart on the mandibular second molar? _____

Permanent
Mandibular
Right
2nd Molar
OCCLUSAL

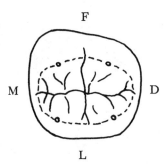

distal

From the occlusal view, the occlusal surface and groove pattern of the mandibular second molar resemble an ellipse with the major axis running in the _____ direction.

Permanent
Mandibular
Right
2nd Molar
OCCLUSAL

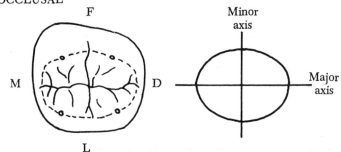

mesiodistal

Examine the drawings and note the differences between the groove patterns of the mandibular first and second molars.

The second molar has a triangular groove to the distal that is absent on the first molar. What is the name of that groove? _____

Permanent
Mandibular
Right
1. 1st Molar
2. 2nd Molar
OCCLUSAL

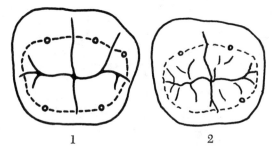

Four triangular ridges, one from each cusp, divide the occlusal surface into three fossae. Similar to the first molar, the fossae are named the ————, ———— and ——— fossae.

Permanent
Mandibular
Right
2nd Molar
OCCLUSAL

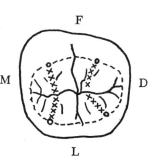

mesial, distal, central

Which grooves are contained (at least in part) within the central fossa? ————

Permanent
Mandibular
Right
2nd Molar
OCCLUSAL

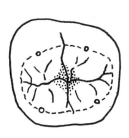

facial, lingual, mesial, distal

Similar to the nomenclature for the maxillary molars and the mandibular first molar, the union of the mesial and distal grooves is called the ———— groove.

Permanent
Mandibular
Right
2nd Molar
OCCLUSAL

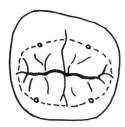

From the facial aspect, the chief characteristics that distinguish the mandibular second molar from the mandibular first molar are . . .

1. the size of the distofacial cusp in relation to the mesiofacial cusp;
2. the number of developmental grooves that descend onto the facial surface;
3. the number of cusps visible;
4. the number of cusps that contribute to the facial surface.

The details of each of these differences have been covered during the discussion of the occlusal aspect. Use your present knowledge and the diagrams provided to complete each of the following statements.

A. On the mandibular first molar, the smaller of the two facial cusps is the ——————— cusp. On the mandibular second molar, how does the size of the distofacial cusp compare with that of the mesiofacial cusp? (larger/equal/smaller) ———————.

B. If X equals the number of developmental grooves that descend onto the facial surface of the mandibular first molar, and Y equals the number of grooves that descend onto the facial surface of the mandibular second molar, then $X^2 - Y^2 =$ —————— (a numerical answer is required).

C. Because of the placement and height of the cusps, five cusps are visible from the facial aspect of the mandibular first molar. For similar reasons, how many cusps are visible from the facial aspect of the mandibular second molar? ———————

D. The facial surface of the mandibular second molar is formed by ——————— (number) lobes.

TURN TO TOP OF PAGE 450 FOR THE CORRECT ANSWERS.

Permanent
Mandibular
Right
1., 3. 1st Molar
2., 4. 2nd Molar
1., 2. OCCLUSAL
3., 4. FACIAL

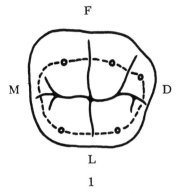

1

Occlusal
Mandibular First
Molar

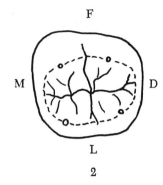

2

Occlusal
Mandibular Second
Molar

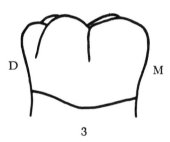

3

Facial
Mandibular First
Molar

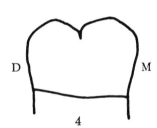

4

Facial
Mandibular Second
Molar

449

In most respects, the mesial and distal surfaces of the mandibular second molar resemble the mesial and distal surfaces of the mandibular first molar. The greatest difference, however, is between the _____ (mesial/distal) surfaces of the two teeth.

Permanent
Mandibular
Right
1., 2. 1st Molar
3., 4. 2nd Molar
1., 3. MESIAL
2., 4. DISTAL

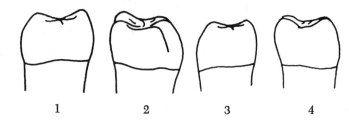

1   2   3   4

distal

Usually, the central fossa of the mandibular second molar is not as deep as the central fossa of the mandibular first molar. The perpendicular distance from the cusp tips to the level of the deepest cut of a developmental groove is greater on the mandibular _____ (first/second) molar.

Permanent
Mandibular
1. 2nd Molar
2. 1st Molar
FACIOLINGUAL
   SECTION

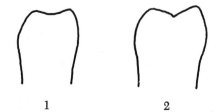

1   2

first

A pit is commonly found at the confluence of two or more grooves. Since occlusal pits are named for the fossa where they are found, the pit labeled (a) is the _____; that labeled (b) is the _____.

Permanent
Mandibular
Right
2nd Molar
OCCLUSAL

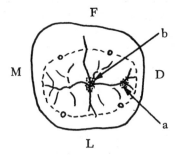

Concerning the cusps, what is the chief difference between the distal surfaces of the mandibular first and second molars? ————.

Permanent
Mandibular
Right
1. 1st Molar
2. 2nd Molar
DISTAL

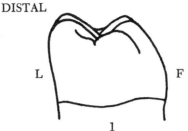

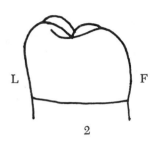

The distal cusp is not present on the second molar.

The crown of the mandibular second molar converges toward the lingual, but the degree of convergence is smaller than that on the mandibular first molar. Therefore, on which of the two molars is the mesiodistal measurement of the facial half of the crown more nearly equal to the mesiodistal measurement of the lingual half? ————

Permanent
Mandibular
Right
1. 1st Molar
2. 2nd Molar
OCCLUSAL

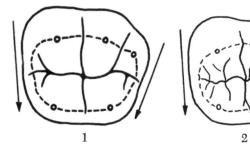

second (molar)

In the occlusocervical direction, the proximal contact areas on mandibular molars (first and second) are located in the ———— third of the crown.

Permanent
Mandibular
Right
2nd Molar
1. MESIAL
2. DISTAL

SECTION 6.1 MANDIBULAR THIRD MOLAR

The mandibular third molar presents a tremendous variety of individual variations. For this reason, it is difficult to define a "typical" mandibular third molar. It most often resembles the tooth immediately mesial to it and therefore usually has _____ (number) cusps.

Permanent
Mandibular
Right
1. 2nd Molar
2. 3rd Molar
OCCLUSAL

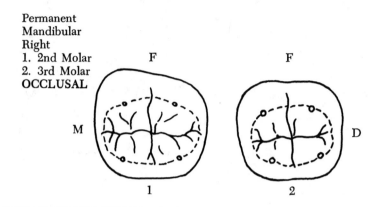

1   2

Although the mandibular third molar may have four cusps, the second most common type is similar to the mandibular first molar and has _____ (number) cusps.

Permanent
Mandibular
Right
3rd Molar
OCCLUSAL

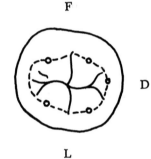

The mandibular third molar is generally smaller and more rounded than the second molar; therefore, one would expect the central fossa on this tooth to be shallow and _____ (size).

Facially, the cusps are short and well rounded and _____ (similar/dissimilar) to the corresponding cusps in the second molar.

Permanent
Mandibular
Right
3rd Molar
FACIAL

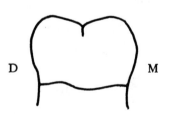

452

With one exception, the maxillary and mandibular molars have two antagonists. When the teeth of the maxillary and mandibular arches occlude ideally, which molar has but one antagonist? _____ _____

_____

SCHEMATIC DRAWING OF
MAXILLARY AND MANDIBULAR
LEFT QUADRANTS

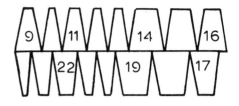

maxillary third molar

With normal occlusion, two of the sixteen mandibular teeth have but one antagonist, the two mandibular _____.

SCHEMATIC DRAWING OF
MAXILLARY AND MANDIBULAR
LEFT QUADRANTS

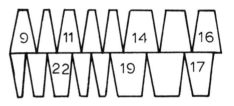

central incisors

GO TO NEXT PAGE FOR MATRIX TEST 6

MATRIX TEST 6

Directions . . .

Place an X in the square that matches the top row with the left hand column.

Mark your answers then *turn to Page 428.*

Mandibular Molars	Mandibular Molars		
	First	Second	Neither
The tooth with three lingual cusps . . .			
The tooth with the more symmetrical form . . .			
The tooth with the smaller measurements in all dimensions . . .			
The tooth with the greater amount of lingual convergence on the mesial and distal surfaces . . .			
The tooth with two developmental grooves of the facial surface . . .			

ANSWERS ON PAGE 428.

REVIEW TEST 6

Make a note of the correct answers. *Turn to Page 429 to check them.*

1. In length, the facial cusps of the mandibular second molar are . . .
   a. shorter than the lingual cusps.
   b. nearly equal to the lingual cusps.

2. The union of the mesial and distal developmental grooves on the mandibular second molar is called the . . .
   a. transverse groove.
   b. central groove.

3. The most common form of the mandibular third molar has ——————— cusps, but the second most common form has ——————— cusps.
   a. five, four.
   b. four, five.

4. The mandibular tooth with only one antagonist is the
   a. third molar.
   b. central incisor.

5. The mandibular molar with the most shallow central fossa is the . . .
   a. second molar.
   b. third molar.
   c. first molar.

ANSWERS ON PAGE 429.

SECTION 7.0 PROXIMAL CONTACTS AND CROWN CONTOURS OF THE MOLARS: A QUICKIE REVIEW

In the region of the posterior teeth, the lingual embrasures are deeper than facial embrasures. This is because the proximal contacts between posterior teeth are toward the _____ (facial/lingual) surface.

Permanent
Maxillary
Right
1. 3rd Molar
2. 2nd Molar
3. 1st Molar
4. 2nd Premolar
5. 1st Premolar
OCCLUSAL

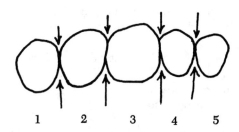

facial

The first, second, and third molars of both arches have their mesial and distal contacts located occlusocervically approximately in the center of the _____ third of the crown.

Permanent
Maxillary
Left
1. 2nd Premolar
2. 1st Molar
3. 2nd Molar
4. 3rd Molar
Mandibular
5. 2nd Premolar
6. 1st Molar
7. 2nd Molar
8. 3rd Molar
FACIAL

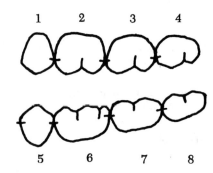

middle

Maxillary posterior teeth have the height of contour in the middle third on the _____ surface.

Permanent
Maxillary
Right
2nd Molar
MESIAL

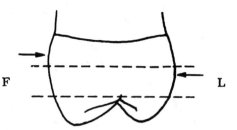

456

All maxillary teeth exhibit facial and lingual contours that measure approximately ½ mm horizontally.

The lingual surface of the maxillary left first molar has its height of contour in the _____ third and its amount of contour measures _____ mm.

The contour on the facial surfaces of mandibular posteriors is similar in both location and measurement to those on the facial surfaces of the maxillary posterior teeth. Mandibular premolars and molars have facial heights of contour in the _____ third and their amount of contour is approximately _____ mm.

Permanent
Mandibular
Left
1. 1st Premolar
2. 1st Molar
DISTAL

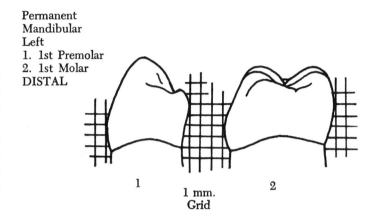

1   2
1 mm.
Grid

The contours of maxillary and mandibular posterior teeth differ basically in the measurement of their lingual surfaces. The mandibulars have lingual amounts of contour that measure nearly double those of the maxillaries. The contour on the lingual surface of mandibular posterior teeth approaches _____ mm in measurement.

Permanent
Mandibular
Right
1st Molar
MESIAL

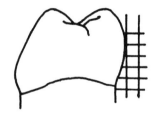

In their position in the oral cavity, teeth are often inclined and the observed height of contour is noticeably different from the anatomical height of contour. The observed height of contour is closer to the occlusal surface and the amount of contour appears greater than the anatomical contour would suggest. As shown in the drawing to the right, the mandibular molars have their crowns tilted toward the _____ (facial/lingual).

Permanent
Mandibular
Right
1st Molar
MESIAL
20°

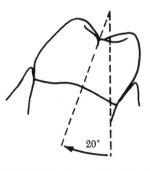

20°

In the discussion of facial and lingual contours, the average or most common tooth form was described. As with most anatomical features, individual deviations from the norm will occur on a specific tooth or a group of teeth.

SECTION 7.1   ROOT ANATOMY OF THE MOLARS: TERMINOLOGY

Some of the significant features of the root anatomy are the number and location of the roots on each tooth, the relative length of the roots, the curvature of each root, and the usual size and location of convex and concave areas on the root surfaces.

A notable crown-root distinction is that variation occurs more frequently on the root than on the crown of a tooth. This variability is more pronounced in the _____ (apical/cervical) portion of the root.

apical

Incisors, most canines, and most premolars are single rooted. Maxillary molars generally have three roots, and mandibular molars have two roots. Of the three teeth assigned the universal code numbers 3, 6, and 13, the triple-rooted tooth is number _____, the _____ _____ _____
(arch)   (quadrant)   (tooth name)

3, maxillary right first molar

When a tooth has three roots, the root portion of that tooth has one root trunk and three _____ _____.

Permanent
Maxillary
Right
1st Molar
1. DISTAL
2. FACIAL

Terminal Root →

Root Trunk →

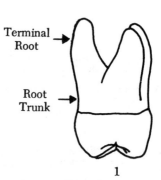
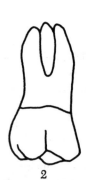

1   2

Although the curved contours of the roots do not present distinct surface boundaries, the terms facial, lingual, mesial, and distal are used to indicate root surfaces and directions. Of the three terminal roots on maxillary molars, one is located toward the lingual and two toward the _____.

Permanent
Maxillary
Right
1st Molar
1. DISTAL
2. FACIAL

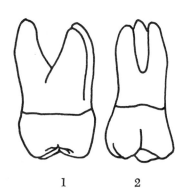

1 2

facial

Terminal roots are named for the position they occupy in relation to the surfaces of the crown. Root (A) is the distofacial root, (B) the _____ root, and (C) the _____ root.

Permanent
Maxillary
1st Molar
Right
1. DISTAL
2. FACIAL

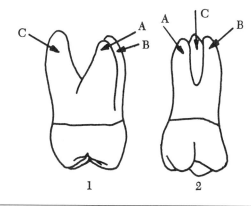

1 2

B. mesiofacial;
C. lingual

Mandibular molars generally have two terminal roots, the _____ and _____.

Permanent
Mandibular
1st Molar
Right
1. FACIAL
2. MESIAL

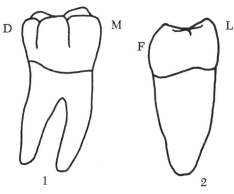

1 2

459

SECTION 7.2 ROOT ANATOMY OF THE MOLARS: MAXILLARY FIRST MOLAR

The root structures of the maxillary first and second molars, discussed next, have a number of similar features. The roots of the maxillary third molar vary more and will be covered separately.

On the roots of the maxillary molars, the level of trifurcation is variable, but the root trunk is almost always short. In the cervico-apical direction, the root trunk will consist of _____ (more than half/less than half) of the total root length.

Permanent
Maxillary
Right
1st Molar
FACIAL

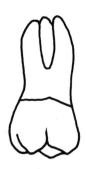

---

less than half

Corresponding to the division of the terminal roots, the three surfaces of the trunk are grooved from the trifurcation nearly to the cervical line. Because of the relative position of the roots, on which three surfaces of the root trunk are these grooves found?

  a. facial, lingual, mesial

  b. mesial, distal, lingual

  c. mesial, distal, facial

Permanent
Maxillary
Right
1st Molar
1. FACIAL
2. DISTAL
3. MESIAL
4. LINGUAL

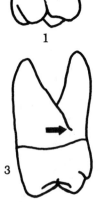

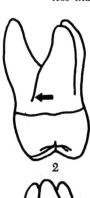

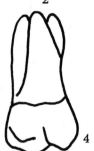

On multi-rooted molars, regardless of the number of terminal roots, a general term is often used to designate the division of the common root trunk into terminal root ends. This general term is **furcation.**

On a maxillary molar, the longest, largest, and strongest of the three roots is the _____ root.

Permanent
Maxillary
Right
1st Molar
1. MESIAL
2. HORIZONTAL
   SECTION

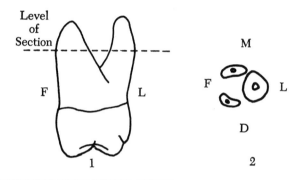

Level
of
Section

M

F   L

F   L

D

1

2

lingual

The two facial roots are nearly the same length, but the more highly developed and sometimes longer of the two facial roots is the _____ root.

Permanent
Maxillary
Right
1st Molar
FACIAL

D   M

In overall size (all directions), how do the three terminal roots order themselves, largest to smallest?

_____ largest

_____ next largest

_____ smallest

Permanent
Maxillary
Right
1st Molar
1. MESIAL
2. HORIZONTAL
SECTION

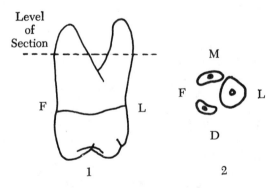

lingual, mesiofacial, distofacial (in that order)

In which of the two horizontal directions are the two facial roots wider?

_____

Permanent
Maxillary
Right
1st Molar
1. MESIAL
2. HORIZONTAL
SECTION

faciolingual

On the lingual root, the relative width in the faciolingual and mesiodistal directions is reversed from that on the two facial roots. In which horizontal directions is the lingual root the widest? _____

The wide lingual surface of the lingual root is sometimes marked by a longitudinal groove that is more pronounced in the cervical than at the apical portion.

Permanent
Maxillary
Right
1st Molar
1. LINGUAL
2. HORIZONTAL
   SECTIONS

Level of Section

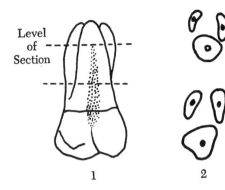

1   2

SECTION 7.3   ROOT ANATOMY OF THE MOLARS: MAXILLARY SECOND MOLAR

One general distinction between the root structures of the maxillary first and second molar is that the terminal roots lie closer together on one of these teeth, the _____ (arch)

_____.
(tooth name)

Permanent
Maxillary
Right
1. 2nd Molar
2. 1st Molar
LINGUAL

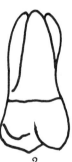

1   2

A second distinction between the maxillary first and second molars is the position of the apex of the lingual root in relation to the crown. In lingual view, the apex of the lingual root is centered over the distolingual developmental groove on the crown of the maxillary _____ molar.

Permanent
Maxillary
Right
1. 2nd Molar
2. 1st Molar
LINGUAL

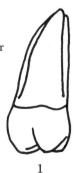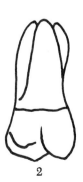

1   2

On the maxillary second molar, the apex of the lingual root is centered over the _____ (mesiolingual/distolingual) cusp.

**Permanent
Maxillary
Right
1. 2nd Molar
2. 1st Molar
LINGUAL**

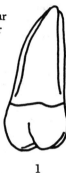
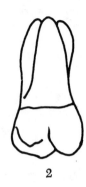

1   2

Fused and crooked terminal roots are two variations occurring on the root structures of the maxillary second molar. Which molar (maxillary first or second molar) has a root form that deviates more often from the average form? _____

The lingual root is somewhat banana shaped viewed from the mesial or distal, but it is straight when viewed from the lingual.

At the apical third, the lingual root changes directions, inclining slightly toward the _____.

**Permanent
Maxillary
Right
1st Molar
1. LINGUAL
2. MESIAL**

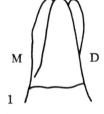
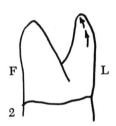

M   D   F   L

1   2

Occasionally, the single lingual root does not change directions at its apical third. When this is the case, it diverges for its entire length in a _____ direction.

**Permanent
Maxillary
Right
1st Molar
MESIAL
1. More Common
2. Less Common**

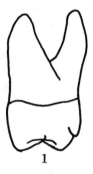
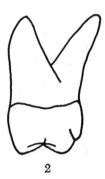

1   2

The terminal roots of the maxillary first molars generally diverge initially but return toward the midline near the _____ third.

Permanent
Maxillary
Right
1st Molar
1. FACIAL
2. DISTAL

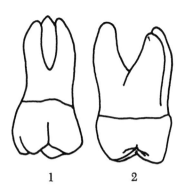

1   2

lingual

---

apical

The facial roots of the maxillary second molar have more surface irregularities (convexities and concavities) than the maxillary first molar. In relation to the first molar, however, the second molar has curvature of the terminal roots that is _____ (more/less) divergent from the midline of the crown.

Permanent
Maxillary
Right
1. 2nd Molar
2. 1st Molar
FACIAL

D 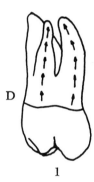 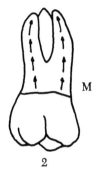 M

1   2

---

less

In facial view, the two facial roots on the maxillary second molar have a slight deflection toward the center axis of the tooth in the apical third. Therefore, the larger of the two facial roots is initially straight, but near the apex it is inclined in the _____ direction.

Permanent
Maxillary
Left
2nd Molar
FACIAL

M 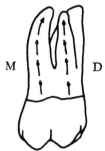 D

465

From the facial view, the apical third of the smaller root, the distofacial, has a slight deviation in the _____ direction.

Permanent
Maxillary
Left
2nd Molar
FACIAL

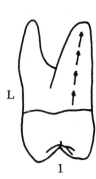

M   D

In proximal view, one of the two facial roots of the maxillary second molar is nearly vertical in the cervico-apical direction. The other has a slight deviation to the facial. Which of the two facial roots is more nearly vertical? _____

Permanent
Maxillary
Left
2nd Molar
1. MESIAL
2. DISTAL

L   F

1   2

In distal view, the distofacial root of the maxillary second molar has a slight deflection in the _____ direction.

Permanent
Maxillary
Left
2nd Molar
DISTAL

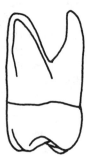

The cervico-apical curvature of the lingual root on the maxillary second molar is roughly similar to that of the maxillary first molar. Using your own words, describe the cervico-apical curvature of the lingual root on the maxillary molar as viewed from the mesial.

Permanent
Maxillary
Left
2nd Molar
MESIAL

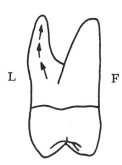

Your answer should indicate that the deviation is initially toward the lingual but straightens to a vertical or slightly facial orientation in the apical portion.

In lingual view, the lingual root may have a slight deflection toward the distal. More generally, however, it can be described as being relatively _____.

Permanent
Maxillary
Left
2nd Molar
LINGUAL

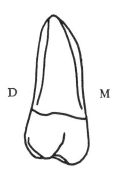

straight (vertical or synonym)

Of the three apexes on the maxillary first and second molars, one is blunt, one slightly blunted, and one pointed. The most blunt apex is on the _____ root; the most pointed is on the _____ root.

Permanent
Maxillary
Left
2nd Molar
DISTAL

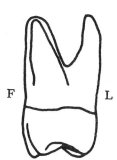

SECTION 7.4   ROOT ANATOMY OF THE MOLARS: MAXILLARY THIRD MOLAR

The maxillary third molar presents too many variations in root form to be precisely described. Generally, however, it is similar to the maxillary first and second molars and has ——————— (number) terminal roots.

Permanent
Maxillary
3rd Molars
FACIAL

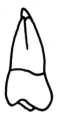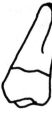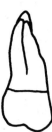

three

Frequently, the roots of the maxillary third molar are fused, forming one large root. Because of the fusion of the root structures, the root trunk of the maxillary third molar is usually ——————— (longer/ shorter) than that on the other maxillary molars.

Permanent
Maxillary
Right
3rd Molar
1. MESIAL
2. HORIZONTAL SECTION

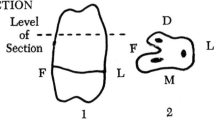

longer

The maxillary third molar may have as few as one fused root or as many as eight terminal roots.

Permanent
Maxillary
Right
3rd Molar
MESIAL

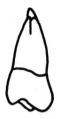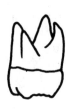

SECTION 7.5 ROOT ANATOMY OF THE MOLARS: MANDIBULAR MOLARS

The root trunk of mandibular molars is divided from lingual to facial and creates two terminal roots: one to the _____ and one to the _____.

---

mesial, distal

The root structures of the mandibular first and second molars have several features in common. Two surfaces of the root trunk have a smoothly contoured developmental depression running from the bifurcation to about the cervical line. These depressions are deep near the bifurcation but become progressively more shallow, fading out near the cervical line. Remembering the location of the terminal roots, on which of the four surfaces of the root trunk do these depressions occur? _____

   a. mesial distal
   b. facial and lingual

Permanent
Mandibular
Right
1st Molar
1. FACIAL
2. HORIZONTAL SECTION

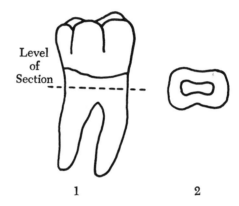

Level of Section

1   2

---

b. facial and lingual is correct

The greater horizontal width on the terminal roots of the mandibular molars runs in the same direction as the bifurcation, in the _____ direction.

Permanent
Mandibular
Right
1st Molar Roots
MESIAL
  (Apical Third)

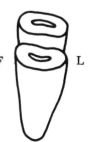

F   L

Each of the terminal roots on the mandibular molars has longitudinal grooves on the mesial and distal surfaces. When these grooves are well developed, a horizontal section appears I-beam in shape. The longitudinal grooves are highly developed on the mesial root, but on the distal root the grooves are less prominent and may be absent. In each of the drawings, which letter names the mesial root? _____ _____
     (Fig. 1)   (Fig. 2)

Permanent
Mandibular
1st Molar
**HORIZONTAL
  SECTIONS**

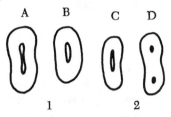

A, D

The drawing show the lingual tilt of the mandibular first molar as it is aligned in the mouth. Comparing the mesial and distal views of a mandibular molar, one finds that one of the terminal roots is slightly narrowed faciolingually and has a sharper cervico-apical taper. Which root is narrower and has the sharper apex? _____

Permanent
Mandibular
Right
1st Molar
1. MESIAL
2. DISTAL

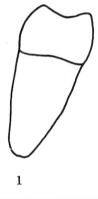
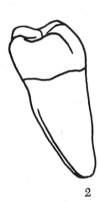

distal

If the apex of the distal root is sharp or pointed, what would be an appropriate term to describe the apex of the mesial root?

_____

Permanent
Mandibular
Right
1st Molar
1. MESIAL
2. DISTAL

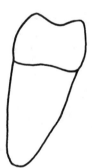
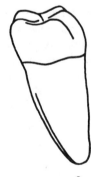

The drawing shows the slight mesial tilt of the tooth in the mouth. This facial view also illustrates the two root lengths. The root with the sharper apex (proximal view) is sometimes very slightly shorter. If one of the terminal roots is longer, which is it likely to be? _____

Permanent
Mandibular
Right
1st Molar
FACIAL

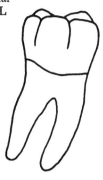

mesial

The cervico-apical curvature of the roots on each of the mandibular molars will be discussed separately. The discussion of longitudinal curvature will consider the appropriate portion of the root trunk as part of each terminal root. The curvature will be described from the facial view.

The mesial root of the mandibular first molar curves in a low arc away from the midline in the cervical half and toward it in the apical half. From the cervical line toward the apex, the mesial root initially curves to the _____ (direction) and then toward the _____.

Permanent
Mandibular
Right
1st Molar
FACIAL

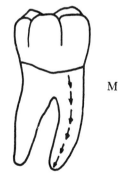

D   M

471

The distal root is nearly straight with a slight deflection away from the midline of the crown.

Permanent
Mandibular
Right
1st Molar
FACIAL

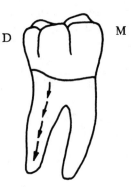

D   M

The apex of the distal root occasionally has a deflection in either direction, in some cases toward the _____ and in others toward the _____.

Permanent
Mandibular
Right
1st Molars
FACIAL

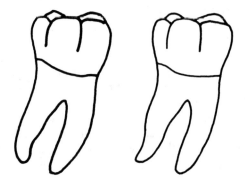

The roots of the mandibular second molar are more variable than those of the mandibular first molar. Mesiodistally, they may spread out wider than the roots of the mandibular first molar, or they may be so close together as to appear fused. Generally, the mesial and distal roots are closer together and more nearly parallel than the roots of the first molar. The cervico-apical curvature of one of the two roots appears to be slightly straighter. The straighter root is the _____.

Permanent
Mandibular
Left
2nd Molar
FACIAL
1. Average form
2., 3. Variations

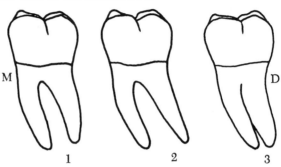

Of the mandibular first and second molars, which tooth has terminal roots that deflect more to the distal?_____

Permanent
Mandibular
Left
1. 1st Molar
2. 2nd Molar
FACIAL

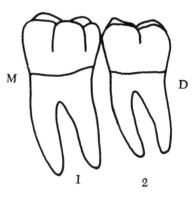

Although single or fused roots are common and extra roots may occur, the roots of the mandibular third molar generally resemble those of the other mandibular molars. What are the names of the roots on the mandibular third molar? _____ and _____.

Similar to the other mandibular molars, on which root are the longitudinal grooves more prominent? _____

Permanent
Mandibular
Left
2nd Molar
FACIAL

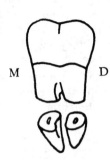

M   D

The roots of the mandibular third molar have irregular curvatures in the cervico-apical direction. However, the over-all curvature shows a deflection that is away from the midline of the mandibular arch. The roots of the mandibular third molar deviate in a _____ direction.

Permanent
Mandibular
Left
3rd Molar
FACIAL

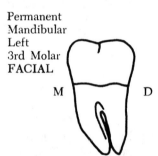

M   D

MATRIX TEST 7

Directions . . .

Place an X in the square that matches the left hand column with the top row.

Mark the answers *and turn to Page 430.*

Molars	Facial	Lingual	Mesial or Mesio-facial	Distal or Disto-facial
Largest root of maxillary first molar.				
Inclination of lingual root apex, maxillary first molar.				
The smallest root of the maxillary first molar.				
Root with the sharpest apex, maxillary second molar.				
Largest root, mandibular first molar.				
Straighter root (occluso-apical direction) of mandibular first molar.				
Inclination of roots, mandibular third molar.				

ANSWERS ON PAGE 430.

REVIEW TEST 7

Write down the correct answers for each question. Check them on Page 431.

1. What is the usual number of terminal roots of the molars in each arch?
   a. Maxillary ——————
   b. Mandibular ——————

2. Which of the following molars is most likely to have terminal roots that are fused?
   a. Maxillary second molar
   b. Maxillary third molar
   c. Mandibular second molar

3. The mandibular first molar has a facial and a lingual root.
   a. True
   b. False

4. The distal root of the mandibular second molar has a cervico-apical curvature that
   a. . . . inclines distally, with the apex usually deviated toward the mesial.
   b. . . . inclines distally, with (usually) no apical deviation.

ANSWERS ON PAGE 431.

SECTION 8.0   PULP ANATOMY OF THE MOLARS: MAXILLARY MOLARS

The maxillary first molar has a pulp chamber with four major pulp horns corresponding to its four major cusps. These are called the _____, _____, _____ and _____ pulp horns.

Permanent
Maxillary
Right
1st Molar
1. FACIOLINGUAL
   SECTION
2. MESIODISTAL
   SECTION

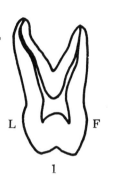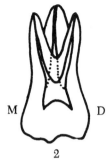

L   F   M   D

1   2

mesiofacial, distofacial, mesiolingual, and distolingual (in any order)

Surprisingly, given the number of roots in a maxillary molar, there are more often _____ (number) root canals.

Permanent
Maxillary
Right
1st Molar
1. FACIOLINGUAL
   SECTION
2. MESIODISTAL
   SECTION

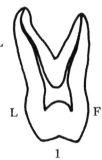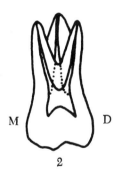

L   F   M   D

1   2

four

The two root canals present (with either one or two foramina) in the mesiofacial root, generally unite near the apical third of the root. A horizontal section showing two root canals in the mesiofacial root probably was taken in the _____ (cervical/apical) portion of the root.

Permanent
Maxillary
Right
1st Molar
1. FACIOLINGUAL
   SECTION
2. MESIODISTAL
   SECTION

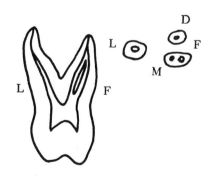

L   F

1   2

About 40% of the time the mesiofacial root is undivided and the total number of root canals is _____.

Permanent
Maxillary
Right
1st Molar
1. MESIODISTAL
   SECTION
2. HORIZONTAL
   SECTION

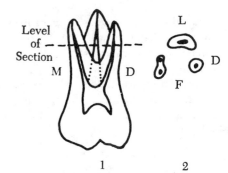

Whether there are three root canals (mesiofacial undivided) or four root canals (mesiofacial divided), the orifice of each major canal serves as a corner of the maxillary first molar pulp chamber. Therefore, the shape of the floor of the pulp chamber is roughly _____.

Permanent
Maxillary
Right
1st Molar
1. MESIODISTAL
   SECTION
2. HORIZONTAL
   SECTION

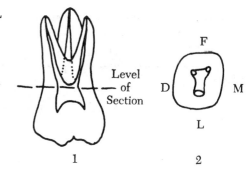

A horizontal section taken at the level of the cervical line usually cuts through the pulp chamber. Therefore, the floor of the pulp chamber of the maxillary molars is generally located somewhere between the cervical line and the _____ of the root structure.

Permanent
Maxillary
Right
1st Molar
MESIODISTAL
   SECTION

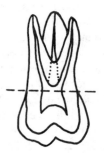

A series of horizontal sections through the lingual root show that the lingual root canal is nearly round at the orifice and near the apex. In the middle portion of the lingual root, the lingual root canal is more elliptical, with the major axis running in the _____ direction.

Permanent
Maxillary
Right
1st Molar
1. MESIODISTAL
   SECTION
2. HORIZONTAL
   SECTIONS

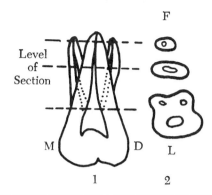

Similar to the pattern of the distofacial root, the distofacial root canal of a maxillary molar is small and tapered. A horizontal section through this root shows it to be almost _____.

Permanent
Maxillary
Right
1st Molar
1. MESIODISTAL
   SECTION
2. HORIZONTAL
   SECTION

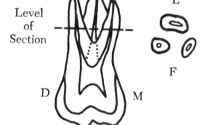

When the mesiofacial root has a single root canal (called the mesiofacial root canal) it is usually flattened. It is widest in the _____ direction.

Permanent
Maxillary
Right
1st Molar
1. MESIODISTAL
   SECTION
2. HORIZONTAL
   SECTION

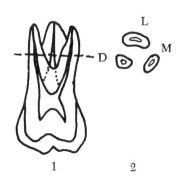

479

The pulp cavity of the maxillary second molar is similar to that of the maxillary first molar. What are the names of the root canals in the most common form of the maxillary second molar? _____, _____, and _____.

Permanent Maxillary Left 2nd Molar
1. MESIODISTAL SECTION
2. HORIZONTAL SECTION

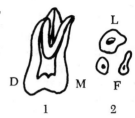

mesiofacial, distofacial, lingual (in any order)

The many different forms of the maxillary third molar make a detailed description of its pulp cavity impossible. Important to remember is that the root canals have the same general shape and number as the _____.

Permanent Maxillary Right 3rd Molars
1. FACIAL
2. HORIZONTAL SECTIONS

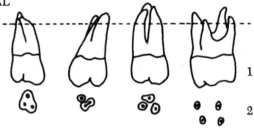

roots

SECTION 8.1 PULP ANATOMY OF THE MOLARS: MANDIBULAR MOLARS

The pulp cavities of the mandibular molars have more variations than those of the maxillary molars. The mandibular first and second molars have a different number of cusps; therefore, the roofs of the pulp chambers of the two teeth have a different number of _____

Permanent Mandibular
1. Right 1st Molar
2. Left 2nd Molar
DISTAL

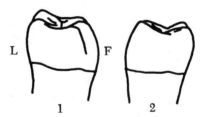

The pulp chamber of the mandibular first molar can be expected to have _____ (number) pulp horns; the second molar will have _____ pulp horns.

Permanent
Mandibular
1. Right
1st Molar
2. Left
2nd Molar
DISTAL

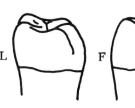

1   2

Here are horizontal sections made just apical to the bifurcation of the roots of the mandibular molars. How many root canals are present in the greatest percentage of the mandibular molars? _____

Permanent
Mandibular
Molars
HORIZONTAL
   ROOT
   SECTIONS

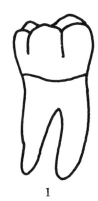

If three root canals are present, the larger, kidney-shaped canal is found in the _____ root, and the smaller, more circular canals are found in the _____ root.

Permanent
Mandibular
Right
1st Molar
1. FACIAL
2. HORIZONTAL
   SECTION

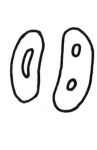

1   2

481

Of the two root canals in the mesial root, one is toward the facial, the other toward the lingual. Because of the location, when three root canals are present in the mandibular molar, they are named the distal canal, the facial canal of the mesial root and the _____ canal of the mesial root.

Permanent
Mandibular
Right
1st Molar
HORIZONTAL
   ROOT SECTION

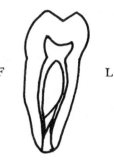

The facial canal of the mesial root and the lingual canal of the mesial root are often connected by small horizontal tunnels running in a _____ (faciolingual/mesiodistal) direction.

Permanent
Mandibular
Right
1st Molar
FACIOLINGUAL
   SECTION

The two mesial canals may have individual apical openings or may unite to form a single canal with a single _____ near the _____ of the root.

Permanent
Mandibular
Right
1st Molar
FACIOLINGUAL
   SECTION OF
   APICAL THIRD

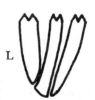
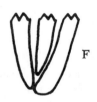

In some mandibular molars, the mesial root canals are not separate. Instead, there is a broad, ribbon-shaped root canal in the mesial root. When this occurs, the root canal is called the _____ root canal.

Permanent
Mandibular
Right
1st Molar
HORIZONTAL
   ROOT SECTION

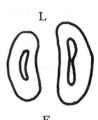

482

The distal root canal in a mandibular molar usually is single and broad in a ———— direction.

Permanent
Mandibular
Right
1st Molar
HORIZONTAL
ROOT SECTION

mesial

L

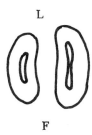

F

faciolingual

In a few cases, the distal root of a mandibular molar may have two root canals (Fig. 3).

Of the three drawings, which illustrates the number of root canals that occurs most frequently in mandibular molars? ————
Which illustrates the number that occurs least frequently? ————

M 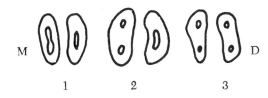 D

1   2   3

Figure 2, Figure 3 (in that order)

The pulp cavity of the mandibular third molar frequently has a form similar to that of the other mandibular molars. If the form is a noticeable variation, then the pulp cavity tends to follow the form of the tooth. If four roots are present, one expects to find ———— root canals.

four

MATRIX TEXT 8

Directions . . .

Write in the correct word(s) in the square that matches the left hand column with the top row.

Write the answers on one of the translucent sheets, then remove the sheet *and turn to Page 432.*

Pulp of Posterior Teeth	Maxillary First Molar	Mandibular First Molar
Most common number of root canals.		
If the tooth has a less common number of root canals, what number of canals would that be?		
Number of pulp horns in pulp chamber.		
Names of usual root canals (if more than one).		

ANSWERS ON PAGE 432.

REVIEW TEST 8

In order to end this chapter on a positive note, we have constructed a single, powerful test item with an interesting result.

1. Complete the following addition problems:
    a. Add the usual number of pulp horns on a mandibular second molar to the number of root canals it usually has.

    _____ + _____ = _____

    b. Add the most common number of root canals that every molar typically shows to the number of major pulp horns usually occurring on the maxillary first molar.

    _____ + _____ = _____

    c. Add the second most frequent number of root canals on mandibular molars to the number of pulp horns on the mandibular first molar.

    _____ + _____ = _____

ANSWERS ON PAGE 433.

5
THE PRIMARY DENTITION

SECTION 1.0   THE PRIMARY DENTITION

Each quadrant of primary dentition consists of two incisors, a canine, and two molars. The total number of teeth in the primary dentition is _____.

In contrast to the permanent dentition, how many premolar teeth are in the primary dentition?

_____

Primary Dentition
Maxillary
Mandibular
OCCLUSAL
(Universal
   Coding System)

Right

Left

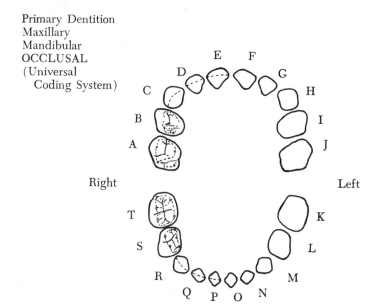

twenty, none

Because the anterior teeth consist of the incisors and canines and the posterior teeth of premolars and molars, each quadrant of the permanent dentition contains three anterior teeth and five posterior teeth. Each quadrant of the primary dentition contains _____ (number) anterior teeth and _____ (number) posterior teeth.

486

Of the two, which dentition has crowns that are more bulbous or balloon-like? _____

Permanent
Maxillary
Right
1. Central Incisor
FACIAL
2. 1st Molar
MESIAL

D   M   F   L

1   2

Primary
Maxillary
Right
3. Central Incisor
FACIAL
4. 2nd Molar
MESIAL

D   M   F   L

3   4

primary

The bulbous shape of the primary teeth is emphasized by a more pronounced constriction in the region of the _____.

cervical line

The "pinched in" region in the area of the cervical line is called a cervical _____.

Primary
Maxillary
Right
1. Central Incisor
FACIAL
2. 2nd Molar
MESIAL

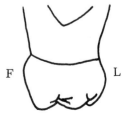

D   M   F   L

1   2

A second feature contributing to the bulbous appearance of the crowns of <u>primary molars is the strong **occlusal convergence** of the facial and lingual surfaces.</u> What effect does the convergence have on the faciolingual measurement of the occlusal surface? _____

Primary
1. Maxillary
Right
2nd Molar
MESIAL
Right
2. Mandibular
1st Molar
MESIAL

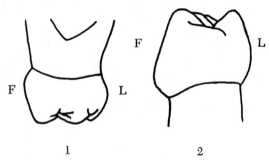

1   2

Makes it smaller (proportionately smaller than permanent molars)

On primary crowns, the height of contour on the facial and lingual surfaces is more prominent than on permanent crowns.

The height of contour on the facial and lingual surfaces of the crown is sometimes called a **cervical** or **gingival ridge**. One term is more anatomically oriented, the other more clinically oriented. Which is more clinically oriented? _____

Primary
Maxillary
Right
1. Central Incisor
MESIAL
2. 2nd Molar
MESIAL

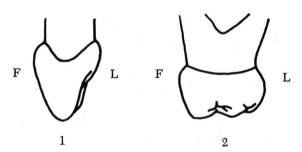

1   2

Compared to a permanent molar, the occlusal table of a primary molar is smaller in two different ways: has less total area and is proportionately smaller in relation to the total crown bulk.

The smaller total area of the occlusal table is the result of a smaller crown size and greater convergence of the facial and lingual surfaces. The proportionately smaller occlusal table on primary molars is related to only one of these two features, the _____.

1. Primary Maxillary Right 1st Molar OCCLUSAL
2. Permanent Maxillary Right 1st Molar OCCLUSAL

greater convergence of the facial and lingual surfaces

	PRIMARY			PERMANENT		
	CENTRAL INCISOR	CANINE	FIRST MOLAR	CENTRAL INCISORS	CANINE	FIRST MOLAR
Root Length*	10	13.5	10	13	17	12 to 13
Crown Length*	6	6.5	5.1	10.5	10	7.5

*Approximate length in millimeters

Examine this table of approximate crown and root length of some of the primary and permanent teeth.

The primary central incisor has a root length of 10 and a crown length of 6. The ratio of these two lengths is 1.66, meaning that the root is, proportionately, one and two-thirds longer than the crown.

The permanent central incisor, on the other hand, has a root length of 13 and a crown length of 10.5. The ratio of root to crown length is, therefore, 1.24. This means that the root is proportionately longer than the crown by only one and one-quarter times.

This relationship between root and crown length in primary and permanent teeth holds true throughout the dentitions.

In which dentition is the ratio of root length to crown length greater?

a. Primary
b. Permanent

489

In which dentition do the roots of the molars have a greater degree of divergence or outward flare?
_____

1. Primary
Maxillary
1st Molar
FACIAL
2. Permanent
Maxillary
1st Molar
FACIAL

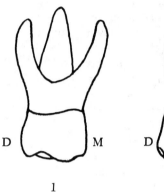
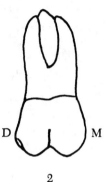

D   M   D   M

1   2

The flare of the roots of primary molars provides space for the developing tooth buds of the _____ premolars.

Write a one or two word response that describes each of the following features of the primary dentition in relation to the permanent dentition.

    A. Gross form of crown _____
    B. Over-all crown size _____
    C. Area of occlusal table in relation to crown size (posterior teeth only) ___

    D. Degree of cervical constriction _____
    E. Root length in relation to crown length _____
    E. Relative amount of outward flare (divergence) of root structure (multi-rooted teeth only) _____

A. *more bulbous; B. smaller; C. proportionately smaller; D. greater; E. proportionately longer; F. greater*

ERUPTION SEQUENCE AND DATES
FOR PRIMARY TEETH*

MAXILLARY AND MANDIBULAR	RANGE OF TYPICAL ERUPTION DATES	
Central Incisors	6 months	— 1 year
Lateral Incisors	9 months	— 16 months
First Molars	1 year	— 1½ years
Canines	1½ years	— 2 years
Second Molars	2 years	— 3 years

MOST COMMON ERUPTION SEQUENCE*					
Maxillary:	CI LI	1M	C		2M
Mandibular:	CI	LI	IM	C	2M

*Adapted from Lunt, R.C. and Law, D.B.A. Review of the chronology of eruption of deciduous teeth. *JADA* 89:872 1974, with permission of Dr. Lunt.

Though the eruption sequence is similar for each arch, the central incisors in the _____ arch normally precede their counterparts in the opposing arch.

mandibular

Which posterior tooth erupts prior to the eruption of one of the anterior teeth in each arch? _____.

first molar

A longitudinal section of a primary tooth reveals three anatomical features of significance in clinical dentistry. In relation to the corresponding features of the permanent teeth, (a) the enamel cap is thinner, (b) pulp cavities are relatively larger, resulting in proportionately thinner dentin, and (c) the pulp horns extend higher. Which of these three features makes the pulp of a primary tooth more susceptible to exposure by decay, cavity preparation, or fracture? _____

Primary
Maxillary
1. Central Incisor
FACIOLINGUAL
LONGITUDINAL
  SECTION
2. 1st Molar
MESIODISTAL
LONGITUDINAL
  SECTION

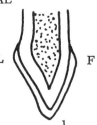

L   F

1

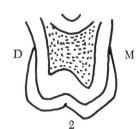

D   M

2

491

The <u>dentin in primary teeth is generally less dense</u> than in permanent teeth. Because a thicker, <u>more dense dentin causes a darker color, will the primary teeth generally have a darker</u> or lighter color than the permanent teeth? _____

The gross morphology of the primary dentition has many features common to that of the permanent dentition. Only the more important forms and critical differences will be described.

SECTION 1.1   PRIMARY MAXILLARY CENTRAL INCISOR

On the facial surface of the primary maxillary central incisor, the mesiodistal width is _____ (greater/less) than the incisocervical length.

Primary
Maxillary
Right
Central Incisor
FACIAL

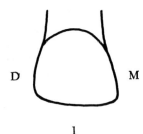

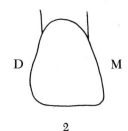

1

2

In other words, the crown of the primary maxillary central incisor is wider mesiodistally than it is long incisocervically. This "squatty," short appearance is characteristic of all primary anterior teeth, and is _____ (similar/dissimilar) to permanent anterior teeth.

1. Primary
Maxillary
Right
Central Incisor
FACIAL
2. Permanent
Maxillary
Right
Central Incisor
FACIAL

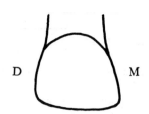

The facial surface of the central incisor is convex in both the incisocervical and mesiodistal directions, but it is more convex in the _____ direction.

Primary
Maxillary
Central Incisor
1. MESIAL
2. INCISAL

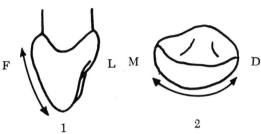

mesiodistal

The lingual features on the crown of a primary maxillary central incisor are smoothly contoured but have the same names as the corresponding features on a permanent central incisor. Identify each of the features labeled.

A. _____
B. _____
C. _____
D. _____

Primary
Maxillary
Right
Central Incisor
LINGUAL

A. mesial marginal ridge; B. lingual fossa; C. cingulum; D. distal marginal ridge

The root of a primary central incisor tends to be nearly circular in horizontal section and evenly tapered toward the apex in the longitudinal direction. Overall, the geometric form of the root can be described as _____ in shape.

Primary
Maxillary
Right
Central Incisor
1. MESIAL
2. HORIZONTAL
   SECTION

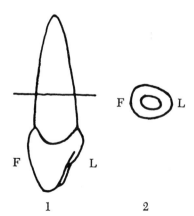

The roof of the pulp chamber in a primary maxillary central incisor has three pulp horns. As with permanent incisor, the facial portion is described as having how many lobes? _____

Primary
Maxillary
Right
Central Incisor
MESIODISTAL
LONGITUDINAL
SECTION

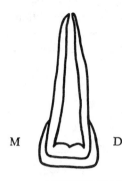

M   D

three

Since the cingulum of the primary incisor represents a single lobe, the tooth can be described as having a total of _____ lobes.

Primary
Maxillary
Right
Central Incisor
1. LINGUAL
2. MESIAL

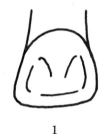 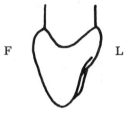

F   L

1   2

four

SECTION 1.2   PRIMARY MAXILLARY LATERAL INCISOR

Of the two primary maxillary incisors, which is wider in the mesiodistal direction? _____

Primary
Maxillary
Right
1. Lateral Incisor
2. Central Incisor
FACIAL

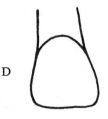 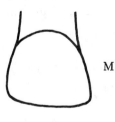

D   M

1   2

What is the incisocervical size relationship between the crowns of the primary maxillary central and lateral incisors? _____

Primary
Maxillary
Right
1. Lateral Incisor
2. Central Incisor
FACIAL

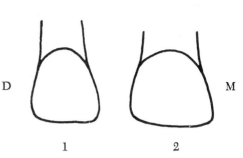

D   M

1   2

On the primary lateral incisor, the facial and lingual features are less prominent than those of the central incisor. Which primary incisor has the more prominent cingulum? _____

Primary
Maxillary
Right
Lateral Incisor
LINGUAL

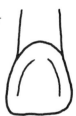

Illustrated is a significant difference between the cervical regions of the pulp cavity of the primary central and lateral incisors. What is the difference? _____

Primary
Maxillary
1. Central Incisor
2. Lateral Incisor
FACIOLINGUAL
LONGITUDINAL
  SECTION

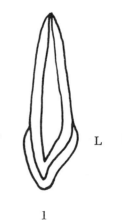
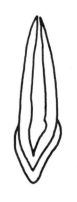

F   L   F   L

1   2

*A cervical constriction of the pulp cavity in the
lateral incisor is absent in the central incisor.*

Apart from this distinction, the root and pulp structures on the primary maxillary lateral incisors and central incisors are essentially _____ (similar/dissimilar).

Primary
Maxillary
1. Central Incisor
2. Lateral Incisor
FACIOLINGUAL
LONGITUDINAL
    SECTION

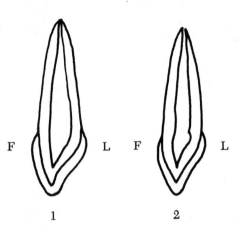

similar

SECTION 1.3   PRIMARY MANDIBULAR CENTRAL INCISOR

What is the size relationship between the maxillary and mandibular central incisors? _____

Primary
1. Maxillary
Right
Central Incisor
LINGUAL
2. Mandibular
Right
Central Incisor
LINGUAL

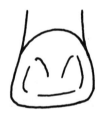 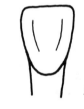

*The mandibular are smaller (the maxillary are
larger)*

Although the facial surface on a mandibular incisor is convex in the mesiodistal direction, the degree of convexity progressively decreases from the _____ (cervical/incisal) border to the _____ border.

Primary
Mandibular
Central Incisor
1. FACIAL
2. INCISAL

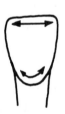 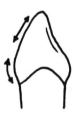

As with the other primary anterior teeth, but unlike the permanent mandibular anterior teeth, the primary mandibular central incisor has its incisal edge _____ (in line with/displaced from) the longitudinal axis of the tooth from a proximal view.

Primary
Mandibular
Right
Central Incisor
MESIAL

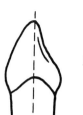

in line with

Similar to the permanent mandibular central incisor, the primary mandibular central incisor has mesioincisal and distoincisal angles that are approximately _____ (45°/right) angles.

Primary
Mandibular
Right
Central Incisor
FACIAL

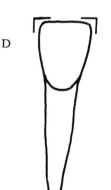

right

Compared to the maxillary incisor, the lingual contours of a mandibular incisor are reduced and smoothly curved. Therefore, the cingulum and marginal ridges will be _____ (distinct/indistinct).

Primary
1. Maxillary
Right
Central Incisor
LINGUAL
2. Mandibular
Right
Central Incisor
LINGUAL

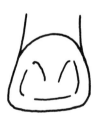

497

SECTON 1.4 PRIMARY MANDIBULAR CENTRAL INCISOR

Of the two mandibular incisors, which crown has the greater incisocervical length? _____

Primary
Mandibular
Right
1. Central Incisor
2. Lateral Incisor
FACIAL

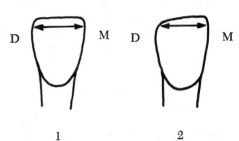

lateral incisor

The crown of the mandibular lateral incisor compared to the mandibular central incisor, is longer and slightly _____ (narrower/wider).

Primary
Mandibular
Right
1. Central Incisor
2. Lateral Incisor
FACIAL

wider

Of the two incisal angles on the mandibular lateral incisor, which is more rounded? _____

Primary
Mandibular
Right
Lateral Incisor
FACIAL

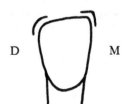

Which incisor has the longer root? _____

Primary
Mandibular
Right
1. Central Incisor
2. Lateral Incisor
FACIAL

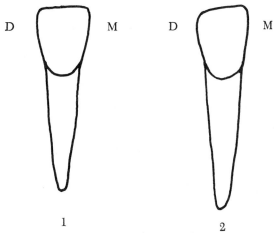

D   M   D   M

1   2

MATRIX TEXT 1

Directions . . .

Place an X in the square that matches the left hand column with the top row. Mark the answers *then turn to Page 510.*

	Both/ Neither	Central	Lateral
Primary maxillary incisor with the wider crown.			
Primary maxillary incisor with the longer crown.			
Primary mandibular incisor with the crown that appears slightly wider.			
Mandibular incisor with a rounder distoincisal angle.			

ANSWERS ON PAGE 510.

SECTION 1.5   PRIMARY MAXILLARY CANINE

The primary canines have considerably _more bulk than the primary incisors_. In the maxillary arch, in which directions are the measurements of the canines larger than those of the incisors? _____ (A/B/C)

A. mesiodistal and faciolingual only
B. mesiodistal and incisocervical only
C. mesiodistal, incisocervical, and faciolingual

Primary
Maxillary
Right
1. Canine
2. Lateral Incisor
3. Central Incisor
a. FACIAL
b. MESIAL

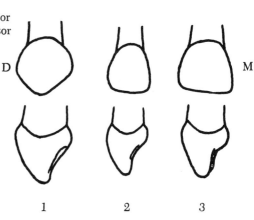

1   2   3

C. (all three directions)

The number and position of the lobes that can be seen on a primary canine are _similar to those of the incisors_. Therefore, the facial portion is described as having _____ (number) lobes and the lingual portion as having _____ (number) lobe(s).

three, one (in that order)

The facial portion of the canine is "_enlivened_" by the well developed central lobe area which forms two characteristic canine features, the _____ and its prominent _____ ridge.

Primary
Maxillary
Right
Canine
1. FACIAL
2. MESIAL

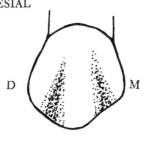

1   2

501

The cusp tip divides the incisal into the mesial cusp ridge and the distal cusp ridge. Which cusp ridge is longer? ————

Primary Maxillary Right Canine FACIAL

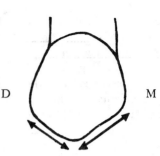

D   M

mesial

On the lingual, the prominent marginal ridges and the lingual fossae have the same names as the corresponding features on permanent canines. Name the features labeled in the drawing.

Primary Maxillary Right Canine LINGUAL

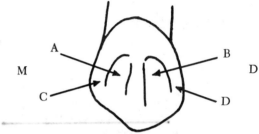

A. ————
B. ————
C. ————
D. ————

A. mesiolingual fossa; B. distolingual fossa; C. mesial marginal ridge; D. distal marginal ridge

In the cervical third of the crown, the lingual ridge blends with the cingulum. The lingual ridge thus becomes less prominent as it runs in a ———— direction.

Primary Maxillary Right Canine LINGUAL

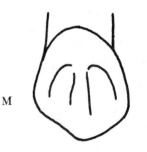

M   D

Why is the following statement false? "The single, relatively <u>long and thick,</u> root of the primary maxillary canine is gradually tapered from the cervical line to the apex."

The statement is false because _____

    a. the root is not relatively long and thick ...... GO TO NEXT FRAME

    b. the root does not have a gradual taper from the cervical line to the apex ...... GO TO TOP OF PAGE 504

Primary
Maxillary
Right
Anterior Teeth
FACIAL

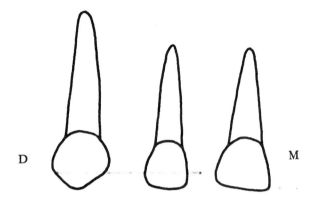

D   M

◗ From preceding frame

a. is incorrect

The curvatures of the root are difficult to detect in a two dimensional drawing. Perhaps the caricature at the right will help.

Primary
Maxillary
Canine
MESIAL

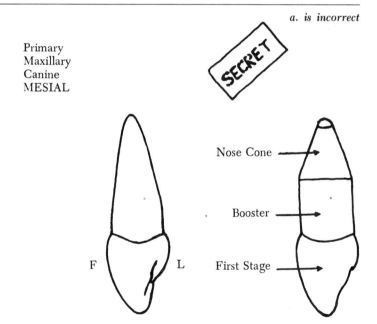

F   L   Nose Cone ⟶

Booster ⟶

First Stage ⟶

RETURN TO THE PRECEDING QUESTION AND SELECT THE CORRECT RESPONSE.

The maxillary canine root is not gradually tapered. There is a very slight increase in diameter just apical to the cervical line. The diameter is fairly constant throughout the ———— half of the root.

Primary
Maxillary
Right
Canine
FACIAL

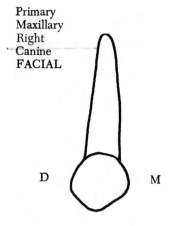

D   M

cervical

The pulp chamber of the maxillary canine has three horns: the distal, central, and mesial. The largest is the ————

Primary
Maxillary
Right
Canine
MESIODISTAL
LONGITUDINAL
    SECTION

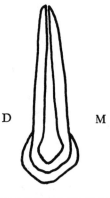

D   M

central

The distal pulp horn is slightly larger and longer than the mesial horn. Rank the three pulp horns in the order of their size (largest to smallest).

———— largest

————

———— smallest

Primary
Maxillary
Right
Canine
MESIODISTAL
LONGITUDINAL
    SECTION

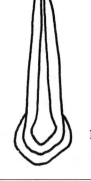

D   M

504

In the maxillary canine, there is little demarcation between the pulp chamber and the root canal. Thus, the pulp cavity of the canine is similar to that of the maxillary _____ incisor.

Primary
Maxillary
Right
Canine
MESIODISTAL
LONGITUDINAL
SECTION

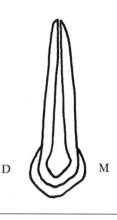

D   M

SECTION 1.6   PRIMARY MANDIBULAR CANINE

The mandibular canine has essentially the same features and characteristics as the maxillary canine. One exception is the relative lengths of the mesioincisal and distoincisal edges (mesial cusp ridge and distal cusp ridge). On the mandibular canine, which incisal edge is longer?

_____

Primary
1. Maxillary
2. Mandibular
Right
Canine
FACIAL

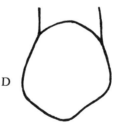

D

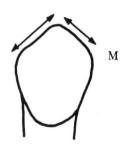

M

Indicate the quadrant to which each belongs (Hint: measure the relative length of the mesial and distal cusp ridges)

1. _____ _____ _____
   quadrant
2. _____ _____ _____
   quadrant

Primary
1. Maxillary
2. Mandibular
Right
Canine
FACIAL

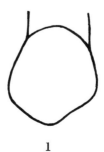

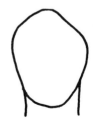

1   2

505

Which of the two canine teeth is wider mesiodistally? _____

Primary
1. Maxillary
2. Mandibular
Right
Canine
FACIAL

D

M

1

2

Compared to the maxillary canine, the lingual features of the primary mandibular canine are less prominent. The marginal ridges blend with the cingulum which is _____ (larger/smaller) than that of the maxillary canine.

Primary
Mandibular
Right
Canine
LINGUAL

M

D

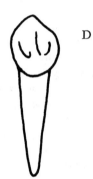

Although less prominent than on the maxillary canine, the usual features are present on the lingual portion of the mandibular canine. Identify each:

A. _____
B. _____
C. _____

Primary
Mandibular
Right
Canine
LINGUAL

M

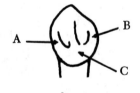

A

B

C

D

506

One difference between the root of the mandibular canine and the maxillary canine is the cervico-apical taper. Which canine has the more tapered root? _____

Primary
1. Maxillary
2. Mandibular
Right
Canine
FACIAL

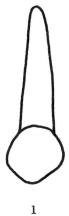
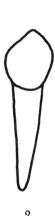

1   2

mandibular canine

The primary mandibular canine has no demarcation between the pulp chamber and root canal. In this regard, the mandibular canine is similar to most other primary anterior teeth except the _____

Mandibular
Right
Canine
1. FACIOLINGUAL
   LONGITUDINAL
   SECTION
2. MESIODISTAL
   LONGITUDINAL
   SECTION

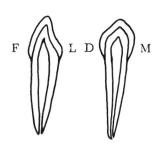

maxillary lateral incisor

The primary canine with a mesioincisal edge longer than its distoincisal edge is found in the _____ arch.

maxillary

507

MATRIX TEXT 2

Directions . . .

Place an X in the square that matches the left hand column with the top row. Mark your answers and *then turn to Page 512.*

	Both/ Neither	Maxillary Canine	Mandibular Canine
Canine with an evenly tapered root.			✓
Canine with the wider crown.		✓	
Canine with five lobes.	✓		
Canine with the less prominent mesial and distal marginal ridges.			✓
Canine with its mesial cusp ridge longer than its distal cusp ridge.		✓	

ANSWERS ON PAGE 512.

REVIEW TEST 1

Make a note of your answers. Check them on Page 511.

1. The molars of which dentition have the more narrow occlusal table (faciolingually) in proportion to the crown size?
   a. Permanent
   b. Primary

2. The greater dimension of the facial surface of the primary maxillary central incisor is the:
   a. incisocervical
   b. mesiodistal

3. There is a conspicuous demarcation between the pulp chamber and the root canal in the:
   a. primary maxillary central incisor
   b. primary maxillary lateral incisor

4. Which of the following is **not** a characteristic feature of the primary dentition?
   a. Thin enamel cap
   b. Thick and dense dentin
   c. Large pulp chamber

5. In which dentition is the ratio of root length to crown length greater?
   a. Primary
   b. Permanent

6. Is this statement true or false?
   Whereas the incisocervical crown length of the maxillary lateral incisor is less than the length of the maxillary central incisor crown, the mandibular lateral incisor crown has a greater incisocervical length than the mandibular central incisor crown.
   a. true
   b. false

ANSWERS ON PAGE 511.

TEST ANSWER SECTION

MATRIX TEST 1
(From Page 500)

If any items were missed, *turn to the page indicated for review.*
If all were correct, *turn to Page 509 for the Review Test.*

	Both/ Neither	Central	Lateral
Primary maxillary incisor with the wider crown.		X (PP. 494– 495)	
Primary maxillary incisor with the longer crown.		X (PP. 494– 495)	
Primary mandibular incisor with the crown that appears slightly wider.		X (P. 498)	
Mandibular incisor with a rounder distoincisal angle.			X (PP. 497– 499)

REVIEW TEST 1
(From Page 509)

CORRECT ANSWERS: 1. b 2. b 3. b 4. b 5. a 6. a

IF YOU GOT ALL QUESTIONS CORRECT, congratulations, you have completed nearly half of this chapter. Before continuing, we would suggest that you take a break and do something fun and interesting that is unrelated to dental anatomy. This will help to clear the cobwebs from the mind, cure what ails you, and help to make the thought of studying a more pleasant one. *Continue on Page 514 when you return.*

IF YOU MISSED ONE OF THE QUESTIONS, read the directions for reviewing below. *Review and then retake the test on Page 509.*

1. IF YOU MISSED QUESTION 1, examine the drawings on Pages 488–489.

2. IF YOU MISSED QUESTION 2, measure the crown dimensions of primary maxillary central incisor on Page 492.

3. IF YOU MISSED QUESTION 3, see the drawings of the pulp chambers and root canals on Pges 495–496.

4. IF YOU MISSED QUESTION 4, see Page 491. Try to remember each of the important characteristics of the primary dentition.

5. IF YOU MISSED QUESTION 5, reread Page 489.

6. IF YOU MISSED QUESTION 6, study Pages 494–495 (maxillary incisors) and Page 498 (mandibular incisors).

IF YOU MISSED TWO OR MORE QUESTIONS you probably know what we are going to say. Yes, *go back to Page 486 and review this section again. When you finish, retake the test on Page 509.* Just think of a situation you'll be in when you see children with "mixed" dentitions and you've got to know what's in there.

MATRIX TEXT 2
(From Page 508)

If any items were missed, *turn to the page indicated for review.*
If all were correct, *turn to Page 509 for the Review Test.*

	Both/ Neither	Maxillary Canine	Mandibular Canine
Canine with an evenly tapered root.			X (P. 507)
Canine with the wider crown.		X (P. 506)	
Canine with five lobes.	X (P. 501)		
Canine with the less prominent mesial and distal marginal ridges.			X (PP. 506– 507)
Canine with its mesial cusp ridge longer than its distal cusp ridge.		X (PP. 505)	

REVIEW TEST 2
(From Page 546)

CORRECT ANSWERS: 1. b 2. a 3. b 4. c

IF YOU GOT ALL THE QUESTIONS CORRECT, congratulations and adulations are in order for finishing this chapter. If you have taken this entire series of five chapters, you deserve to find yourself an appropriate self-reward for completing all the hundreds of questions in this book. The research done on this program indicates that, even though you may not feel it is so right now, you have learned a tremendous amount that you did not know before. Best of luck in applying that knowledge in the future. We would suggest that if you review the material in these chapters at a future date you may find the indexes helpful but, most importantly, you should retake the Matrix and Review Tests as an objective measure of your retention. These tests will direct you to pages for review. Question-answering is more helpful in review than simply rereading all the words.

IF YOU MISSED ONE OF THE QUESTIONS, review the pages indicated below.

1. IF YOU MISSED QUESTION 1, see Pages 525–526.

2. IF YOU MISSED QUESTION 2, examine the occlusal view on Pages 527–528 and the lingual view on Page 529 to find the groove.

3. IF YOU MISSED QUESTION 3, reread Page 532.

4. IF YOU MISSED QUESTION 4, study the cusps on Page 539 and the grooves on Pages 539–540.

IF YOU MISSED TWO OR MORE OF THE QUESTIONS, review from Page 525 and then retake the review test on Page 546. It happens to the best of us.

The maxillary first molar usually appears 3-cusped or 4-cusped. In any case, the geometric outline of the occlusal view is roughly _____.

Primary
Maxillary
Right
1st Molar
1. 3 cusps
2. 4 cusps
OCCLUSAL

triangular

Since the convergence of the triangular form is toward the lingual, which part of the crown is wider in the mesiodistal direction? _____ (facial/lingual)

Primary
Maxillary
Right
1st Molar
1. 4 cusps
2. 3 cusps
OCCLUSAL

facial

The cusps of the different forms of the maxillary first molar have similar names: (a) mesiofacial, (b) distofacial, (c) mesiolingual, and (d) distolingual. The more common 3-cusped form does not have a _____ cusp.

Primary
Maxillary
Right
1st Molar
1. 4 cusps
2. 3 cusps
OCCLUSAL

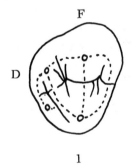
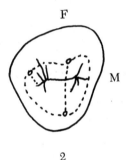

Name each of the three cusps of the 3-cusped maxillary first molar.

a. _____

b. _____

c. _____

Primary
Maxillary
Right
1st Molar
OCCLUSAL

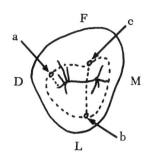

a. distofacial; b. lingual; c. mesiofacial

On the 4-cusped form, the smallest, least developed is the _____ cusp.

Primary
Maxillary
Right
1st Molar
1. OCCLUSAL
2. LINGUAL

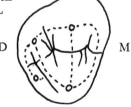

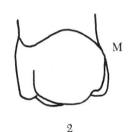

distolingual

Similar to the permanent molars, the occlusal surface (occlusal table) of a primary molar is surrounded by cusp ridges and the mesial and distal _____.

Primary
Maxillary
Right
1st Molar
OCCLUSAL

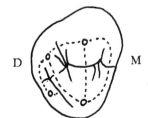

The **oblique ridge** that is characteristic of maxillary molars in the permanent dentition is also present on the maxillary molars of the primary dentition (Fig. 2). However, on the 3-cusped form of the primary maxillary first molar (Fig. 1), the oblique ridge blends with the _____ _____ ridge.

Primary
Maxillary
Right
1st Molar
1. 3 cusps
2. 4 cusps
OCCLUSAL

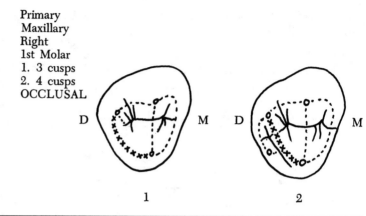

1   2

On either the 3-cusped or 4-cusped form of the primary maxillary first molar, the oblique ridge runs in an oblique direction, uniting the _____ and the _____ cusps.

Primary
Maxillary
Right
1st Molar
1. 3 cusps
2. 4 cusps
OCCLUSAL

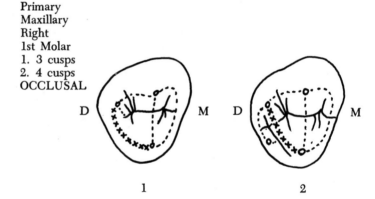

1   2

Of the two teeth adjacent to the maxillary first molar, the facial end of the oblique ridge is closest to the _____.

Primary
Maxillary
Right
1st Molar
1. 3 cusps
2. 4 cusps
OCCLUSAL

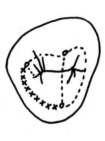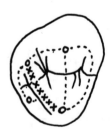

1   2

On the occlusal surface of the 3-cusped form, the mesial and central pits mark the confluence of **developmental grooves**. The confluence of the distal, facial, and mesial grooves is marked by the ⎯⎯⎯⎯⎯ pit.

Primary
Maxillary
Right
1st Molar
OCCLUSAL

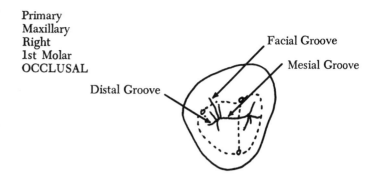

The pit at the mesial end of the mesial groove is called the ⎯⎯⎯⎯⎯ pit.

Primary
Maxillary
Right
1st Molar
OCCLUSAL

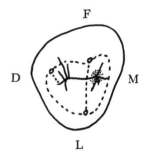

The three grooves that originate in the central pit are named for the direction they run from that pit. As labeled, these grooves are the A. ⎯⎯⎯⎯⎯, B. ⎯⎯⎯⎯⎯, and C. ⎯⎯⎯⎯⎯ developmental grooves.

Primary
Maxillary
Right
1st Molar
OCCLUSAL

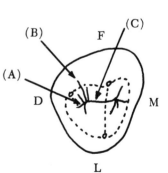

517

The mesial pit marks the confluence of four developmental grooves: the mesial, mesiofacial triangular, mesial marginal, and mesiolingual triangular. The groove running between the mesial and central pits is the _____ groove.

Primary
Maxillary
Right
1st Molar
OCCLUSAL

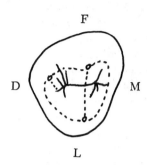

mesial

The groove that originates at the mesial pit and ascends the slope of the mesial marginal ridge is the _____ groove.

Primary
Maxillary
Right
1st Molar
OCCLUSAL

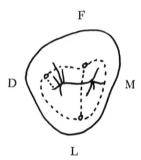

mesial marginal

The mesiolingual triangular and mesiofacial triangular grooves originate at the mesial pit and run in the direction of the mesiolingual and mesiofacial line angles.

    Name the developmental grooves labeled A, B, C and D:

A. _____
B. _____
C. _____
D. _____

Primary
Maxillary
Right
1st Molar
OCCLUSAL

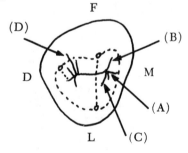

A. mesial marginal; B. mesiofacial triangular; C. mesiolingual triangular; D. facial

The distal groove extends distally from the _____ pit, becoming indistinct as it reaches the _____.

Primary
Maxillary
Right
1st Molar
OCCLUSAL

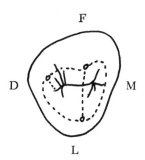

central, distal marginal ridge

On the 4-cusped form of the primary maxillary first molar, three occlusal pits are present: mesial, central, and distal. The oblique ridge cuts across the occlusal surface and passes between the _____ and _____ pits.

Primary
Maxillary
Right
1st Molar
OCCLUSAL

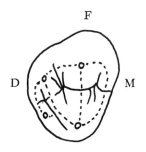

central, distal

With one exception, the four grooves that meet at the distal pit are named similar to those meeting at the mesial pit. The distolingual groove is not a triangular groove. Name the grooves in the drawing.

A. _____
B. _____
C. _____
D. _____

Primary
Maxillary
Right
1st Molar
OCCLUSAL

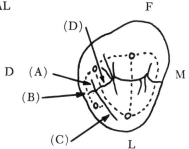

Which groove on the 4-cusped form partially
interrupts the oblique ridge? _____

Primary
Maxillary
Right
1st Molar
OCCLUSAL

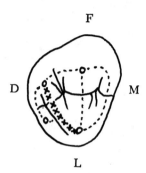

The most common occlusal pattern found on the primary maxillary first molar is the _____-cusped form.

From the facial view, the mesiofacial cusp
exhibits greater development than the distofacial cusp. When the mesiodistal width of
the facial surface is divided into thirds, the
mesiofacial cusp extends across the mesial
_____ (⅓, ⅔) of the facial surface.

Primary
Maxillary
Right
1st Molar
FACIAL

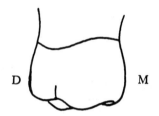

In addition, the mesiofacial cusp has a
greater development in the occlusocervical
direction. This cusp development gives the
cervical line a skewed curvature and causes
the greatest occlusocervical length on the facial surface to be located in the _____
half of the crown.

Primary
Maxillary
Right
1st Molar
FACIAL

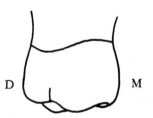

Occasionally, a developmental groove may cross the faciocclusal line angle and extend onto the facial surface, separating the mesiofacial and distofacial cusps. This groove is called the _____ groove.

Primary
Maxillary
Right
1st Molar
FACIAL

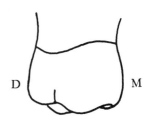

The mesial and occlusal views of the primary first molar illustrate the prominent height of contour on the facial surface (**faciocervical ridge**). The prominence of this ridge is characteristic of primary first molars, particularly the added thickness of this ridge toward the _____ (mesial/distal).

Primary
Maxillary
Right
1st Molar
1. MESIAL
2. OCCLUSAL

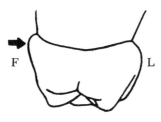

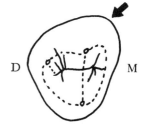

1

2

Compared to the mesiodistal width of the facial surface of this tooth, the lingual surface is _____.

Primary
Maxillary
1. Left
2. Right
1st Molar
1. LINGUAL
2. FACIAL

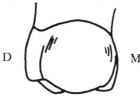

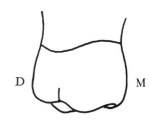

1

2

The lingual portion of the maxillary first molar contains the largest cusp on the tooth, the ———.

Primary
Maxillary
Left
1st Molar
LINGUAL

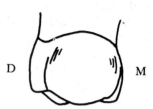

D ... M

mesiolingual

When a small distolingual cusp is present, it is partially separated from the mesiolingual cusp by a groove originating at the distal pit, the ——— groove.

Primary
Maxillary
Left
1st Molar
LINGUAL

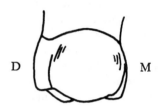

D ... M

distolingual

The roots of the primary maxillary first molar have the same names and relative positions as those of the permanent maxillary first molar. Name the roots in the drawing.

Primary
Maxillary
Right
1st Molar
FACIAL

A. ————————
B. ————————
C. ————————

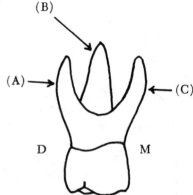

(A)→ ←(C) (B)

D ... M

The roots of the primary maxillary first molar are flared. This provides room for the **tooth bud** of which permanent tooth? _____

Primary
Maxillary
Right
1st Molar
FACIAL

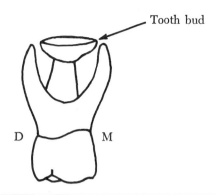

Tooth bud

D   M

maxillary first premolar

The mesiofacial root is second in size. List the three roots in the primary maxillary first molar in order of decreasing size.

_____ largest
_____
_____ smallest

Primary
Maxillary
Right
1st Molar
FACIAL

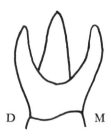

D   M

lingual, mesiofacial, distofacial (in that order)

The roof of the pulp chamber follows the general form of the occlusal surface of the crown. Corresponding to the cusps, the primary maxillary first molar may have either _____ or _____ (number) pulp horns.

Primary
Maxillary
Left
1st Molar
MESIODISTAL
  SECTIONS
1. LINGUAL
2. FACIAL

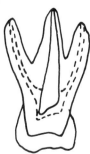
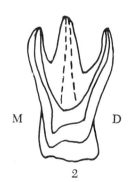

M   D

1   2

The pulp chamber of the primary maxillary first molar has a greater development facially than lingually, mesially than distally. Therefore, the largest and longest pulp horn is the _____.

Primary
Maxillary
Left
1st Molar
MESIODISTAL
  SECTIONS
1. LINGUAL
2. FACIAL

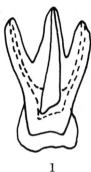
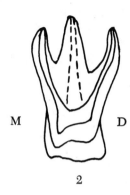

M   D

1   2

mesiofacial

The names of three pulp horns of the 3-cusped maxillary first molar are

_____ largest
_____ smallest

Primary
Maxillary
Left
1st Molar
MESIODISTAL
  SECTIONS
1. LINGUAL
2. FACIAL

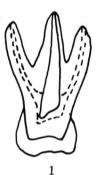
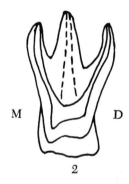

M   D

1   2

mesiofacial, mesiolingual, distofacial

Give a short answer (one or two words) to these questions about the primary maxillary first molar.

1. How many cusps are present on the most common form? _____
2. Name the largest cusp. _____
3. Name the largest pulp horn. _____
4. How many developmental grooves meet at the central pit? _____
5. Of the facial and lingual end of the oblique ridge, which is located more toward the mesial? _____
6. A characteristic of this tooth is the development of the faciocervical ridge (buccogingival ridge) especially on one half of the crown. Which half? _____
7. The root canals correspond to the roots, one canal per root, making a total of _____ (number).

SECTION 2.1 PRIMARY MAXILLARY SECOND MOLAR

Morphologically, the primary maxillary second molar strikingly resembles the permanent molar that erupts adjacent to it, the

_____ _____
  (dentition)   (arch)

_____.

  (tooth names)

1. Primary
Maxillary
Right
2nd Molar
OCCLUSA
2. Permanent
Maxillary
Right
1st Molar
OCCLUSAL

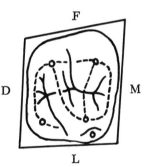

permanent maxillary first molar

In occlusal outline, the primary maxillary second molar is approximately rhomboid in appearance. However, as with the permanent maxillary first molar, the faciolingual measurement of the crown is _____ (greater/less than) the mesiodistal measurement.

Primary
Maxillary
Right
2nd Molar
OCCLUSAL

greater

Of the two primary maxillary molars, which is larger? _____

Primary
Maxillary
Right
1. 2nd Molar
2. 1st Molar
OCCLUSAL

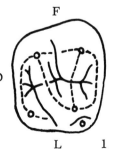

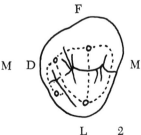

A small cusp is sometimes present on the lingual portion of the mesiolingual cusp. Thus, the number of cusps on the primary maxillary first molar is either _____ or _____; but the second molar has either _____ or _____.

Primary
Maxillary
Right
1. 2nd Molar
2. 1st Molar
OCCLUSAL

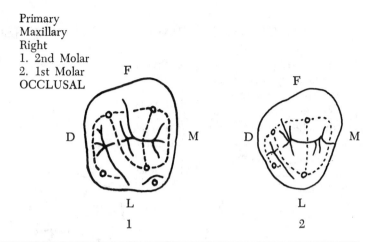

three, four; four, five (in that order)

The small fifth cusp, the **Carabelli cusp,** and the four major cusps are named in a manner similar to those of the permanent maxillary first molar. Name the cusps of the primary molar:

A._____
B._____
C._____
D._____
E._____

Primary
Maxillary
Right
2nd Molar   (E)
OCCLUSAL

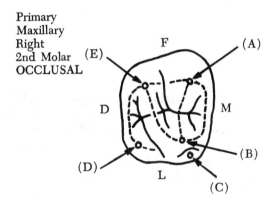

A. mesiofacial; B. mesiolingual; C. Carabelli cusp; D. distolingual; E. distofacial

Of the four major cusps of the primary maxillary second molar, the widest is the _____.

Primary
Maxillary
Right
2nd Molar
OCCLUSAL

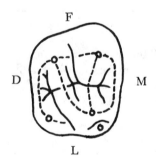

The smallest of the four major cusps, also on the lingual portion of the crown, is the _____.

Primary
Maxillary
Right
2nd Molar
OCCLUSAL

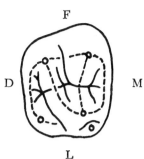

Three pits mark the intersections of the developmental grooves on the occlusal surface. As on the four-cusped form of the first molar, they are the _____, _____, and _____ pits.

Primary
Maxillary
Right
2nd Molar
OCCLUSAL

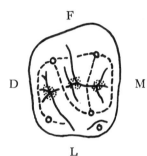

distal, central, mesial, (any order)

The primary maxillary second molar has eleven developmental grooves. All but the three most lingually located (the distolingual triangular, distolingual, and mesiolingual) are positioned in a manner similar to those on the four-cusped primary maxillary first molar. Name the grooves labeled in the illustration:

A. _____
B. _____
C. _____
D. _____

Primary
Maxillary
Right
2nd Molar
OCCLUSAL

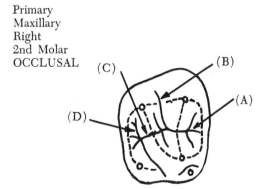

Of the distolingual, distolingual triangular, and mesiolingual grooves, only the triangular groove does not separate two cusps. Name the labeled grooves:

Primary
Maxillary
Right
2nd Molar
OCCLUSAL

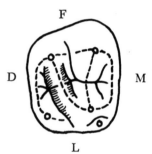

A. _____
B. _____
C. _____

On the primary maxillary second molar, the characteristic ridge of maxillary molars is well developed. It unites the _____ and _____ cusps and is named the _____ ridge.

Primary
Maxillary
Right
2nd Molar
OCCLUSAL

Of the four cusps on the primary maxillary second molar, three are nearly equal in height. They are the _____, _____, and _____.

Primary
Maxillary
Right
2nd Molar
1. FACIAL
2. LINGUAL

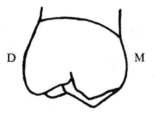

1   2

The mesiolingual is the _____ (longest/shortest) of the four major cusps on the maxillary second molar.

Primary Maxillary Right 2nd Molar
1. FACIAL
2. LINGUAL

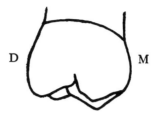 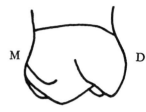

1   2

longest

From the facial and lingual views, three developmental grooves mark the boundaries of the lobes in the occlusal portion of the crown. Name these grooves.

A. _____
B. _____
C. _____

Primary Maxillary Right 2nd Molar
1. FACIAL
2. LINGUAL

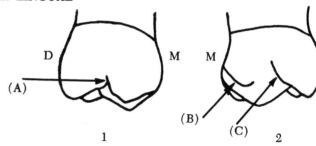

1   2

A. facial; B. mesiolingual; C. distolingual

Similar to the other maxillary molars (primary and permanent), the primary maxillary second molar has three roots: the _____, _____, and _____.

Primary Maxillary Right 2nd Molar FACIAL

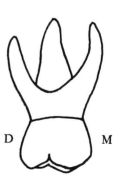

The pulp cavity of the primary maxillary second molar has one pulp horn that corresponds to each cusp and one root canal that corresponds to each root. Therefore, it has _____ (number) root canals and either _____ or _____ pulp horns.

Primary
Maxillary
Right
2nd Molar
1. SECTION THROUGH
   DISTOFACIAL &
   LINGUAL ROOTS
2. SECTION THROUGH
   MESIOFACIAL &
   LINGUAL ROOTS

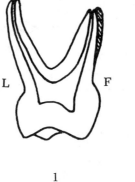

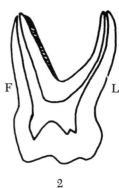

L   F   F   L

1   2

three, four, five

Similar to that of the primary maxillary first molar, the pulp cavity of the second molar shows more development facially and mesially. As a result, the largest and longest pulp horn is the _____.

Primary
Maxillary
Right
2nd Molar
1. SECTION THROUGH
   DISTOFACIAL &
   LINGUAL ROOTS
2. SECTION THROUGH
   MESIOFACIAL &
   LINGUAL ROOTS

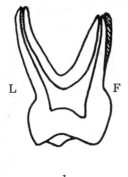

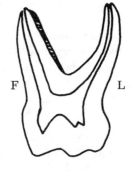

L   F   F   L

1   2

Give a short answer to these questions about the primary maxillary second molar.

1. What tooth in the human permanent dentition has a morphology similar to this tooth? _____
2. If a cylindrical object, such as a pencil, is inserted into the mouth in a roughly anterior to posterior position, is the object more nearly parallel or perpendicular to the oblique ridge? _____
3. Name the widest and longest cusp. _____

SECTION 2.2 PRIMARY MANDIBULAR FIRST MOLAR

Because of the extreme occlusal convergence of the facial surface, the occlusal table of the mandibular first molar is narrow in the _____ direction.

Primary
Mandibular
Right
1st Molar
1. OCCLUSAL
2. MESIAL

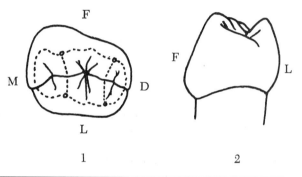

1   2

From the mesial aspect, the prominent faciocervical ridge appears as a bulbous "overhang" and serves as an identifying feature. Which label (a or b) identifies this ridge in the drawing to the right? _____

Primary
Mandibular
Right
1st Molar
MESIAL

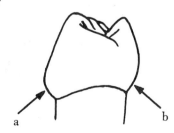

The facial view of this tooth is unusual. The faciocervical ridge is much more prominent at its _____ end.

Primary
Mandibular
Right
1st Molar
FACIAL

D

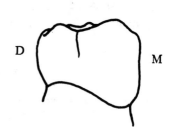

M

mesial

Of the two facial cusps (mesiofacial and distofacial) one is considerably wider but only slightly higher than the other. Which facial cusp is higher in the occlusocervical direction? _____

Primary
Mandibular
Right
1st Molar
FACIAL

D

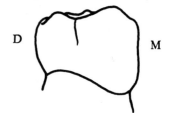

M

mesiofacial

The facial groove may or may not be evident from the facial aspect. Whether or not the groove is present, the intersection of the facial lobes is suggested by the shallow, smoothly contoured facial concavity between the cusps. Because of the cusp development in the mesiodistal direction, the facial concavity is located in the _____ half of the crown.

Primary
Mandibular
Right
1st Molar
1. FACIAL
2. OCCLUSAL

D

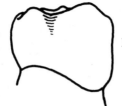

M

F

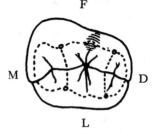

M

D

L

1

2

From the facial aspect, the skewed curvature of the cervical line is caused by the prominent mass formed by the highly developed _____.

Primary
Mandibular
Right
1st Molar
FACIAL

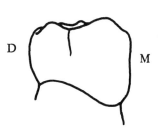

D

M

Seen from the mesial aspect, the occlusocervical curvature of the facial surface, from faciocervical ridge to cusp tip, is nearly _____ (convex/flat)

Primary
Mandibular
Right
1st Molar
MESIAL

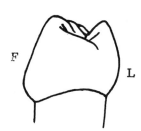

F

L

Two cusps are evident on the lingual portion of the crown of the mandibular first molar. Similar to the facial cusps, the wider and longer of the two lingual cusps is located toward the _____.

Primary
Mandibular
Right
1st Molar
LINGUAL

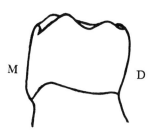

M

D

The relative sizes of the four cusps are shown in occlusal view. The two mesial cusps are larger than the distal cusps, the mesio- _____ cusp being slightly larger than the _____ cusp.

Primary
Mandibular
Right
1st Molar
OCCLUSAL

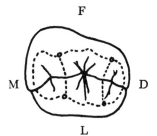

F

M

D

L

The distal portion of the occlusal surface has a deep **occlusal sulcus.** However, the mesial portion is marked by a distinct **transverse ridge** which runs across the occlusal surface between the _____ and _____ cusps.

Primary
Mandibular
Right
1st Molar
OCCLUSAL

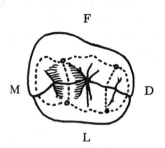

In the maxillary arch, the ridge that crosses the occlusal surface of the molars is the _____.

On the primary mandibular first molar, the ridge crossing the occlusal surface is the _____.

Primary
1. Maxillary
Right
2nd Molar
OCCLUSAL
2. Mandibular
Right
1st Molar
OCCLUSAL

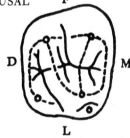

1

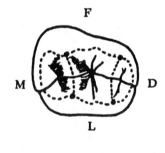

2

Three pits are formed by the intersection of the developmental grooves of the occlusal surface: the mesial, central, and distal pits. The transverse ridge divides the occlusal surface into two fossae, one containing the _____ pit, the other the _____ and _____ pits.

Primary
Mandibular
Right
1st Molar
OCCLUSAL

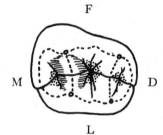

The facial, mesial, lingual, and distal development grooves originate at the central pit. Name the following grooves:

A. _____

B. _____

C. _____

D. _____

Primary
Mandibular
Right
1st Molar
OCCLUSAL

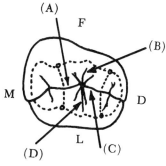

A. mesial; B. facial; C. distal; D. lingual

In addition to the distal groove, three grooves intersect at the distal pit: the distofacial triangular, distal marginal, and distolingual triangular. Name the grooves in the drawing.

A. _____,

B. _____,

C. _____

Primary
Mandibular
Right
1st Molar
OCCLUSAL

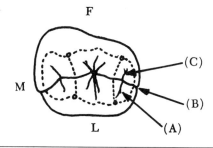

A. distolingual triangular; B. distal marginal; C. distofacial triangular

The mesial groove is shallow and may fade out on the mesial and distal slopes of the _____.

Primary
Mandibular
Right
1st Molar
OCCLUSAL

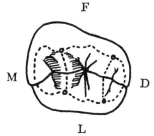

535

Groove (A) is the _____, and groove (B) is the _____.

Primary
Mandibular
Right
1st Molar
OCCLUSAL

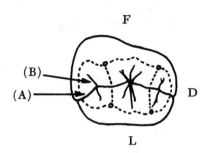

A. mesial marginal; B. mesiofacial triangular

Similar to the permanent mandibular molars, the primary mandibular molar has two roots, the _____ and _____ roots.

Primary
Mandibular
Right
1st Molar
1. FACIAL
2. MESIAL

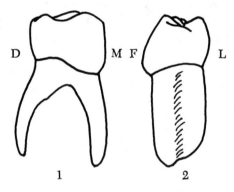

---

mesial, distal

As was true on the roots of permanent mandibular molars, the mesial and distal roots of the primary mandibular first molar are narrow and convex in the _____ direction, but broad in the _____ direction.

Primary
Mandibular
Right
1st Molar
1. FACIAL
2. MESIAL

The pulp cavity of the primary mandibular first molar has three root canals. The larger of the two roots, corresponding to the two largest cusps, contains two canals. Following the established pattern for naming an entity of dental anatomy, the names of the three root canals are —————, —————, —————.

Primary
Mandibular
Right
1st Molar
1. LINGUAL
2. HORIZONTAL SECTION

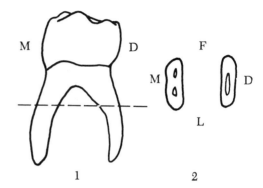

1   2

Corresponding to the number of cusps, the roof of the pulp chamber in the primary mandibular first molar has ————— (number) pulp horns.

Primary
Mandibular
Right
1st Molar
FACIOLINGUAL
   SECTIONS

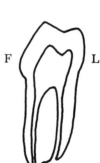
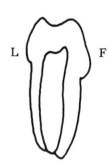

Corresponding to the relative sizes of the cusps, the largest and second largest pulp horns are the ————— and —————.

Primary
Mandibular
Right
1st Molar
FACIOLINGUAL
   SECTIONS

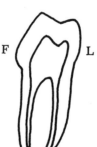
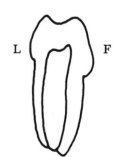

SECTION 2.3   PRIMARY MANDIBULAR SECOND MOLAR

The primary mandibular second molar has a morphology that closely resembles that of the permanent mandibular first molar. Specimens of the two teeth can be distinguished by their relative sizes and by the bulbous quality of the primary tooth. Although the drawing does not permit a size comparison, the primary molar is represented by drawing number _____ because it has the more _____ shape.

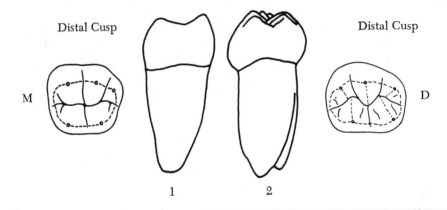

Distal Cusp   M   D   Distal Cusp

1   2

Additional distinctions between the morphology of the primary mandibular second molar and the permanent mandibular first molar include:

1.   The relative size of the distal cusp (see above).
2.   Some slight differences in the groove patterns of the occlusal surfaces.
3.   The ratio of the faciolingual to mesiodistal crown diameter.

On which of the two teeth (shown at the top of this page) is the mesiodistal crown diameter greater than the faciolingual diameter as seen from an occlusal view? _____ (primary/ permanent/both).

Two sets of names are in common use for the cusps of the primary mandibular second molar:

Mesiofacial ———————A———————Mesiofacial
Distofacial ———————B———————Middle facial
Distal ————————————C———————Distofacial
Mesiolingual ——————D———————Mesiolingual
Distolingual ——————E———————Distolingual

The problem arising from the two sets of names is knowing which cusp is referred to by the term ————.

Primary
Mandibular
Right
2nd Molar
OCCLUSAL

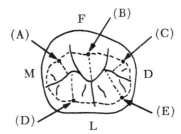

This program uses the names mesiofacial, distofacial, and distal. Therefore, cusp (A) is the ———— cusp and cusp (B) the ———— cusp.

Primary
Mandibular
Right
2nd Molar
OCCLUSAL

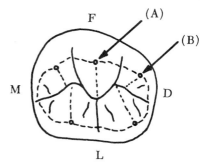

Each cusp has a well developed triangular ridge running from the cusp tip to the central portion of the ————.

Primary
Mandibular
Right
2nd Molar
OCCLUSAL

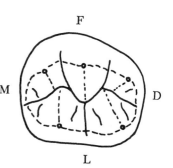

The three major grooves that meet at the central pit are the lingual, mesiofacial, and distofacial. In the drawing, the mesiofacial groove is labeled _____; the lingual groove is labeled _____.

Primary Mandibular Right 2nd Molar OCCLUSAL

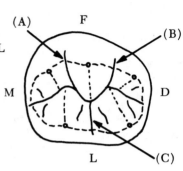

A, C (in that order)

The mesial (A) and distal (B) grooves of the primary mandibular second molar do not originate at the central pit, but branch from the _____ and _____ grooves.

Primary Mandibular Right 2nd Molar OCCLUSAL

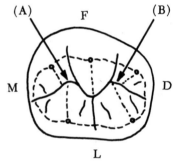

mesiofacial, distofacial

The mesial and distal grooves do not link the mesial and distal pits with the central pit. The mesial groove connects the _____ and the _____.

Primary Mandibular Right 2nd Molar OCCLUSAL

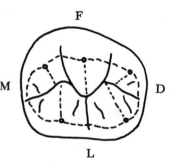

Similarly, the distal groove runs from the _____ to the _____.

Primary
Mandibular
Right
2nd Molar
OCCLUSAL

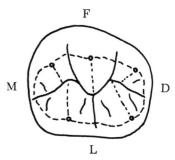

Six other grooves are evident:

Mesiofacial triangular
Mesial marginal
Mesiolingual triangular
Distofacial triangular
Distal marginal
Distolingual triangular

Each of the six originates at either the mesial or distal pit. Name the four grooves labeled in the drawing:

A. _____
B. _____
C. _____
D. _____

Primary
Mandibular
Right
2nd Molar
OCCLUSAL

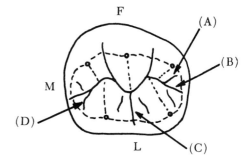

As seen from the facial and lingual views, the highest of the five cusps is the _____.

Primary
Mandibular
Right
2nd Molar
1. FACIAL
2. LINGUAL

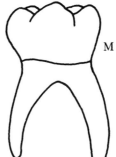
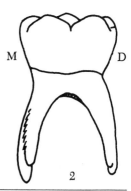

How do the two lingual cusps compare for height and size? _____

Primary Mandibular Right 2nd Molar
1. FACIAL
2. LINGUAL

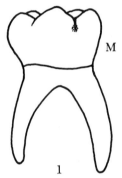

nearly equal (or similar answer)

In the occlusal portion of the facial and lingual surfaces are extensions of the developmental grooves that separate the cusps. The terminal end of the mesiofacial groove is often marked by a small, pointed depression called a _____.

Primary Mandibular Right 2nd Molar
1. FACIAL
2. LINGUAL

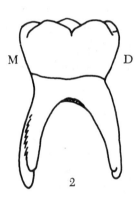

pit

The facial pit on the primary mandibular second molar is generally located between the _____ and _____ cusps.

Primary Mandibular Right 2nd Molar FACIAL

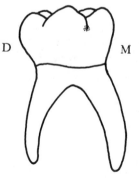

On the primary mandibular second molar, the characteristic bulbous form of the primary dentition is emphasized by the strong occlusal convergence of the facial surface. This convergence makes the _____ ridge more prominent.

Primary
Mandibular
Right
2nd Molar
MESIAL

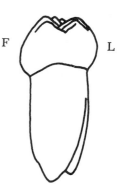

The flared roots provide space for the developing tooth bud of the permanent second premolar. The primary mandibular second has two roots: the _____ and _____.

Primary
Mandibular
Right
2nd Molar
1. LINGUAL
2. MESIAL

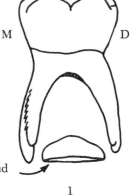

Tooth Bud

The roots of the primary mandibular second molar are generally similar to those of the mandibular first molar but _____ in size.

Primary
Mandibular
Right
1. 1st Molar
2. 2nd Molar
FACIAL

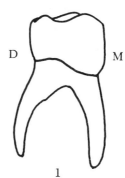
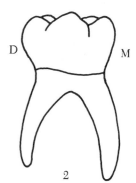

The pulp cavity of the primary mandibular second molar has either three or four root canals. In either case, the mesial root has _____ (number) root canals.

The number of root canals in the distal root of the primary mandibular second molar is either one or _____.

Primary
Mandibular
Left
2nd Molar
HORIZONTAL
   SECTIONS

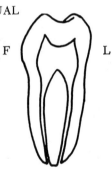

The mesial portion of the pulp chamber in the primary mandibular second molar is larger than the distal portion. The mesial horns are larger and higher than the distal horns; also, the mesial marginal border of the chamber is high and convex. This relative mesial to distal size differential of the pulp chamber is _____ (similar to/the opposite of) that in the primary mandibular first molar.

Primary
Mandibular
Right
2nd Molar
FACIOLINGUAL
SECTION
1. MESIAL
2. DISTAL

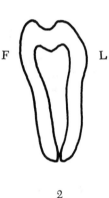

As suggested by the number of cusps, the roof of the pulp chamber in the primary mandibular second molar has five _____.

Primary
Mandibular
Right
2nd Molar
1. FACIAL
2. LINGUAL

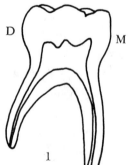
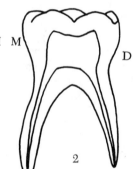

Give a short answer to each of these questions concerning the primary mandibular molars.

1. How many cusps are present on each tooth?
   a. First molar ———————————————————————
   b. Second molar ———————————————————————

2. Name the roots on a primary mandibular molar.

3. Which primary mandibular molar has a prominent transverse ridge that unites the mesiofacial and mesiolingual cusps? ——————.

4. Which permanent tooth does each of the primary second molars most resemble?
   a. Maxillary second molar ———————————————————————
   b. Mandibular second molar ———————————————————————

If you missed one of the questions, review on the page indicated.
1. (a) four (Page 533)
   (b) five (Page 539)

2. Mesial and distal (Page 536, 544)

3. First molar (Page 534, 540)

4. (a) Permanent maxillary first molar (Page 525)
   (b) Permanent mandibular first molar (Page 538)

REVIEW TEST 2

Make a note of your answers and check them on Page 513.

1. The fifth cusp often found on the primary maxillary second molar is the . . .
   a. distal cusp.
   b. Carabelli cusp.

2. The lingual surface of the primary maxillary second molar has two major cusps (distolingual and mesiolingual) spearated by the . . .
   a. distolingual groove.
   b. mesiolingual groove.

3. The most prominently convex portion of the faciocervical ridge on the primary mandibular first molar is the . . .
   a. distal.
   b. mesial.

4. On the primary mandibular second molar, the distal cusp is separated from the distofacial cusp by the . . .
   a. distal groove.
   b. buccal groove.
   c. distofacial groove.

ANSWERS ON PAGE 513.

TABLE OF CODE CONVERSION
Universal and International Tooth Identification Codes

1	1-8 or 18	A	5-5 or 55
2	1-7 or 17	B	5-4 or 54
3	1-6 or 16	C	5-3 or 53
4	1-5 or 15	D	5-2 or 52
5	1-4 or 14	E	5-1 or 51
6	1-3 or 13		
7	1-2 or 12	F	6-1 or 61
8	1-1 or 11	G	6-2 or 62
		H	6-3 or 63
9	2-1 or 21	I	6-4 or 64
10	2-2 or 22	J	6-5 or 65
11	2-3 or 23		
12	2-4 or 24	K	7-5 or 75
13	2-5 or 25	L	7-4 or 74
14	2-6 or 26	M	7-3 or 73
15	2-7 or 27	N	7-2 or 72
16	2-8 or 28	O	7-1 or 71
17	3-8 or 38	P	8-1 or 81
18	3-7 or 37	Q	8-2 or 82
19	3-6 or 36	R	8-3 or 83
20	3-5 or 35	S	8-4 or 84
21	3-4 or 34	T	8-5 or 85
22	3-3 or 33		
23	3-2 or 32		
24	3-1 or 31		
25	4-1 or 41		
26	4-2 or 42		
27	4-3 or 43		
28	4-4 or 44		
29	4-5 or 45		
30	4-6 or 46		
31	4-7 or 47		
32	4-8 or 48		

INDEX

Non-centric cusps, 86, 303
Nonsuccedaneous, 12, 249, 358
Number of cusps, 69, 70
Number of lobes, 69, 70
Number of roots, 27
Number of teeth, 12, 13, 486

Oblique ridge, 363, 516
Occlusal, 10, 11
   convergence, 489
   embrasures, 91, 335, 336
   fossae, 307, 308
   groove pattern, 319
   plane, 80
   ridge, 516
   sulcus, 258, 534
   table, 20, 489
   third, 24
Occlusion, 82, 303
Occlusocervical dimension, 97, 336−338
-odont, 12
Odontoblasts, 38, 60
Oral mucosa, 73
Orifice, 41
Orthodontic alignment, 58
Osteoblasts, 58
Overbite, 84
Overjet, 84

Papilla, 90
Papillary gingiva, 64
Passive eruption, 78
Periodontal ligament, 58, 61
Permanent, 12
Permanent vs. primary teeth, 486−492
-phyo, 12
Pit
   distal, 261
   lingual, 127−129
   mesial, 261
Point angle, 246
Polyphyodont, 12
Posterior, 10
Premolars, 2, 6−8
Primary, 12
Primary dentin, 60
Primary vs. permanent teeth, 486−492
Proximal, 20, 21
Proximal contacts, 88, 97, 335−337, 456

Proximal contacts (cont'd.)
   Review Test on, 350
Pulp, 38
Pulp anatomy, 236−242
   mandibular canine, 242
   mandibular first molar, 480−483, 537
   mandibular first premolar, 353−355
   mandibular incisor, 238, 239
   mandibular second molar, 480−483, 544
   mandibular second premolar, 354, 355
   mandibular third molar, 483
   Matrix Test on, 243, 356, 484
   maxillary canine, 239−241, 504, 505
   maxillary central incisor, 236, 237
   maxillary first molar, 477−480, 523, 524
   maxillary first premolar, 351, 352
   maxillary lateral incisor, 237
   maxillary second molar, 480, 529−531
   maxillary second premolar, 352, 353
   maxillary third molar, 480
   Review Test on, 244, 357, 485
Pulp cavity, 38−43
Pulp chamber, 38, 39
Pulp horns, 38−43

Quadrant abbreviations, 18
Quadrant, 11−13, 486
Quadrant symbols, 18

Recession, 78
Resorbtion, 77
Review Tests
   Chapter 1, 9, 26, 36, 46, 66, 81, 95, 113
   Chapter 2, 130, 146, 184, 211, 220, 235, 244
   Chapter 3, 263, 279, 286, 317, 334, 350, 357
   Chapter 4, 374, 387, 402, 416, 443, 455, 476, 485
   Chapter 5, 509, 546
Ridges, 126, 247
   distal cusp, 173, 247
   distal marginal, 126
   facial, 177, 247
   lingual, 178, 205, 206, 247
   linguocervical, 126, 140
   linguoincisal, 139, 140, 141
   marginal, 126, 246
   mesial cusp, 173, 247
   mesial marginal, 126, 140, 206, 207
   transverse, 305
   triangular, 254